Health in France
2002

Haut Comité de la Santé Publique
Ministère de l'Emploi et de la Solidarité
8, avenue de Ségur
75350 Paris 07 SP, France
Tel.: 01.40.56.79.80
email : hcsp-secr-general@sante.gouv.fr
http://www.hcsp.ensp.fr

Editions John Libbey Eurotext
127, avenue de la République
92120 Montrouge, France
Tel.: 01.46.73.06.60
e-mail : contact@john-libbey-eurotext.fr
http://www.john-libbey-eurotext.fr

All rights reserved. No part of this publication may be reproduced or transmitted in any form, or by any means, electronic or mechanical, including photocopy, recording, or any information storage or retrieval system, without permission in writing from the publisher.

ISBN: 2-7420-0466-1
© John Libbey Eurotext - Paris, 2003 for the english version

© La Documentation française - Paris, 2002 for the french version
© Haut Comité de la Santé Publique for both versions

Ministry of Employment and Solidarity
High Committee on Public Health

Health in France 2002

February 2002

High Committee on Public Health

President: The Minister of Health

Ex-officio members: The Director-General for Health, The Director for Hospitalisation and Care Logistics, The Director of Social Security, The Director of the National Health Insurance Agency for Salaried Workers, The Director-General of the National Institute for Health and Medical Research, The Director of the National School of Public Health.

Members: Maryvonne Bitaud-Thépaut, Jean-François Bloch-Lainé, François Bonnaud, Yves Charpak, Jean-Pierre Claveranne, Alain Coulomb, Daniel Defert, Jean-François Dodet, Isabelle Durand-Zaleski, Isabelle Ferrand, Francis Giraud, Odette Grzegrzulka, Pierre Guillet, Jacques Lebas, René Roué, Roland Sambuc, Simone Sandier, Anne Tallec, Denis Zmirou.

Vice-President: Roland Sambuc

General Rapporteur: Anne Tallec

General Secretary: The Director-General for Health

Deputy General Secretary: Geneviève Guérin

Preface

Ten years after its creation in 1991 and in accordance with its remit, the High Committee on Public Health (HCPH) is publishing its third Report on "Health in France".

In the last ten years, significant changes have been made to the way in which questions of public health are addressed, notably by the creation of several new agencies and institutions, including the French Agency for Safe Health Care Products (Afssaps, *Agence française de sécurité sanitaire des produits de santé*), the French Agency for Safe Food (Afssa, *Agence française de sécurité sanitaire des aliments*), the recently established French Agency for Environmental Safety (Afsse, *Agence française de sécurité sanitaire environnementale*), the Institute for Public Health Surveillance (InVS, *Institut de veille sanitaire*) and the National Agency for Health Accreditation and Evaluation (Anaes, *Agence nationale d'accréditation et d'évaluation en santé*, formerly Andem, *Agence nationale pour le développement de l'évaluation médicale*). Moreover, in order to ensure that public health policy responds more closely to real needs, and to help identify priorities in a system whose strong and weak points are fairly well delineated, the National and Regional Health Conferences have been created. Strategic choices are currently being formulated in a Social Security Funding Bill to be presented to Parliament, a Bill in which overall spending limits are proposed for health insurance. However, we know that imposing strict limits on health care expenditure can compromise the global quality of health care provision and preclude equitable access to medical progress. The solution to this is to shift the focus of the discussion to public health.

Over the last ten years, the light shed by the HCPH has made an enormous contribution in the formulation of strategic choices, an ongoing contribution embodied in this Report in which the Committee's analyses and proposals are organised around three main themes:
– how to reduce inequality in the matter of health,
– how to optimise the allocation of resources,

Preface

– how – with the overriding ambition of promoting democracy in health – to place users (patient, sick person) right at the heart of the health care system: how to provide them with the information that they need, and how to involve them in decisions concerning their own treatment and care.

This approach was presented as the main theme in the discussions of health policy at the National Health Conference meeting in Strasbourg in February 2001.

This policy is embodied in the Bill currently before Parliament pertaining to "patients' rights and the performance of the health care system". This legislation sets out to address some of the legitimate concerns expressed by the French people in the context of the 1998 Consultative Assembly on Health, calling for more account to be taken of their opinions, more participation, more prevention and more support.

Recognition that patients have rights is a first step but is not an end in itself. Such recognition can do no more than correct some of the system's problems (notably inequality) and even then, such rights can only be respected if there is a wholehearted commitment to co-operate on the part of the professionals.

The recognition that patients have rights – by health professionals as well as citizens – will contribute towards democratisation of the health care system so that each and every member of society has the same access to care and prevention. Moreover, each and every patient must be given the chance to understand the relevant health-related issues, without which understanding they can never be in a position to make rational decisions from an informed perspective.

Policy in this area must pay heed to every individual's freedom to behave as he or she wants as long as their choices are freely made and their actions do not endanger others. What risks to take in life is a choice that everyone has to make, and the priority for policy makers is to learn how to help people make informed decisions and then respect their choices. Making their contacts *risk-aware* in this way constitutes one of the most important components of the work of today's health care providers.

As an inevitable transformation takes place in our health care system (which remains one of the best in the world, if not the very best), questions about the medical decision-making process come up ever more frequently: "Who is to make the decisions?", "With what objectives in mind?" and "At what level of risk, either imminent or in the future?"

At this time of unprecedented technical and medical progress, ethical questions seem to be more numerous, more complex and more urgent than ever before. Such questions require ongoing discussion between health care professionals, patients and community representatives. Current priorities include questions of responsibility in the case of disability, iatrogenic problems and, most recently, potential problems stemming from progress in predictive medicine.

In its conclusions and recommendations, the HCPH has tried to emphasis those issues which will dominate the future picture: how to present useful information, how to re-establish confidence, and clarification of responsibilities.

Exactly one-hundred years ago in 1902, the new "Grand" public health law laid the foundations of a novel approach to public health, an approach which held sway throughout the last century.

Today, at the dawn of the 21st Century, we have a whole new set of issues to confront. A new law to address these issues is currently under discussion, and we will have to find a way to implement its provisions which are intended to bring citizens and politicians together to formulate public health policy in a collaborative and democratic process, both at the national and the regional level.

From now on, the Government's health policy will be debated every year (up until now, such policy has only been regularly discussed in the context of Social Security funding).

To nourish this debate, the Government will compile a preliminary report and submit it to a revamped National Health Conference.

In this deliberation and evaluation process which has generated novel ideas and helped consolidate the idea of democracy in health, the High Committee on Public Health has over the last ten years contributed to political decisions by reviewing the situation and offering advice in the matter of health.

I would like to express my thanks and admiration for the quality of the work of the committee, and the commitment of its members, both of which are in ample evidence in this report on "Health in France".

Bernard Kouchner
Minister of Health

CONTENTS

	Preface	5
	Foreword	11
Recommended strategic directions **The French paradox**	Overall positive results make certain situations all the more difficult to accept	18
	Health care issues to be addressed in the medium-term	22
	Health policy issues: short-term objectives	30
Part one **Data about health status**	Composition of the Working Group	42
	Introduction	43
	Summary and issues	46
	Methodology	55
	Young people of under 15 years of age	63
	People of between 15 and 44 years of age	83
	People of between 45 and 74 years of age	103
	Those of 75 and over	124
	Annexe	142
Part two **Health inequalities and disparities in France**	Composition of the Working Group	144
	Introduction	145
	Socially-based inequality in health	147
	Geographical inequalities in health	160
	Socio-geographical inequality in health	178
	Understanding and correcting socially-based inequality in health	181
	Public policy to mitigate inequality in health	203
	Summary and recommendations	215
Part three **Resource allocation in the health system**	Composition of the Working Group	220
	Introduction	221
	Health system resources: the current situation	223
	How resources are estimated and allocated	234
	Discussion	249
	Recommendations	255
Part four **The user, a player in the health care system**	Composition of the Working Group	264
	Introduction	265
	Participation in the formulation of public health policy	276
	Involve users in the running of institutions	287
	Ensure balance in the patient/care provider relationship	299
	Recommendations	310

Contents

Part five **A critical, prospective analysis of the way the health system is organised**	Composition of the Working Group	314
	Introduction	315
	Is the way the health care system currently works based on genuine priorities, and does it cater to people's needs?	316
	Is the health care system organised in a strategic, functional way?	320
	Are questions of health dealt with in democratic processes in which the general public can participate?	327
	Is the health care system organised in such a way as to enable it to respond to future challenges?	333

Acknowledgements 339
References 340
Abbreviations 353
List of tables 357
List of figures 359
List of inserts 362
Table of contents 363

Foreword

Every three years since its creation in 1991, the High Committee on Public Health has published "Health in France", a report on the health status of the French people and an analysis of changes in the health care system. Preceding reports were published in 1994 and 1998.

The 2002 Report owes a great deal to Gilles Brücker who was Vice-President of the HCPH during most of the work, and also to the initial deliberations of the steering committee chaired by Yves Charpak. The Report is composed of five parts, each contributed by a different working group appointed by the High Committee. The first part deals with data about health status and, in the following three parts, specific aspects of how health care in France could be improved are tackled in depth, namely inequality, the allocation of resources, and the place of the user in the system. The final part gives a prospective view of the logistics of the French health care system.

For its tenth anniversary Report, the Committee has extended its global analysis with an editorial component which, on the basis of a review of apparently paradoxical features of our health care system, identifies the issues which will become priorities in the future, proposes targets to aim for in these areas, and points out directions to follow in the short term to ensure successful change in a rapidly evolving field.

In terms of the way in which data on health status are analysed, this Report differs substantially from its predecessors.

The first Report published in 1994 outlined the system's strong and weak points in order to define public health targets. In so doing, the High Committee produced, for the first time, a structured review of how public health policy is formulated.

The 1998 Report described and analysed trends as evidenced by changes in certain key indicators, mainly on the basis of mortality figures.

Foreword

The present Report puts mortality figures into perspective by integrating them with data from three other sources which shed light on morbidity and usage of the health care system. These data are notably based on information about the patterns of prescription by independent physicians (General Practitioners and specialists in private practice) and hospital admissions (PMSI data).

Finally, it was decided to break the analysis down into four different age brackets which yields results that are more conducive to the formulation of targeted policy. Somewhat unconventional age brackets were defined on the basis of social realities and the fact that the biological ageing process has considerably slowed down in recent decades.

Life expectancy at the age of 65 is higher in France than in any other European country. However, not only is the life expectancy of men still significantly lower than that of women, but there are also major differentials between regions: socially-based inequalities in health remain a priority.

Inequality and premature mortality (*i.e.* death before 65 years of age) are still important areas for improvement in our system. Without any doubt, remedying these problems will depend more on action in the sphere of prevention than improving curative treatment modalities. Changes necessary to promote health education and improve the efficacy of preventive measures are discussed in the Report, notably the need to integrate psychosocial parameters into the models used to analyse high-risk behaviour patterns.

With respect to economic parameters, the High Committee is quite aware that massive resources are allocated to the health care system but questions can be put in a number of areas: about the complexity of the system's accounting practices; about the absence of any clear relationship between funding and health policy; about setting targets in a context of funding which has to be renewed every year or every few years. The standard of care provision still varies from region to region and this situation may deteriorate in the future as the number of practising professional health care providers decreases, a possibility which needs to be anticipated and dealt with in good time. In the Report, a whole series of proposals is made about various questions concerning the allocation of resources.

The place of users in the health care system and, more specifically, the extent to which they are represented in the running of institutions, is going to be enhanced in the Bill now before Parliament pertaining to patients' rights and the performance of the health care system. Providing patients with more information – especially about matters and decisions that directly concern them – can only engender a better relationship between patient and doctor by conferring on both an active role in the therapeutic process. The Report also proposes ways of bringing members of the community into the formulation of public health policy to promote "democracy in health", an ideal which depends on an informed public with a sound knowledge base about health in general and how the health care system works in particular.

The last part is a critical, prospective analysis of the health care system based on comparisons of the actual situation and the results of the analysis. A series of questions are addressed, notably: "Is the system addressing people's needs and priorities?", "Is the system organised appropriately?", "Is it democratic?" and "Is it fit to deal with the important issues, both present and future?".

Since publication of the first HCPH Report, various legislative, regulatory and logistical changes have been made to correct certain weak points identified in the French health care system: regional health policy has been harmonised and regional health programmes have been established; forums for the discussion of health-related priorities have been set up in the form of the National and Regional Health Conferences, and the Consultative Assemblies on Health; great advances have been made in treatment modalities (including pain management) and care provision in general; access to care has been enhanced as a result of Universal Health Insurance Coverage (CMU, *Couverture Maladie Universelle*); and mass screening programmes for certain forms of cancer are now up and running.

Nevertheless, there are still major defects – unnecessary complexity, lack of co-ordination – of which the public (and even some intimately involved in the system) are unaware. The persistence of an unacceptable level of premature death and serious inequalities, and the need to confront new issues (notably the ageing of the population) require urgent action in the matter of public health.

Any health care system operates in a changing world and flexibility must be one of its primary characteristics if improved health is to be guaranteed. The recommendations made by the High Committee in this Third Report address exactly this objective: how to encourage change and expand the capacity for change in the French health care system, and how to do it quickly.

Roland Sambuc
Vice-President

RECOMMENDED STRATEGIC DIRECTIONS

The French paradox

Recommended strategic directions

This text was compiled by

Rapporteur Bertrand Garros, The President of the National Prevention Committee

Roland Sambuc, The Vice-President of the High Committee on Public Health
Marc Duriez, General Secretariat of the High Committee on Public Health
Anne-Carole Bensadon, General Health Directorate
William Dab, General Health Directorate
Isabelle Durand-Zaleski, High Committee on Public Health
Francis Giraud, High Committee on Public Health
Geneviève Guérin, General Secretariat of the High Committee on Public Health
Pierre Guillet, High Committee on Public Health
Jacques Lebas, High Committee on Public Health
René Roué, High Committee on Public Health
Simone Sandier, High Committee on Public Health
Anne Tallec, High Committee on Public Health

Since its creation, the High Committee on Public Health has concluded each of its three terms of office with the publication of a Report on "Health in France". The first, published in 1994, made a major contribution to developing a new approach to – indeed a whole culture of – public health in the country, introducing the various parties concerned in the system to the idea of targets and priorities. It also introduced hitherto unfamiliar concepts such as premature and avoidable death.

The second Report, published in 1998, reviewed the changes which had occurred since the first Report, both in terms of the evolution of certain key indicators and general trends in the health care system. The ability to monitor and evaluate trends in this way illustrated the value of the HCPH approach.

For this third Report, the Committee has sought to maintain continuity and, at the same time add new elements: continuity in the review of health status, and new elements in terms of presentation and the focus of the HCPH's contribution.

The job of reviewing the status of health of the French people was split between five working groups (made up of members of the HCPH and external contributors) which addressed respectively "Data about health status", "Health inequalities and disparities", "Resource allocation in the health system", "The user, a player in the health care system", and finally, "A critical, prospective analysis of the way the health system is organised". Each group identified themes which were then discussed in the course of a series of plenary sessions of the HCPH.

The High Committee also took into consideration a number of recently published reports dealing with the same or related themes, *e.g.* the revamping of independent practice to mention one of the more recent reports. Its deliberations also covered the

Recommended strategic directions

Bill pertaining to patients' rights and the performance of the health care system now before Parliament after years of preparation, and the Social Security Funding Bill in 2002. In so doing, the members of the HCPH sought to make a positive contribution that would complement the work of the five working groups and nourish discussion in the public arena.

These recommendations constitute neither a summary of the Report as a whole, nor a conclusion to it. Rather, they represent the views of the members of the HCPH as to which are the key issues and objectives in health policy after a broad, global review of the current situation. The High Committee's proposals fall into two different time frames, the medium term and the short term (although most of the recommendations to be implemented in the short term are nevertheless intended to be long-standing). Although it recognises that stability can be a virtue in effective health care policy, the High Committee is also sure that certain, rapidly implemented measures could lead to significant progress. Such measures are necessarily regarding the fact that the ground has to be prepared for major reforms which are inevitable (although somewhat virtual at this point in time). At a time when questions about our health care system are becoming ever more urgent with pessimism often dominating the discussion, it is worth remembering that sometimes it is possible to act immediately.

Overall positive results make certain situations all the more difficult to accept

Good overall health indicators

With a life expectancy of 78 years at birth, the French people (considering both men and women together) are not the longest-lived nation in the world but they are well ahead of others living in many countries at a comparable level of development. In the European Union, France comes fourth (the Swedes living the longest).

Infant mortality is extremely low (mainly because of an impressive reduction in the incidence of Sudden Infant Death syndrome): of every 1,000 babies born in France, about 995 will celebrate their first birthday (with nearly all of the other five dying in the first few days of life).

Similarly, the life expectancy of a 65-year-old is now high, 16 years for a man and 20 years for a woman, figures which are the highest in Europe.

Overall positive results make certain situations all the more difficult to accept

Among the other good health indicators, cardiovascular mortality in France is far lower than anywhere else in Europe.

Positive trends

Over the last few years, many positive changes have been observed in both health status and the working of the health care system.

Alcohol consumption has continued to drop, although some young people are participating in new forms of high-risk behaviour. Cardiovascular mortality has also continued to drop as a result of the management of risk factors and therapeutic, medical and surgical progress. Death resulting from falls has dropped, especially amongst the elderly and finally, the introduction of tritherapy has dramatically reduced AIDS mortality.

The generalisation of cataract surgery, joint replacement and peridural anaesthesia during deliveries has significantly improved the quality of life of many people. And finally, mass screening programmes for certain forms of cancer (either already running or about to be put into operation) may bear fruit in the future as long as the level of participation is high enough and the efficacy of the tests is such as to outweigh the possible adverse effects.

In parallel to these medical advances, significant improvements have been made in recent years in terms of the working of the health care system. Access to the system has been greatly improved by the introduction of Universal Health Insurance Coverage (CMU), and the idea of democracy in health has been consolidated by the establishment of the Consultative Assembly on Health (an idea which is to be further reinforced by the upcoming law on patients' rights and the performance of the health care system).

A significant fraction of the Gross National Product is invested in health

In 2000, the French spent more than 140 billion euros on health, a sum which corresponds to 10% of the Gross National Product. In 1998, France was fourth among OECD countries in terms of the fraction of the GNP devoted to health care. However, if *per capita* expenditure is considered rather than the ratio to the GNP, France is much lower (11th among OECD countries).

Between 1995 and 2000, health care expenditure rose by an average of 1.5% per annum in real terms (taking inflation into account) with a higher rate of increase at the end of this period than at the beginning. The National Health Insurance Expenditure Target (Ondam, *Objectif national des dépenses d'assurance maladie*) is regularly exceeded. Therefore, it cannot be claimed that

Recommended strategic directions

health care costs are being tightly restrained. However, because of the introduction of activity quotas which are often tied to the quality of the services, shortages may occur in certain areas (*e.g.* nursing and physical therapy) or at certain times of the year (during the summer and Christmas holidays).

Paradoxical situations

In the light of the excellent results referred to above coupled with the fact that significant resources are devoted to health and health care, certain paradoxical situations emerge, most of them quite unacceptable. Although France has the highest life expectancy at 65 in Europe, it is also the country in which (together with Portugal) life expectancy at birth is reduced to the greatest degree by death before 65. If no French men died before the age of 65, life expectancy at birth would be increased by 7 years. Rather than being due to curable disease, most deaths before 65 – or "premature deaths" – are associated with more or less preventable causes, *e.g.* excessive smoking and drinking, traffic accidents, suicide or AIDS.

Premature death is also a component of the problem of inequality – between the sexes, between different social classes, and between different regions. Recent research has shown that the differentials in France in this context are greater than those observed in comparable European countries for which the relevant data are available. Thus, the life expectancy of men is 7.5 years less than that of women, and the life expectancy at 35 of men in the managerial class is over 6 years greater than that of unskilled workers. Similarly, major differences emerge between geographical regions, even at a very small scale (*e.g.* between different cantons and industrialized areas). The life expectancy of boys born in the Region of Nord-Pas-de-Calais is a little over 71 years, a figure already reached in the southern Region of Midi-Pyrénées twenty years ago (where it is now about 76 years).

Despite a dense network of physicians all over the country and a relative readiness on the part of French people to seek medical advice, vaccine coverage is poor, *e.g.* many have never been vaccinated against mumps, measles and rubella. Elective abortion is likewise very common, evidence of failure to use contraception.

Other paradoxical situations emerge. Bacterial resistance to antibiotics is particularly common in France, a situation which often complicates patient care and which in part results from the abusive prescription of antibiotics. In order to overcome resistance, increasingly potent (and expensive) drugs are required and, above and beyond the resultant increased expenditure, the ultimate effect is a public health problem in that therapeutic failure is all the more likely.

The way the health care system works also gives rise to aberrant situations, such as the fact that hospitals are often overwhelmed when independent practitioners – who could take care of many of the patients admitted for emergency treatment without any problem – are plentiful (at least in urban settings).

Outmoded strategies and logistics

The paradoxical situations outlined above – as well as the good overall results – largely stem from the strategies followed to improve the nation's health.

Since the Second World War, treatment has been considered by all involved (decision-makers, professional care providers, patients, etc.) as the key issue in health. Increasing care provision and improving accessibility (notably by removing economic obstacles) have been seen as the foundation stones of health policy. It took the advent of AIDS to bring about the realisation that other determinants could be important and that other strategies might be more profitable in certain circumstances. In other words, for a long time (and still to a large extent today, despite significant progress in thinking), French health policy consisted of enhancing care provision rather than enhancing health. It is therefore perfectly logical that the most impressive improvements have been observed in those diseases which respond best to treatment (*e.g.* cardiovascular disease) and the worst results in those in which therapeutic intervention is less effective (*e.g.* cirrhosis of the liver, lung cancer and cancer of the upper airways or digestive tract). This gap between true health determinants and the simplistic nature of the strategies implemented (notably the over-riding emphasis on treatment) is indubitably a factor in both the major problems of today's health care system, namely inequality and the high level of premature death.

This lack of consistency between the strategies adopted and epidemiological realities is compounded by inadequacies in the way in which the health care system is funded. Budgets are always organised on an annual basis with all the counters being put back to zero at the end of the financial year. However, with the changing pattern of disease, the situation is no longer dominated by infectious diseases which strike in the form of short-lived epidemics, with outcomes – either positive or negative – evident in the very short term. Today, the health picture is dominated by chronic diseases which take many years to develop so that sufferers – even those who are already seriously ill – may be able to remain independent and live with their disease for a significant period of time. In other words, our current risk management modalities are structured to deal with short-term problems which are in fact in the minority these days. The idea of an annual health

Recommended strategic directions

budget or expenditure target is therefore based on an outmoded concept rather than the current reality. This year-by-year structure imposes an accountant's philosophy in which the way the health care system is funded has nothing to do with the longer-term dynamic underlying today's health care problems.

Finally, no critical appraisal of the way in which health care is organised would be complete without an examination of the extraordinary complexity and compartmentalisation within the system. With every new reform, new structures have been tacked onto existing ones without genuinely replacing them. The distribution of power has likewise been allowed to get out of hand: the process of decentralisation failed to abolish the deeply entrenched vertical hierarchy and, at the same time, it added horizontal components and brought in external players, a superposition which only led to increased overlap and intricacy with, as a corollary, the multiplication of "steering", "co-ordinating" "harmonisation" and "management" committees. Although the French State no longer has the same power as before decentralisation in certain fields, local structures are not entrusted with the same degree of responsibility as their European counterparts. This very French process has resulted – very subtly, it must be said – in less transparency and a major loss of efficiency. Neither the professionals nor the people now know exactly where they stand and, in the years to come, this situation in which more and more time has to be devoted to co-ordinating a proliferation of different individual players, structures and institutions is going to have to be reconciled with an across-the-board reduction in human resources in the health care system.

Health care issues to be addressed in the medium-term

Dealing with increased life expectancy and an ageing population

As in all developed countries, the proportion of the French population of over sixty-five years of age is sharply increasing. According to National Census figures, from 13.5% in 1975, it had grown to 16.5% by 1999. Initially, this trend was mainly due to lower reproduction rates but today, the main underlying factor is increased life expectancy, *i.e.* an extremely positive phenomenon.

However, the inexorable expansion of the elderly population raises a number of questions about how to keep the very old in reasonable health and how to cope with increasing dependency. "Pessimists" predict that an increasing number of elderly subjects will have a more or less linear effect on the overall requirement for health care resources, whereas "optimists" reject this scenario, tending to emphasise the progress already made in terms of increased disability-free life expectancy.

In fact, the number of elderly people who have lost their independence is not rising as fast as the number of elderly people in general, largely because of the ability to manage many chronic diseases these days, especially certain forms of cardiovascular disease. For example, between surgery and drug treatment, subjects with serious heart failure can now live and be kept independent for far longer. However, "independent" does not mean that they do not need care. A key corollary to the prolonged survival of patients with chronic disease is establishing effective and flexible monitoring systems, notably aimed at forestalling loss of independence. In other words, when it comes to dealing with an ageing population, the primary concern, for the benefit of everyone, is to prevent or delay the onset of age-related problems, notably the development of chronic disease and the loss of independence. And helping French people to live longer and in better health will necessarily involve implementing preventive measures throughout life, including at advanced age.

Thus, as soon as an elderly subject appears to be beginning to lose independence, his or her global care strategy should be reviewed, and measures devised to provide help and support above and beyond simply dealing with the patient's current health problems, *i.e.* with an ageing population, health care policy must address the consequences of disease as well as its management. This will involve novel approaches in the framework of a continuum, a modus operandi for which our current, highly stratified health care system is poorly adapted. The first thing to be overcome is the sharp institutional segregation between "social" and "health care" services, a structural division which is quite incompatible with caring for the elderly. Moreover, age should not be used as a criterion to direct people towards any specific organisation or instrument, and nor should it exclude anyone from any particular form of care. Less compartmentalisation would also make it easier to co-ordinate actions and institutions, both at the national and the local levels.

The ageing of the population is also giving rise to novel social issues. While these arguments are by no means confined to health, care-related questions are often a central element. At issue is how to foster new forms of cross-generational solidarity, both at the institutional level (social coverage funding, etc.) and at a more personal level (within the family, between neighbours, etc.). Individuals' and patients' rights take on a special resonance in this context, as do a whole host of ethical questions related to the end of life.

Recommended strategic directions

Cut down premature death and promote equitable health

As pointed out above, both premature death and inequitable health remain serious problems in France to a quite unacceptable extent and their mitigation must be a primary objective of public health policy. The bias towards strategies based on curative medicine has been at the expense of other potentially effective strategies aimed at preventing health problems developing in the first place.

For a sick person, the most important considerations are the accessibility and performance of the health care system and therefore it is quite logical that every effort be made to optimise these parameters. However, in many diseases, treatment is a relatively limited option without any hope of eventual cure. For example, although a patient with type II diabetes needs to be treated and cared for, how much more effective it would be to prevent the disease developing, *i.e.* cut down its incidence. Excess body weight is a major risk factor for type II diabetes and it is known that obesity is far more common among the poor, so this example provides a perfect illustration of how the most effective strategy to reduce an instance of inequality in health does not just involve improving care modalities, but needs to include a component to tackle the factors which are causing the health problem. The proof of this is the fact that, despite major improvements in both the accessibility and the performance of the health care system over the last twenty-five years, inequality is still as deeply entrenched as ever. Today, social and geographical inequality applies more to access to preventive measures than to treatment, given the major progress registered in the latter area. Across the board, insufficient attention is paid to environmental factors, working conditions and lifestyle considerations, all key determinants when it comes to good health.

Here, it is essential to bear in mind the major role of smoking and heavy drinking in not only premature death but also social and geographical inequalities. Cutting these high-risk behaviour patterns down would have a significant effect on both parameters but a policy aimed at this end, if it is not to be over-simplistic and therefore ineffective, must be based on an in-depth understanding of why smoking and heavy drinking are more common in certain social groups than in others. Analysing social expectations in this respect is another important factor.

Inequality in health needs to be considered from a perspective of images and determinants if policies which are more rational and more functional from an epidemiological point of view are to be formulated. More account needs to be accorded to certain key determinants, including cultural background, level of social integration, and the capacity to adapt to new living conditions. Furthermore, when phenomena associated with poverty are being addressed, special attention needs to be paid in a number of areas, including why certain social groups do not see health as a priority, why seeking medical help is sometimes left to the last minute, cultural barriers, the remoteness of health care institutions and professionals, and the lack of appropriate training programmes for professionals.

Prepare for reduced numbers of health professionals

Over the last few months, attention has been drawn to the possible consequences of the decrease in the number of doctors practising due to occur over the next ten to twenty years. As was the case for the ageing of the population, some of the projections are highly alarmist, suggesting that there will be a serious shortfall in the number of physicians in the near future – or even that one exists already. This has to be taken in the context of a few established but apparently inconsistent facts:
– never have there been so many qualified doctors in the country,
– the concentration of doctors is higher in France than in many economically comparable countries.

Yet:
– some hospital posts cannot be filled so that foreign doctors have to be brought in, especially to staff emergency services,
– in certain fields (both in and out of hospitals), there is already an impression of shortage, notably in terms of the length of time it takes to be given an appointment,
– in certain geographical areas (both urban and rural), the number of physicians leaving is greater than the number incoming.

Finally:
– the total number of practising physicians will drop within the next ten years,
– this problem does not just apply to doctors but also to other professional health care providers – and even to the population as a whole in which the number of people retiring over the next few years will significantly exceed the number coming onto the job market.

It is therefore clear that no real shortfall exists yet, but that problems do exist with respect to certain specialties, certain geographical areas, and certain types of practice. Extrapolating from the situation today may help us predict tomorrow's problems which will no doubt be on a larger scale. The short-term priority consists therefore of finding ways to make care provision more flexible to allow the system to respond to a demand which will be both greater and more diverse. At the same time, the flexibility of the system should also be increased so that it is more capable of integrating the latest medical and technological advances.

In any case, the number of students admitted into medical school will have to be reviewed, without forgetting the lag time due to the

Recommended strategic directions

long duration of medical training. In the end, parallel measures will probably be necessary, *e.g.* revision of how tasks and responsibilities are shared between physicians and others, and between General Practitioners and specialists. Logistical changes may also help the situation, *e.g.* simplifying procedures and cutting down the number of meetings would free up a significant fraction of professional health care providers' time.

In the same vein, human resources could be better exploited if there were more flexibility between different occupations, if not at the individual level then at least between institutions, *e.g.* sharing personnel. This could be achieved without damaging the interests of those affected.

Another danger is that a fall in the number of physicians will compound the problem of geographical inequality, either between the urban and rural settings or between different neighbourhoods in big cities.

The general public will have to be kept informed about any measures taken, and told if they need to change the way they act in order to respond to the changes. In practice, one of the most effective ways of dealing with falling numbers of doctors would be to reduce the number of inappropriate consultations and solicitations of the health care system; education is the way to achieve this, but care must be taken that the income of professional health care providers is not compromised as a result.

In general terms, when anticipating the possible effects of a decrease in the number of practising physicians and establishing the correct number of students to be admitted into medical school, rather than treating the issue as a terrible problem, we should see it as an opportunity to rationalise the system and improve its performance, including in terms of the quality of care provided.

Take local dynamics into account

The administrative region has become a far more important component in regulation of the French health care system in recent years. Numerous regional institutions have been created with a view to more efficient resource allocation. Health care priorities, identified by Regional Health Conferences on the basis of local needs, have been embodied in the directions adopted by the ARH and the Urcam structures, although each of these distinct organisations reacts and makes proposals according to its own agenda.

The way the system is currently organised is incompatible with resolving the issues that are currently emerging as the most important of all:
– first and foremost, a global view of health and health care, in which actions in the name of both the cure and prevention of

disease constitute a *continuum*, and are based on the principle of what is avoidable,
– subsequently, the need to co-ordinate prevention and treatment, a need which will entail co-ordination between the various regional institutions.

In this respect, the soon to be created Regional Health Councils should provide a framework for co-ordination although they will have no real decision-making power. Nevertheless, going forward will necessarily entail consolidation of democratic control by elected assemblies in order to ensure a balance of power.

The administrative region does not constitute the only geographical entity in which local issues and dynamics can be raised, and several recent laws passed in the context of town and country planning tend to promote co-operative initiatives between the various different basic French administrative units. For example, groups of neighbouring communes (the municipal body which is the smallest entity in the French administrative hierarchy) are joining together to form "communautés de communes", a change which actually represents a profound if silent revolution, and one which is going to mean a shift in the power balance at both the communal and department levels. These new geographical entities will be where horizontal policies are defined. Health policies and programmes will have to be integrated into these new structures, in exactly the same way as planning policy. This can only foster synergy between the institutions and players on the ground, in a context in which all health determinants are taken into account.

Improve performance in the health care system

The World Health Organisation ranked the French health care system as the best in the world, although the high level of premature death and major health inequalities are serious problems which illustrate that there remains great room for improvement.

Any attempt to measure the efficiency of a system comes up against problems associated with the validity of the indicators, the availability of information, and the appropriateness of the methodology used. Even if the overall resources allocated to the various sectors of care provision are known in a general way, this information cannot be compared with an estimate of needs, nor with results in terms of health status. Improving the performance of a health care system therefore depends on a better understanding of the strategies implemented, the resources allocated, and the results obtained. This applies particularly to differences between regions. For example, why are mortality rates so different? In the absence of a clear answer to that question, we continue to focus on care provision as a way of remedying the

Recommended strategic directions

situation, even though the results so far have been far from convincing. Is each region using the resources put at its disposal with the same degree of efficiency? To tell the truth, no-one knows.

Therefore, reliable indicators have to be developed to make it possible to compare the performance of the health care system in different regions (or other sub-regional geographical entities). The type of data needed is analogous to that used by the National Education system to compare the performance of different areas or schools. In this case, result indicators (*e.g.* success rate for the "Bac" [higher education's final diploma]) need to be interpreted in the context of external factors such as students' social background: it may turn out that schools with relatively low marks are actually performing better than other, more prestigious educational establishments once social conditions which are known to affect academic success have been taken into account.

The same type of approach could be applied to the health care system to compare regions or smaller geographical entities. To understand why life expectancy at birth varies so significantly from region to region, it would be very useful to be able to distinguish between the contributions of various components, *e.g.* social factors, inadequate resources, or inefficient exploitation of the resources. The conclusions to be drawn in terms of health care policy and resource allocation evidently depend on the relative importance of these factors, among others.

Enhancing the performance of the health care system depends also on changing professional practices and patient behaviour patterns. Predicted demographic changes (which will apply to health care professionals as well as the general population) are going to make operational improvement inevitable. Better quality can be the aspiration that unites everyone, including those seeking to improve the quality of their professional life. Efficacy and the quality of the medical services provided should be evaluated by both patients and professionals, especially in the context of resource allocation. The need to eliminate useless or even dangerous consumption habits is even more urgent today than before, but access to genuinely innovative modalities should be facilitated and distributed equitably. The level at which certain forms of treatment (dental and ophthalmologic) are reimbursed should also be stepped up significantly.

In a general way, the most important modification to be made in terms of behaviour and practices will consist in every involved party taking up a position in a *continuum* going all the way from action on the primary factors which determine health status to post-treatment follow-up care. Preventive and curative medicine should not be set against one another, and everyone should be asking themselves at all times what behaviour is likely to preclude the appearance of disease. If, notwithstanding, a health problem arises, the priorities must be how to manage it as quickly as possible and how to minimise its impact on daily social, professional and family life.

The quest for quality founded on an idea of what is avoidable can only be realised if the French health care system is simplified, and improvement will not be possible unless more account is accorded to the opinion of the man in the street, and more attention paid to satisfying him. This involves finding solutions to the problem of long waiting lists, improving the information given to patients by physicians, respecting patients' dignity and ensuring continuity in care provision. It will also mean cutting down the number of different organisations involved in the system, the accumulation of such organisations having been more a historical accident than a result of necessity (*e.g.* the multiplicity of health insurance schemes).

Promote community involvement and democracy

The return of old diseases together with the emergence of new ones has tarnished the image of medicine as being an all-powerful science in which progress is inexorable. Furthermore, acceleration in the rate of medical progress and technological innovation not only poses the problem of how these advances are to be financed, but also that of how they are to be implemented and how to deal with the new relationships that are engendered between professional health care provider and patient. Finally, social changes – notably those related to the new poverty – raise questions about the capacity of the system to cope with novel needs. At the same time as exercising the experts and managers of the system, these phenomena have also raised the consciousness of all the players in the collective arena concerning questions of health. It is in this sense that health has "come back" into the public eye.

But the formulation of public health policy must be founded first and foremost on health priorities rather than economic imperatives; this necessitates a double legitimacy, *i.e.* both social and technical. Not only must all points of view be broached and discussed, but also everyone should be given the chance and the knowledge necessary to contribute to the dialogue, a condition with an obvious cultural component. Information must be circulated and made available to as many people as possible, in terms of both material availability and comprehensibility. Real democratic debate is only possible if the key current issues are thoroughly understood by all concerned. At the moment, many topics are only understood by a small group of specialists and experts so that even the majority of professional health care providers – not to mention the vast majority of the general public – are insufficiently informed to make any real contribution to the discussion.

Recommended strategic directions

After consolidation of the patient's right to access to personal medical information, it is necessary to define a collective right of the population to know the level of its health status, the determinants of this status, and associated inequalities. The right to be informed about the working of the system should also be recognised. In all cases, information should be provided in a suitable format or medium and should be comprehensible to everyone rather than only to specialists and professionals.

But to participate in a debate, it is not sufficient to understand the underlying issues and arrive at an opinion: it is also necessary to be given the chance to voice that opinion. The rulings of April 1996 established a number of procedures and structures to guarantee some degree of user representation. Experience has shown that, although these initiatives were a step in the right direction (the Regional Health Conferences, etc.), much remains to be done. The law on patients' rights and the performance of the health care system currently being debated in Parliament should significantly enhance the situation but, more important than specific procedures, the best chance of making progress in promoting "democratic expression" will probably be through all political and generalist social bodies taking into account the "health" dimension.

Health policy issues: short-term objectives

All concerned are more or less in agreement that how the French health care system is organised and run needs to be completely overhauled, although, naturally, opinions diverge on exactly how to resolve the various difficulties and operational problems. Measures can be taken immediately or in the relatively short term to pave the way for later, more comprehensive changes. The first step is to identify preliminary measures to launch the transformation process without precluding any lines of action in the future, *i.e.* measures which will pave the way forward, whatever the options ultimately selected. Five series of proposals are presented in this perspective, for each of which reference is made to concrete situations.

Health policy issues: short-term objectives

1. Provide information about the situation and explain the issues

This means enumerating the various reasons why the health care system needs to be reformed, and explaining why new ways of operating have to be introduced. The objective is to foster as rational a public debate as possible based on more than simply emotional arguments. It is also to promote a climate of confidence between the community and health professionals. In this context, two measures could be implemented in the very near future.

Organise national and regional debates

The law on patients' rights and the performance of the health care system provides for regular debates to be organised by the National Health Conference and Regional Health Councils in the very near future. Moreover, numerous provisions of the law on democracy of proximity (passed by the National Assembly in June 2001) could be applied in this context, in particular the establishment of Neighbourhood Councils or the creation of bodies to disseminate information and perform evaluations at the instigation of at least one-fifth of the elected members for any question of communal, departmental or regional interest.

Include systematic evaluation of the impact on health in the public decision-making process

In order to foster a culture of public health at the same time as taking all health determinants into account in the decision-making process, a systematic evaluation of the impact on health should be carried out prior to the making of any decision (analogous to the systematic evaluation of the environmental impact of any public decision). For example, when deciding whether to keep or get rid of a branch railway line, the possible impact on access to the health care system should be taken into account, *i.e.* a perspective based on more than purely financial considerations. Such a procedure – above and beyond any positive results in terms of the quality of the decisions arrived at – would lead to a more global perception at all levels of society of the role of different health determinants. This proposal complements the provisions of the democracy of proximity Bill which pertains to public participation in building and renovation projects with significant impact on either the environment or regional development.

2. More recognition to restore confidence

For a number of years now, professional health care providers have been feeling increasingly undervalued and misunderstood. They do not feel that they are sufficiently involved in decisions on the working of the health care system. Moreover, they feel that they are mistrusted, and that they are always the ones who have to "carry the can" when some aspect of the care system fails. Nevertheless, any change in the health care system will depend on the recognition of their contribution, necessitating the large-scale support of the professionals as well as that of other players,

Recommended strategic directions

including the people. Three concrete measures can be implemented in the near future to improve this situation.

Improve mutual understanding of how the institutions and health care professionals operate

Numerous misunderstandings arise from false – and sometimes absurd – ideas that professionals have about the institutions and the way in which they operate. And similarly, the way in which professionals are represented by those in the institutions is also often caricatured, simplistic and inaccurate. More comprehensive information needs to be presented to all concerned at all levels – initial training, ongoing training, in the universities, at the National School of Public Health (ENSP, *École nationale de la santé publique*) and at the National Social Security Study Centre (Cness, *Centre national d'études de la sécurité sociale*). The current review of the medical training curriculum provides an excellent opportunity for integration of such a component.

Otherwise, meetings and joint training exercises could be organised to include professionals operating in different sectors, *e.g.* independent practitioners and those working for health insurance companies (both medical and administrative personnel). The ultimate objective would be to allow the various types of professional to exchange information about the possibilities and limitations of their respective professional practices.

Develop new avenues of individual communication between different professionals

Communication between different players in the health care system is often either too informal or too rigid and administrative. Between verbal exchange (which is flexible but often nothing is put in writing), the official form (which is uncongenial and often over-simplified) and collective communication (more or less attractive and detailed), there is a place for new avenues of individual communication which are simple at the same time as being relatively formalised.

Interviews with health professionals could be subject to more structured protocols. Thus, the management of type II diabetes mainly relies on regular "fraternal" meetings – following a stipulated protocol – between physicians in independent practice and physicians working for the health insurance scheme.

Exploitation of the possibilities offered by the new information and communication technologies should also be investigated and developed. E-mail represents a fast, effective and simple tool to encourage communication between professionals and the various administrations: it can be used to facilitate direct relationships between two individuals or to get information to specifically targeted groups of people in a cheap and fast manner.

Health policy issues: short-term objectives

Help players make the most of their skills and their institutional affiliations

For a number of years now, a major effort has been made to bring professionals and users together in the making of decisions in the field of health. The usual measures taken involve ensuring their representation on the various councils, commissions and working groups involved in the process. If these representations are not to be merely formal in character, professionals and users must be given the opportunity to acquire sufficient mastery of the questions involved to enable them to form a valid opinion. Therefore, training and education sessions need to be organised before any actual meeting in the presence of representatives of the relevant administrative bodies. This is why the law on patients' rights and the performance of the health care system makes provision for time off work for this type of education, and a right to training. There are many different ways of encouraging participation in this field, *e.g.* certain hospitals have begun making the most of the users' representatives on their administration councils. Such actions need to be expanded to as great an extent as possible with adequate resources, notably in the matter of reimbursing lost revenue.

Simplify the instruments and clarify responsibilities

The logistical complexity of the health care system results in serious energy loss and massive wastage of human resources. Of course, simplifying the instruments will entail deep, long-term reforms but, in the meantime, measures can be implemented which do not necessitate major legislative changes but rather depend on a shared willingness to improve the situation.

Cut down the redundancy of procedures

Skills are split between different institutions in many fields in today's health care system. Each institution, for either regulatory reasons or on its own initiative, has created its own structure for consultation or advice (and its own commissions and working groups etc.), with different institutions trying to outdo one another in this respect in some cases. However, it is often the same local players who find themselves on these different bodies of which a good proportion could be merged, if only with the purpose of cutting down on the number of meetings which have to be attended. This should be one of the concrete objectives for the Regional Health Councils.

Encourage the centralisation of services

The principle of centralised services is being generalised to facilitate daily life, *e.g.* in the case of the simultaneous payment of both the social security and mutual insurance components of reimbursement for treatment. On the other hand, to finance projects, professionals are often still obliged to solicit several different administrative departments or even different offices of the same department, each time having to fill out a separate form. Notwith-

Recommended strategic directions

standing, "one-stop shopping" is a practical option in almost all cases and it is just a question of organising it. Already in place in certain cases, this mode of organisation should be rapidly made systematic.

Exploit existing administrative means to enhance budgetary flexibility

The multiplicity of different budgets not only complicates the lives of health care professionals but also compromises the consistency of actions. Resources should therefore be allocated according to a global rationale to optimise the use of the different sources of funds available in order to avoid the compartmentalisation of instruments due to administrative factors which are incompatible with the continuity of the health care process. Initiatives undertaken in some of the regions show that, with a will, progress can be made on this front.

Create institutional mediators to implement health-related programmes and actions

The development of health policy at the regional, departmental or local level is often accompanied by the appointment of a "project leader" whose essential role is to supervise and co-ordinate the various working groups and commissions necessary to formulating policy. After a given policy has been adopted, the more operational executive functions should be transferred to a "mediator" appointed by agreement on the part of all the concerned institutions. Mediators would have a stipulated term of office to be renewed after a given lapse of time. This corresponds to progressing from the consensual type of procedure conducive to the formulation of policy to the more structured type of organisation necessary for its implementation.

Increase the transparency of the procedures which regulate the relationship between the State and the health insurance system

The question of the respective roles of the State and the health insurance will naturally be at the heart of the coming reforms. The stakes in this context are considerable. It is not surprising that the relationship between the two is a complex one. In the regions, for example, in the context of collaborations between the Drass and the Urcam bodies, local players try to limit the impact of difficulties stemming from nationally-based problems as effectively as possible. Nevertheless, as a result of these difficulties, the players on the ground often suffer from the interruption of administrative functions, in particular delays in the decision-making process or in the transfer of funds. Until this problem is resolved by in-depth reform, the State and the health insurance system should stabilise and regularise their procedures in the short term in order to afford players in the health care system better visibility in the exercise of their jobs and duties.

4. Develop logistics and introduce more flexibility into resource management

Since the first three-yearly High Committee Report was published in 1994, the will to develop a genuine public health policy founded on real public health priorities at both the national and regional level has manifested in the establishment of new procedures and instruments, in particular the Health Conferences and health programmes. Certain organisational problems have arisen as a result of the accumulation of different bodies but it will be possible to resolve these difficulties in the context of a general rationalisation of the architecture of the system. Another question concerns the ideal logistics for conducting health policy. What instruments are necessary? The experience of the last few years has clearly shown that it is now necessary to change from a "militant" approach based on highly committed individuals to a more sustained kind of rationale which is less dependent on individuals. It is no longer possible to propose ambitious policies and programmes based entirely on the good faith of concerned individuals because the logistical resources that individuals have at their disposal are limited. Moreover, new skills and knowledge bases are required since routine administrative procedures are not always ideal for running projects. The fact that in the years to come the number of people retiring is going to exceed the number coming onto the job market will result in not only a reduction in the proportion of the population as a whole in work but also a parallel loss in the number of practising specialists at a time when their services will be needed more than ever. To resolve some of the resultant difficulties, more flexibility in working practices in the health care system will be necessary. Four measures to promote such flexibility could be implemented immediately without waiting any longer.

Develop and harmonise information and assessment systems

The corollary to the multiplicity of decision-makers, funding bodies and players, is a multiplicity of information-gathering services, the scope of different service often corresponding to a certain institution's particular field of action or remit. As a result it is sometimes difficult to get an overall picture of the situation, *e.g.* of health status or of how efficiently resources are being utilised.

Most of the time, the existing data pertain to either care provision or reimbursement. On the other hand, there is not enough data available to get a real idea of the relationship between results and the resources invested. As a result, resources are allocated today on incomplete bases and are dedicated without a hope of being able to make a precise assessment of the efficiency with which they are being utilised. Moreover, the consequences of changes in care provision (*e.g.* failing to replace departing physicians, the closing of hospital departments, etc.) on people's health or accessibility to treatment cannot be thoroughly evaluated.

Recommended strategic directions

At neither the national nor the regional level are sufficient means dedicated to analysing such data, although there has been some progress in this respect in recent years. Generating more useful information means harmonising indicators and adopting, to at least some extent, a common approach based on pooled skills and funding. Making the most of the information already available and extending it to make it possible to compare the way the system is performing in different contexts could derive from the establishment of national and regional information programmes to be co-ordinated by the Regional Health Councils in accordance with the perspectives opened in the new law on patients' rights and the performance of the health care system which provides for the co-ordination of regional surveys and statistics.

Promote the design and running of projects by establishing regional logistical support units

The development of health policy and associated programmes involves mobilising new skills. The horizontal dimension of the action, the co-ordination of institutions on a non-hierarchical, contractual basis, and the mobilisation of professionals, elected officials, users and the people will require a capacity to co-ordinate a great number of different institutions and individuals. It will not be enough just to design – it will also be necessary to explain and convince. The current training of management in the Civil Service, the health insurance system and local authorities, and indeed the training of professionals who are likely to become involved in public health projects in general, fails to prepare them to deal with these situations. Specific training in how to run health-related projects or implement health policy is required, in the form of initial and ongoing programmes for both newcomers into these professions and those already occupying the positions. At this time, the experts in this area are often those who have learnt by painful experience acquired by "getting their hands dirty". Unfortunately, at this point in time, these precious skills are unrecognised and undervalued. They should be brought together in a regional centre and made available to all, independently of whichever specific structure the professionals concerned happen to work for.

Otherwise, conducting regional health care programmes and other procedures such as those pertaining to the networks or Funds for the Improvement of the Quality of Independent Care (FAQSV, *Fonds d'amélioration de la qualité des soins de ville*) involves appeals for a maximum of commitment on the part of the players "on the ground". Past experience shows that sometimes such projects are approved even before they have been sufficiently thought out. It also happens that – as is the case for the FAQSV – the number of acceptable projects is far below the number for which funds are available (and the differential can be huge). This situation results partly from the absence of logistical support for the design and management of such projects. Because of a lack of time or ignorance of various technical and administrative aspects, the professionals on the ground are not always in a position to propose projects which will yield sufficiently reliable results. Notwithstanding, their opportunities for access to structured aid are extremely limited.

Following the example of enterprise zones, every region should establish an analogous "project unit", a collaborative structure to offer sponsors tailor-made help with the design and running of projects. Apart from improving the feasibility of projects and the reliability of their results, such a structure would help avoid the funding institutions becoming financially involved and materially implicated in a project which, at a later date, they will be called upon to assess, *i.e.* such a structure would separate judge and jury.

tablish common structures in the form of flexible, innovative legal instruments

If resources are to be shared, common modes of organisation and management practices will have to be established in the context of flexible, innovative legal instruments. Taking refuge in the status of a non-profit-making organisation too often constitutes an easy solution to manage funds in a more pragmatic manner. Non-profit-making organisations tend to multiply as projects and actions proceed which leads to fragmentation of human resources and scattering of funding, neither of which makes for efficacy. Moreover, this formula has the major disadvantage of demanding little financial commitment from its members which is the reason for the lack of institutional security of many associations. It is true that certain alternative formulae such as that of the public interest group are more difficult to establish and operate. Special formulae adapted on the legal and regulatory fronts could be devised. Moreover, other possibilities could be explored: economic interest groups, employers' associations, social economy unions, collective interest co-operative societies, etc. While collaborative formulae multiply between local authorities or health care establishments, it would not be normal to exclude most players in the health care system from these innovative possibilities.

o allow genuine obility between the public and ivate sectors or tween different levels of the administrative structure

If the institutional organisation of the health care system is today extremely fragmented, the same is true of professional grades, despite the frequency of mixed practice: salaried employees, independent contractors, public sector and private sector employees, different public positions including a multitude of civil servants or, in the private sector, conventions leading to highly variable situations. This complexity is now resulting in differences which can, for example, lead some doctors to prefer the conditions of practice in private hospitals, and nurses to prefer conditions in the public sector.

Recommended strategic directions

Apart from this type of malfunction, the rigidities thus introduced are incompatible with the current obligation to make the most of available skills, which may be in the private or the public sector but not always both at the same time. It is therefore urgent to find formulae which will allow any health professional with the required skills to occupy a post not provided for in the public sector as in the private sector. There is no simple procedure in existence today which allows for the appointment, on the basis of experience, of private sector employees to posts with public sector responsibilities, although the inverse is possible: the recruitment of directors of regional hospitalisation agencies outside of the framework of routine civil service procedures has shown that this type of innovation is quite possible as long as the political will exists.

5. Anticipate

We are very poor at anticipating at this point in time, with the result that many problems have to be resolved retrospectively even though they could have been foreseen. During its first term of office, the High Committee focused on problems associated with complementary insurance coverage resulting from economic difficulties affecting part of the population, and successive plans intended to slow down the rate of increase in health insurance expenditure. It was necessary to wait until the situation became quantitatively and socially unacceptable before basic complementary coverage could be established in the form of Universal Health Insurance Coverage. This problem could have been foreseen and help provided from the outset to those in financial difficulties, as was done by certain health insurance companies and mutual companies. Two series of measures are proposed to favour the anticipation of problems.

Extend vigilance procedures and structures by exploiting the knowledge of the players on the ground

It is a common phenomena that, before a new problem is generally perceived as such, there is a phase during which players on the ground are aware of the problem but are unable to appreciate its scale. In certain cases, monitoring instruments exist to collect isolated observations to put them into context, *e.g.* is there an epidemic underway or not? Such watchdog structures also exist for adverse reactions to drugs (pharmacovigilance) and domestic accidents caused by products and equipment. More watchdogs should be created, particularly in a social context (sociovigilance). These networks could also address adverse effects associated with the working of the health care system in the social and economic contexts, involving all professionals and even the people.

Develop prospective reflection and multidisciplinary approach

Planning initiatives such as those of the Regional Health Organisation Schemes (Sros, *schémas régionaux d'organisation sanitaire*) have resulted in an approach which aims more towards correcting current operational problems rather than adopting a prospective attitude which is likely to be able to predict future problems and prevent them from occurring.

As evidenced by the recently compiled National Collective Health Services Scheme *(Schéma national des services collectifs de santé)*, truly prospective measures necessarily involve a multidisciplinary approach. In practice, the capacity to see into the future is not the sole preserve of any single group of professionals or any single social class. It is by sharing a horizontal vision and by allowing a synergy to develop based on different points of view that there can be hope of demonstrating enough creativity and realism to construct reliable projections of how needs, expectations and response capacities are likely to evolve in the future.

All the measures proposed above can be implemented or prepared for in the short term and the High Committee does not believe that any of them are dependent on major institutional changes (although they will help pave the way for the serious reforms to come). Nevertheless, these measures can only be fully effective if general approach in the French health care system is regularised in three main areas:
– prevent the occurrence of avoidable health problems by devoting more resources to strategies which are aimed at affecting key determinants other than treatment;
– shift the focus to longer-term strategies which are not required to produce annual results and are not based on financial equilibrium;
– promote a more global approach to health problems and their determinants by breaking down barriers between social factors, medicosocial factors and health care.

Declaration by the High Committee on Public Health, adopted at the plenary session on November 20 2001.

PART ONE

Data about health status

Part one Data about health status

Composition of the Working Group

President Anne Tallec, High Committee on Public Health

Rapporteur Gérard Badéyan, Directorate of Research, Studies, Evaluation and Statistics, Ministry of Employment and Solidarity

Members François Bonnaud, High Committee on Public Health
Yves Charpak, High Committee on Public Health
Hubert Isnard, Institute for Public Health Surveillance
Eric Jougla, National Institute for Health and Medical Research, CépiDc
Bernard Junod, National School of Public Health
Marie-Claude Mouquet, Directorate of Research, Studies, Evaluation and Statistics,
Ministry of Employment and Solidarity
Martine Ruch, General Health Directorate,
Ministry of Employment and Solidarity
Catherine Sermet, Centre for Research and Documentation on the Economics of Health

Co-ordination Claudine Le Grand, General Secretariat of the High Committee on Public Health

The Working Group wishes to thank for their contributions Nathalie Bajos, National Institute for Health and Medical Research U292
Jean Bousquet, National Institute for Health and Medical Research U454
Gérard Bréart, National Institute for Health and Medical Research U149
Jean-François Dartigues, National Institute for Health and Medical Research U330
Christiane Dressen, French Committee for Health Education
Emmanuelle Fleurence, Intercommunal Hospital Centre, Créteil
Marcel Goldberg, National Institute for Health and Medical Research U88
Denis Leguay, Mental Health Centre, Angers
Henri Leridon, National Institute for Health and Medical Research U292
Joël Ménard, UFR Broussais-Hôtel-Dieu, Paris
Sylvie Sander, Clinique Sourdille, Nantes
François Tuffreau, Pays de la Loire Regional Health Surveillance Centre
Alain Weill, National Health Insurance Agency for Salaried Workers
Xavier Zanlonghi, Clinique Sourdille, Nantes

Introduction

To set out to describe the state of health of the French nation is an ambitious endeavour which necessarily involves making choices. The choices made in the compilation of this new HCPH report are substantially different from those implemented for preceding versions. This is because of the realisation that the nature of the data on which such a description is based has significantly changed in recent years. The first triennial HCPH report was published in 1994 in a context in which information was relatively lacking (although this first report was broader in scope than similar reports published previously under the auspices of Inserm or the government), and the main objective of the second report published in 1998 was to document the changes that had taken place since 1994.

Now, the information available on health is more comprehensive and more reliable. Many different institutions are collecting data on a permanent or *ad hoc* basis in the name of various approaches to health issues, and many high-quality studies have been conducted in the intervening years. The priorities now are to make the information which is available more accessible, to integrate data from different sources in order to make the most of the work that has already been done, and to try to identify with as much objectivity as possible the most striking observations and the most important findings pertaining to the state of health of the French people.

The decision to try to integrate data taken from diverse sources led the Working Group to opt for an approach based on specific age brackets rather than a global analysis of the population as a whole. This is justified since age is such a key factor in health and because fundamentally different problems arise at the various

Part one Data about health status

stages of life. An age-based approach rather than a disease-based one is also more helpful when it comes to devising policies targeting specific groups in the community. Nevertheless, there are obvious limitations due to the fact that the state of health of an individual – and that of a group – is a *continuum* with extensive interdependence between all ages.

The population has been divided into four age brackets: 0 to 14, 15 to 44, 45 to 74 and 75 and over. Thus, the traditional boundaries of 35 and 65 have been ignored.

The first bracket, that of 0 to 15, represents a period of both physical and psychological growth, a time of learning during which behaviour patterns and representations are being structured. This sub-population is dependent on others – the vast majority of children of under 15 years of age live with their parents –, and attendance at school is obligatory throughout most of the period concerned. Health care for this population comes under the specialism of paediatrics, both in and out of the hospital setting.

The second bracket – 15 to 44 – corresponds to young adults. This can be considered as the period during which experience and knowledge are exploited, the time when risks are taken. It is a time of upward mobility in both professional and social life (notably covering the child-bearing years in the case of women).

Traditionally, the next phase of life used to be closed at 65 in order to coincide with common changes in social life and, most importantly, with retirement. Today, however, the end of working life in the population as a whole spans a far broader time frame with retirement for some at 60, early retirement for others, gradual withdrawal from professional activity, etc. There is not the same abrupt break as previously. Added to this is the fact that most 65-year-olds are now in relatively good health and are still completely independent. Therefore, it was decided to shift the boundary from 65 to 75, *i.e.* fix the age bracket at 45 to 75, the period during which most of the serious health problems to be dealt with by the health care system are going to arise.

Finally, the 75 and over bracket can be considered as that of the elderly, a population which poses specific problems when it comes to care, not only health care but care in general.

Five diverse but complementary sources of information were selected on the basis of availability and the capacity of those that generate the data to provide the figures: mortality data (from the medical registry of causes of death managed by the CépiDc of Inserm); hospital admissions (the PMSI registry of the Drees); consultations with physicians in independent practice (the IMS-Health Ongoing Medical Prescription Monitoring Survey used by the Credes); declared morbidity (the Insurance Coverage and Health Survey of the Credes); and the reasons for recognition of

Introduction

a long-term condition (LTC) (figures compiled by the Cnamts on the basis of a defined list of long term conditions). For data from sources other than mortality, a great deal of work was carried out to compile figures for groups of diseases (which was done for mortality on the basis of the S9 summary list which breaks causes of death down into 110 different categories) to ensure that the most common diseases or situations were selected with as much rigour as possible.

The overall rationale of the Working Group was iterated at the beginning of this chapter for clarity. What follows is a presentation of details about the methods used to interpret the indicators, together with a description of the sources. Then, there are sub-chapters dealing with each of the four age brackets. For each age group, the indicators are dealt with in order: declared morbidity; reasons for medical consultations outside a hospital setting; reasons for admission into hospital; reasons for admission for long term conditions; and causes of death. Each sub-chapter also includes a section entitled "The Main Issues" which seeks to highlight the most striking observations concerning health in that age bracket on the basis of not only data from the five main sources but also from complementary sources. In this section, certain specific problems will be dealt with in greater depth and presented in special boxes.

Finally, to maintain continuity with the preceding reports, the evolution of certain general indicators is shown in two Tables presented as an Appendix.

Part one   Data about health status

Summary and issues

A detailed description of the state of health of the French people and their health care system – together with all the available data – would be a mammoth document, bulky and no doubt difficult to digest.

The High Committee on Public Health has therefore been obliged to make certain choices, as was the case for the previous reports: the choice of sources, of which data to use from each source, of the most relevant analysis methods, and of how to interpret the results. All are necessarily subjective choices, although an effort has been made to systematise and standardise the approach. A different Working Group or institution might have selected other key items or other ranking systems for the problems under consideration.

One of the reasons for this situation is that the role of the HCPH is to present to the decision-makers (*i.e.* the Minister of Health and the French Parliament) those elements it considers important, without any specifications having been stipulated beforehand. However, with respect to quantitative data (as with any other kind of information), it is necessary in general that the right questions be posed to produce relevant answers.

Analysing the state of health of a nation and assessing the efficiency of a health care system requires a minimum of basic knowledge and understanding of the relevant biological, medical, epidemiological and economic models as well as of the mechanisms which interconnect state of health and health care institutions. This familiarity with the subject cannot be supplanted by any ten-minute Powerpoint presentation or sound bite-filled "performance", nor by individual experiences of poor health, nor even by composite indicators, however sophisticated they may be. The unquestioning esteem of life expectancy as a universal indicator of health and of the efficiency of the health care system reveals a cultural inadequacy in our society in this respect. Although useful, in practice this figure gives an idea restricted to the duration of life without any qualitative component, *i.e.* no assessment of degree of disability or overall quality of life, both of which are issues to which a large fraction of health care resources are dedicated these days and which warrant profound consideration when it comes to assessing the performance of any health care system.

Summary and issues

This situation is at the root of a common criticism from which the HCPH Working Group responsible for compiling this chapter on Data and Results cannot entirely dissociate itself, namely "It is the experts who ask the questions and then give the answers".

If the community as a whole and decision-makers need a tailored description of the health of the French people to enable them to make informed choices, they will have to make more of an effort to acquire a minimum understanding of the underlying mechanisms and models so that they can identify the right questions to put to the experts.

The analysis presented in this chapter leads the members of the HCPH Working Group to recommend that the emphasis be put on the following issues:
- improving the working of the health information system, especially developing the monitoring of effects,
- making the community and decision-makers more familiar with the key issues in public health,
- capitalising on and consolidating the considerable progress made in terms of health, and making every effort to ensure that this progress is equitably accessible to all,
- escalating the fight against avoidable causes of premature death, both within and outside the remit of the health care system,
- promoting the development of tertiary prevention modalities, above all for the elderly.

Improving the working of the health information system

In 1994, the first HCPH *Health in France* report drew attention to numerous flaws in the French health information system: its fragmented nature; the lack of any broad perspective; the large number of players involved, each with a different logic; the poor medical content of the information; and the inadequacy of the resources dedicated to analysis and exploitation of the data, once collected.

Considerable progress has been made in recent years. At the end of 1998, the Health Minister transformed the Sesi (Statistics and Information Systems Department) into the Drees (Department of Research, Studies, Evaluation and Statistics), a change which spurred a new dynamic resulting in a more integrated approach to the health care system, especially concerning areas of overlap with social issues. The creation in 1999 of the *Institut de veille sanitaire* (Institute for Public Health Surveillance) under the auspices of the *Réseau national de santé publique* (National Public Health Network) and, more specifically, the extension of its remit to cover "Health and Work" and "Chronic Disease and Injury", represents a definite step forward. Nevertheless, the team at this latter department is small given the size of this field which largely consists of ground as yet unbroken. Otherwise, the ORSs (Regional Health Surveillance Centres) have, in the context of their Federation, consolidated their position at the regional level by establishing collaborative projects and harmonising their methods. The possibility of on-line access to the vast *Score Santé* (Health Score) data base represents another step forward in making information on health care and social indicators more available. Many other structures are also actively participating in this development, notably Inserm and Credes.

Among the new information collecting modalities, the establishment in hospitals of the *Programme de médicalisation des systèmes d'information* (Hospital Medical Information Systems Programme) is making a major contribution to the evaluation of the morbidity that is being managed in hospitals (even if this was not one of the explicit objectives of this programme); for this programme, the decision was taken to make an exhaustive compilation which entails the deployment of enormous resources to collect data on all of the fifteen million hospital stays every year in France. Finally, certain specific actions in areas hitherto poorly covered are proving informative, including the HID (Handicap, Disability and Dependency) survey and the surveys conducted on a three-year basis of the health of 6-year-old, fifth grade and ninth grade children.

Overall incidence figures for cancer (both in France and by region) have been compiled on the basis of extrapolations made from mortality data on the one hand, and incidence data taken from cancer registries on the other. Similarly, a better impression of the impact of ageing has been made possible by the determination of figures on disability-free life expectancy.

However, given the seriousness of the stakes in human, social and economic terms, the current health information apparatus remains inadequate: of insufficient size and, more importantly, not well organised enough to contribute the insight which is absolutely required if an evolving health care system is to be managed properly, especially in the current climate of the combined exigencies of reducing health care expenditure and, at the same time, developing an ambitious but coherent public health policy.

The work carried out to formulate this report brought to light – again – a number of problems:

- The data sources of information are numerous and heterogeneous, and managed by diverse public and private institutions, with different objectives which range from the administration of institutions to the production of scientific data on health. Integrating data from these different sources is often difficult, partly because of a lack of homogeneity in the gathering process (the instruments used, coding systems, validation procedures, etc.)

Summary and issues

and analysis methods (*e.g.* categories and classification systems), and partly because of the absence of common statistical identifiers. For example, knowing that it is impossible to establish a link between two different hospital stays on the part of the same patient, it is not surprising that it is difficult to find out about the specific social or health care services solicited by a certain beneficiary of a disability allowance, and even more difficult when it comes to discovering the cause of his handicap or about the history of his handicap as a child (if applicable). This is because all these pieces of information are managed by different institutions. The only approach which can be attempted at this point in time is simple combination of the data from different sources without any linkage between the statistical units. This is the approach underlying the analysis reported later in this chapter and even this reduced procedure requires an enormous amount of work to harmonise, re-code and reanalyse the data in order to make any kind of comparison possible. Although it may be unreasonable to expect a completely centralised data collection system (or even centralised analysis), it is indispensable that the main institutions responsible for information about health at least work together to harmonise the instruments and methods used to collect data, and use consistent classification systems so that data collected by diverse agencies can be used to best effect.
The question of making it easier to establish links between different sources or different pieces of information by means of common identifiers raises problems of confidentiality, privacy and the rights of the individual, problems which should not be dismissed, although the debate could at least be opened.

- The fragmented nature of information on health means that certain areas remain obscure, and these areas are by no means necessarily the least important or those associated with less expenditure. The example of cardiovascular disease – for which our knowledge is largely based on isolated mortality data – is an eloquent example, but there are also huge gaps in our understanding of nosocomial infections, the causes of disability, mental health, and the state of health of institutionalised, elderly subjects.

- Whereas significant resources have been made available in certain areas (like the PMSI as mentioned above), those allocated to the analysis and presentation of data, and to inter-institutional initiatives remain sadly inadequate, a situation which leads to under-exploitation of data that has already been collected. In the specific case of the PMSI, this under-valuation leads to lack of motivation and even mistrust on the part of those responsible for data collection, a situation which is obviously going to compromise the quality of the data generated. Moreover this lack of confidence appears in a climate of general reticence when it comes to surveys which are frequently commissioned but often poorly co-ordinated, *e.g.* between regional and national programmes. The inadequacy of the resources allocated to analysis also accounts for the lack of conceptual work in this field because the qualified experts involved rarely have enough time to conduct methodological investigations or apply the methods developed by others (*e.g.* the WHO *Global burden of disease* approach).

- Finally, there is a serious division between studies conducted by clinical specialists and those carried out by the institutions. More often than not, one group is unaware of the other's results despite the fact that, in many cases, extremely complementary issues are being addressed.

This criticism of information systems takes on a particular relevance at a time when major changes in health care provision – with a view to reducing the rate of increase in expenditure – are either underway or in the pipeline. These changes concern most areas of health care provision: the hospital system of course with major restructuring work on the way, but also independent practitioners, with notably changes in medical demographics and the establishment of activity quotas for certain paramedical care providers such as nurses and physical therapists.

A large fraction of the most frequent complaints of the French population (which account for a high proportion of medical consultations) are rarely mentioned, probably because the health care system performs "effectively" or at least "at an acceptable level" in these areas. It is of course important to be on the lookout for ways of improving the efficacy and safety of the corresponding care modalities, but it also seems important to establish indicators to monitor these complaints and how they are being dealt with in order to identify potential problems before they result in deterioration in the way in which these common complaints are being managed.

A strategic and political approach to information systems remains to be adopted. Such an approach would exploit to the full what already exists while, at the same time, paving the way for the systems that are being developed and that will become available in the future. Clear responses to a number of questions are required: Who should be generating what? With what purpose in mind? With what resources? Where are the gaps that need filling? What areas of redundancy are inevitable?

Summary and issues

Providing the general public and decision-makers with a more accurate picture of key public health issues

Ranking health problems is obviously difficult although there is a clear discrepancy between the frequency of different diseases and the amount of media coverage they attract. Various reasons underlie this discrepancy.

Firstly, because certain common disorders are being managed relatively well, they are treated as commonplace. In contrast, the question of the safety of treatment modalities for certain problems has become a media issue, with undue attention sometimes being drawn to rare incidents. While this may incite professional health care providers to concentrate on the quality of their work, the zero risk objective imposed by media pressure may eventually compromise the "average" level of care. Resisting this pressure and promoting reasoning based on an integrated analysis of costs, risks and benefits is one of the current priorities in our health care system.

Other conditions are covered less by the media for reasons of cultural acceptance, *e.g.* acute upper airways infections in young children, diseases related to heavy drinking, and impaired vision and hearing in the elderly. As a result, insufficient importance is attached to such problems in the community. However, representations can evolve very fast, as illustrated by the example of pain which is seen as far less acceptable these days than it was in relatively recent history.

The media weight of certain health problems can also be intensified by the activities of interested parties, be they patient support groups or commercial organisations.

Finally and most importantly of all, the media reflect society and tend to give the general public what it wants to hear, often highlighting events charged with emotion and downplaying the common and commonplace.

Although the media spotlight can sometimes effectively draw attention to under-estimated problems, permanent distortion of the relative importance of different diseases can have a serious impact on the decision-making process, and give rise to imbalance in the allocation of human and financial resources.

The answer is not of course to control, pressure or even criticise the media, but rather to identify effective ways of broadcasting reliable information in order to give the decision-makers the chance of handling "media hype" more effectively.

This depends on a fostering a more accurate perception of the true relative importance of the key manifold health risks and issues among both the general public and decision-makers. Experts in public health need to be brought into the decision-making process and encouraged to play a greater role in the evaluation of the consequences of decisions implemented.

Capitalising on and consolidating the considerable progress made in the matter of health, and making every effort to ensure that this progress is equitably accessible to all

In recent years, awareness has increased of the true dimension of the problem of avoidable, premature death in France (a problem which is very much still with us and is the subject of the next paragraph). The imbalance between the resources allocated to care (which has been favoured for decades) and to prevention (which has traditionally been under-valued and under-resourced) led to under-estimation of the considerable progress made in the matter of overall health in the HCPH's previous reports which – it is true – tended to concentrate on care.

Certain advances translate as improvement in indicators or measurable changes in high-risk behaviour patterns, including the following non-exhaustive list of examples:
– alcohol consumption in France is down, although the country remains poorly placed and it is important to be vigilant about high-risk among the young;
– cardiovascular mortality has dropped, largely as a result of preventive measures vis-à-vis certain risk factors which arise in the second half of life (notably hypertension and hyperlipidemia), advances in interventional treatment modalities, and improved ways of preventing recurrences;
– fall-related mortality has decreased, although it is not known whether this is due to falls being fewer and/or less serious, or rather due to improved care;
– infant mortality as a whole has considerably decreased, largely due to progress in neonatology and in the prevention of Sudden Infant Death Syndrome;
– by virtue of tritherapy, mortality due to AIDS has dropped, and the onset of the symptoms of the disease is being delayed.

Other advances have not given specific effects which can be measured, mainly because they do not affect mortality, the indicator for which the most comprehensive, long-term data exist. But there has been progress in terms of disability-free life expectancy and even simple quality of life. This applies, for example, to the generalisation of cataract surgery, the increasingly widespread implantation of prostheses, and the development of epidural anaesthesia during childbirth.

Still other advances are too recent to have yet had any effect on indicators of mortality or morbidity, *e.g.* mass screening for breast cancer.

These advances are the fruit of considerable effort, both financial and human, individual and collective. Recognising the value of all these efforts – which now affect all aspects of health and health care to a greater or lesser extent – is essential if the benefit is to be sustained. And such recognition will provide positive reinforcement for both health care professionals and the population as a whole.

All this does not mean to say that there is no room for improvement. Ways of improving quality and safety always exist and need

Summary and issues

to be actively sought (*e.g.* improving compliance in patients with high blood pressure).

Ensuring equitable access to these advances must also represent a priority so that the serious discrepancies which exist between different regions and different social groups – inequalities which are dealt with in the second part of this report – can be reduced or, at least, not allowed to get any worse. In practical terms, following changes means analysing mean values of the relevant indicators, an approach which often means that data which would make it possible to investigate whether all sub-populations are benefiting equally is simply not available.

This can be addressed by analysing the available data in an appropriate way, by devising suitable *ad hoc* data collection instruments, or by developing strategies to specifically answer the question of equitable access.

For example, it would seem essential to know exactly who are the 50% of women who fail to take advantage of the organised breast cancer screening programs in those regions where such programs are running. Are they well informed women who deliberately opt not to take part and organise their own screening on a private basis? Or are they poorly informed women who are never screened at all?

Similarly for the elderly, it would be useful to know whether the reduction in mortality associated with falls is purely due to the sub-population with assiduous home care; and whether cataract and hip replacement surgery are equitably offered to all those who need them.

Finally, advances often engender ethical problems. Physicians are increasingly brought to asking themselves about the extent to which they should intervene at a time when technical limitations do not always constitute the most relevant obstacle.

Escalating the fight against avoidable causes of premature death, both within and outside the remit of the health care system

The enviable position of France in global mortality figures compared with other countries of a similar level of economic development is largely accounted for by low mortality amongst the elderly. When it comes to "premature" mortality, *i.e.* death before 65, the position of France is not nearly as impressive: within the European Union, the risk of a man dying before this age is only frankly higher in Portugal with France ranking close to Finland, Germany and Denmark.

Analysis of the various components of premature mortality reveals the preponderant causality of certain behavioural patterns, notably drinking and smoking. This mainly applies to men who are more likely to die young. Dealing with this problem inevitably depends on consciousness-raising about health and other educational measures which are inadequate in our country. Few professionals are specifically allocated to this end, and this in a complex field which is particularly difficult to tackle since it necessitates changing representations and modifying behaviour patterns.

If prevention is to be effective, a concerted effort needs to be made by many different actors in a multi-faceted attack both within and outside of the scope of the health care system. Such a plural approach is necessarily difficult to implement and depends on the existence of a strong, political will. Of course, this necessarily applies not only to the simple question of avoidable premature death but rather encompasses all aspects of prevention.

Even within the health care system, compartmentalisation results from serious fragmentation of skills, instruments and budgets. How to finance health care networks which involve expenditure both within and outside of hospitals (for which the accounting modalities are completely different)? How to ensure complementarity between preventive measures financed from a special fund and the same individual acts financed by the social security system?

Above and beyond this, the risks associated with occupational exposure to asbestos or animal meal (which may transmit bovine spongiform encephalopathy), debates centred on the automobile or tobacco industries, or even questions concerning school calendars, all illustrate the dichotomy between the various health-related concerns of people and other social dynamics. Mechanisms to communalise problems and knowledge together with concerted initiatives will not relieve all tensions but ought to make it possible to take health-related issues into account in a more global fashion. For example, the multi-faceted approach adopted towards the problem of substance abuse – under the auspices of the Interdepartmental Mission for the Fight against Drugs and Drugs Addiction (Mildt, *Mission interministérielle de lutte contre la drogue et la toxicomanie*) – is now being seen to be bearing fruit; similarly for food-related risks – under the auspices of the French Agency for Safe Food (Afssa, *Agence française de sécurité sanitaire des aliments*) – and the diverse recommendations of the National Nutrition and Health Plan.

Promoting the development of tertiary prevention modalities, notably for the elderly

When complete cure is impossible, the response is often a fatalistic one with the patient being more or less excluded from the health care system. However, in many circumstances, tertiary prevention – meaning the mitigation of disease-induced functional disability – can significantly enhance a patient's quality of life.

With increasing longevity and the rising incidence of certain chronic conditions such as diabetes and asthma, this aspect of health care is too often undervalued and thus represents a priority area for action. All the various sub-groups within the population are concerned in this in some way or another, but a particularly important group in this context is that of the elderly in whom the key issue is the preservation of independence.

The elderly – who are increasingly numerous and also tending to get older – still have a significant life expectancy: ten years for a 75-year-old man, and thirteen years for a woman of the same age. However, with the existence and, above all, the accumulation of deficits (visual, auditory, motor, etc.), there is a tendency among this population to withdrawal from daily life with the concomitant risks of isolation, depression, malnutrition and, as a result of all this, accelerated loss of cognitive function. The ultimate consequence is reduced quality of life, not only for the elderly subject but also for his or her family, not to mention the major social costs.

Such deficits are often considered as inevitable consequences of ageing and it is difficult not to be surprised at the paucity of resources allocated in this area, *e.g.* to physiotherapy, functional re-education, palliative therapy and, more generally, to facilitating adaptation to changing conditions of life. All this is ultimately a result of the disdain of society at large and the medical community for anything which is not curative. The observation similarly applies to institutions dedicated to looking after the elderly, in which respect, attention should be drawn to the lack of reliable, recent data on the health of subjects living in such establishments.

Methodology

Interpreting health indicators

For a full description of someone's health, regularly updated details concerning a number of different parameters would be ideal:
– health data (test results, physical examinations, details of symptoms, areas of disability, etc.), all measured and presented in a standardised way,
– social, demographic and occupational characteristics,
– details about habits, lifestyle, and health-related perceptions,
– treatment history (care inside and outside of hospitals, self-medication, etc.), including individual preventive modalities (immunisations, counselling, etc.),
– "exposure" to collective safety initiatives (health education and information, preventive programs aimed at other societal issues such as the safety of food, the safety of machines, etc.).

Part one   Data about health status

With all these data, it would be possible to interrelate any health problems with all their causes and consequences. Of course, the reality is quite different because the amount of available data is restricted as a result of limitations following on from the way the health care system and its institutions are organised. Such data are often compiled for purposes other than the assessment of state of health, and no global assessments are made of collective and societal initiatives on health. Moreover, not all of the above information is ever collected (happily for our privacy). We must therefore do with what we have, necessarily bearing in mind throughout any analysis the limitations that the incompleteness of the data imposes.

One of the most important limitations is the difficulty of interrelating data from different sources, *e.g.* investigating the links between death and life styles or behaviour patterns, between the consumption of care resources and disability, between perception of a recognised health care problem and consumption of resources, between hospital care and care in other settings, or between hospital admissions and patients' circumstances (social, familial, occupational, etc.).

One indicator which is readily available is mortality. For every death in France, a medical certificate must be filled in by a physician, recording the relevant details (notably the initial, intermediate and immediate causes of death, and any intercurrent conditions). These certificates are eventually sent to Inserm for processing and statistical analysis. The accuracy of the declared cause of death is dependent on the physician's knowledge of the patient's medical history, and also on his or her understanding of the concept of initial cause of death (*i.e.* which corresponds to the underlying morbid process). Moreover, in many cases, the idea of causality is not a simple one and a single cause of death is not easy to define (*e.g.* a traffic accident associated with a suicide, myocardial infarction, stroke, a side effect of a drug, etc.).

In France, there are about 700,000 births and 530,000 deaths per annum. Since the ultimate probability of dying is 100%, the number of deaths can only rise, at least in the long term. When judging the efficacy of a health care system on the basis of this parameter therefore, the key issues are the age of death, quality of life, and the circumstances of death (which is ideally devoid of suffering and with adequate support structures in place).

The French are dying less at all ages. A good health care system could be one that simply delays death without affecting the causes: the same causes but at a more advanced age. Saying that *"As many people still die of cardiovascular disease"* does not point up any failure of the health care system if patients are dying twenty years older. And this is probably partially true for

Methodology

myocardial infarction and strokes. This is why mortality figures are always presented "for a given age bracket" or in an "age-specific" form (a statistical method which makes it possible to take age-related differences into account and follow trends in this area).

No formal declaration is mandatory when it comes to morbidity (descriptions of diseases and their consequences) apart from a few specific cases (mostly infectious diseases). Therefore we have to resort to indirect sources based on encounters with the health care system, or alternatively, surveys of samples of the population.

The "path" leading from the onset of a health problem to use of the system (*i.e.* care consumption) can be schematically outlined. Any problem must be perceived before it can be defined, and if it is to lead to use of the health care system, there must exist some "solution" that is both financially acceptable (feasibility) and available (provision). This outline should be borne in mind when analysing and interpreting the information which follows.

For example, care consumption for venous problems is no indicator of the frequency of such problems in the population as a whole. Consumption merely means that the problem has been perceived by the person concerned, and then recognised and diagnosed by a doctor who has identified a possible therapeutic strategy which has in turn been defined as acceptable (in both financial and social terms) for the institutions involved as well as the patient. Therefore, any change in the frequency with which the care system is solicited for venous problems does not necessarily mean that the frequency of the problem has changed. More likely is that it is the level of solicitation which has changed.

Taking another example, there may exist major discrepancies between the real frequency of mental problems and the frequency with which such problems are declared, because the victims are not always aware of their problem, or, if they are, they are "ashamed" of it. And variable diagnostic practices between different physicians may introduce further distortion of the true picture.

The frequency in the population of Alzheimer's disease as measured by diagnosis rates has enormously increased, both because of the development of specific treatment modalities and because of massive media coverage of the disease's consequences. This has led to a change in the way family members perceive symptoms. Moreover, the existence of effective treatment modalities has entailed standardisation of diagnostic methods (*i.e.* an increase in the level of recognition of the problem by doctors) and a change in terms of the extent of "recognition of a treatable problem". All this may be enough to account for an apparent rise in frequency.

Part one Data about health status

The popular term is frequency, whereas public health experts make a distinction between incidence, prevalence at a certain point in time, and lifetime prevalence. Health statistics may deal with the frequency of a problem at a given point in time (prevalence), the frequency at which new cases appear over a given time frame (incidence, usually annual), or their existence at some – any – point in life (lifetime prevalence). These measures are interconnected, in particular by virtue of the duration of the disease and the phenomenon of temporary remission: for two diseases with exactly the same incidence, the one that tends to persist longer will be more prevalent. Any treatment modality which extends survival without diminishing the frequency with which a disease appears (its incidence) is going to increase that disease's prevalence. This leads to the paradoxical effect that effective treatment increases the number of patients with the disease who are alive at a given point in time. If a treatment modality induces a certain percentage of remissions, the prevalence of the disease concerned will decrease although not its lifetime prevalence. These ideas are crucial when it comes to interpreting the relationship between care consumption and the underlying health problems. Certain procedures are associated with incidence (*e.g.* the initial diagnosis of a disease and the treatment of acute conditions) whereas for others, prevalence is the more relevant parameter (*e.g.* drug consumption by patients with chronic diseases).

Another drawback with these data sources is that they deal with different "statistical units". The unit may be the individual (*e.g.* mortality) or, in other cases, it may be based on the number of disease-related episodes (*e.g.* one patient may consult a physician – or several different physicians – or be admitted into hospital many times, even in a single year), in which case, one individual will be counted more than once. Prudence is always indicated when defining the denominator (*e.g.* the French population) in a given statistic: if one man sees his doctor once every week for a specific problem, this will appear as 52 different consultations and, if the data collection system cannot assimilate the fact that only one patient is concerned, this could appear as 52 episodes of the disease during the year in question. This applies notably to much PMSI and IMS Health EPPM data, as well as most of the sources on care consumption. As a general rule, the more frequent the interactions with the health care system that are entailed by a disease, the more likely it is that the frequency of the disease will be overestimated by analyses of health care institutions.

Methodology

The data sources used

The Credes Health and Social Coverage Survey (ESPS, *Enquête Santé protection sociale*)

The Health and Social Coverage Survey is a two-yearly enquiry conducted to collect data on health status, medical consumption and the insurance coverage of individuals. State of health data is collected by means of a questionnaire filled out by the subjects of the survey themselves. It consists of a list of thirty diseases broken down into broad groups of pathologies (cardiovascular, respiratory, endocrine, etc.).

The 1998 Survey covered a sample of 7,949 households in mainland France with at least one member affiliated with either Cnamts (National Health Insurance Agency for Salaried Workers), MSA (Agricultural Employees Health Insurance Agency) or Canam (National Health Insurance Agency for the Self-Employed). These households are representative of 95% of the population living in ordinary households. Excluded were people living in institutions or collective housing (*e.g.* workers' hostels), in religious communities, and prison inmates. A total of 23,000 people were interviewed in two cycles, one in the Spring and the other in the Autumn. The survey was based on the questionnaire together with a telephone interview (or a face-to-face interview with the investigator for those without access to a telephone).

The diseases identified in this survey are declared diseases which may or may not have been diagnosed by a physician. Whether or not a disease is deemed to be declarable involves numerous factors, including deliberate or involuntary omission and the variability of perception between different strata of society and people of different cultural background, as well as people's level of knowledge and their concept of what constitutes normal and what constitutes pathological.

IMS-Health Permanent Survey of Medical Prescription (EPPM, *L'Enquête permanente sur la prescription médicale*)

The main purpose of the IMS-Health Permanent Survey of Medical Prescription is to monitor how doctors are prescribing treatments and determine the relationships between diagnosis and prescription practice. By means of a form filled out for each visit with details of the diagnosis established together with reasons for the treatments prescribed, morbidity details are gathered for every patient examined.

The survey is conducted every three months for a sample which, in 1998, included 835 physicians (400 General Practitioners and 435 specialists). One quarter of the panel is replaced every year. The survey is representative of all independently practising physicians in mainland France (General Practitioners, cardiologists, dermatologists, gastroenterologists, gynaecologists, neurologists, psychiatrists and neuropsychiatrists, ophthalmologists, otorhinolaryngologists, paediatricians, pneumologists, rheumatologists, endocrinologists and phlebologists). It does not cover doctors who devote more than 25% of their time to certain paramedical practices (*e.g.* homeopathy or acupuncture). Each participating physician is monitored for seven days and is expected to

Part one   Data about health status

supply details for every single patient seen in the context of his or her independent, outpatient practice. These include the patient's social and demographic characteristics, information on the reasons for consultation, details of the diagnosis, and information on the expected outcome of any drug treatment prescribed. In addition, the physician provides duplicate copies of all prescriptions issued to the patients concerned. In 1998, a total of about 240,000 consultations were documented.

In this survey, the unit is the visit to the doctor. Only those who have consulted a doctor at least once in the year are included in this sample, and the more frequently a patient seeks medical advice, the more likely he or she is to be included. Therefore, this does not by any means constitute a representative sample of the population, nor even of physicians' clients as a whole, but rather reflects the breakdown of physicians' consultations.

Hospital Medical Information Systems Programme (PMSI, *Programme de médicalisation des systèmes d'information*) – Short-term MSO care

The Hospital Medical Information Systems Programme (PMSI) is an instrument designed to measure medical and economic parameters of hospital activity. It consists of a standardised record based on the collection of narrowly defined administrative and medical data. Hitherto, the system routinely operated in services providing short-term care in the fields of medicine, surgery and gynaecology/obstetrics (MSO) but it has recently been expanded to cover units and establishments providing follow-up care and physical therapy (FUPT). How to further expand it to cover psychiatric facilities is currently under consideration.

All the information is encoded according to standard classification systems, notably Version Ten of the World Health Organisation (WHO) International Classification of Disease (ICD) with respect to diagnoses, and these data are used to analyse the reasons for hospital admissions. However, it should be noted that the results are actually expressed in terms of the main diagnosis established for the overall treatment: this is defined at the end of the patient's stay as the specific problem which entailed the major part of the care provided (and which does not therefore necessarily correspond to the initial diagnosis).

The measured unit in the MSO-PMSI instrument is the stay and not the patient. Every stay is recorded but no distinction is made between the hospital stays of two different patients and two different stays of a single patient in the course of one year.

In 1998, this system covered 95% of public sector establishments and 87% of establishments in the private sector. The results analysed in this book are those for 1998 and include all stays into both private and public sector services providing short-term MSO care in mainland France and its overseas departments. Admissions for outpatient procedures such as dialysis, chemotherapy and radiotherapy are not dealt with in the statistical analysis.

Methodology

Groups of ICD classifications have been pooled to constitute reasons for stays and then these reasons have been classified according to frequency. Stays for the main diagnosis of "mental problems" represent only stays in short-term MSO departments and do not include stays in psychiatric facilities.

Recognised long-term conditions

Those covered by the social security system and their dependants can obtain exemption from the patient-payable part of care charges if they suffer from any of the thirty long-term conditions (LTCs) stipulated by decree. If the LTC corresponds to the criteria specified by the High Social Security Medical Committee *(Haut Comité médical de la sécurité sociale)*, the request for recognition of the condition is submitted by the patient or his or her personal physician, and is subject to approval by a physician assigned by the health insurer.

The data presented in this report only concern LTCs admissions requested during 1998 on behalf of patients covered by the national health insurance system (which includes 83% of the entire French population). They are taken from the Medicis data base which compiles data – the patient's age and sex, and disease according to ICD 10 – from all the local agencies.

The number of new LTCs recognised can be used to estimate the incidence of the most serious diseases (cancer, AIDS, psychosis, etc.) and, for certain problems, it represents the only source of data on morbidity (including multiple sclerosis, rheumatoid arthritis, Crohn's disease and certain mental problems). Since these data are available for the whole of France, including overseas departments, they can be very useful when it comes to analysing geographical disparities.

Nevertheless, this system has certain limitations, largely due to the fact that the data are actually compiled for administrative purposes. Certain factors tend to lead to under-estimation: some patients never submit a request for LTC recognition because they have adequate complementary health insurance, some are exempt from the patient-payable charges for special reasons (*e.g.* those benefiting from Universal Health Coverage and those with occupational disability or disease), and in some cases, the specific case does not meet the stipulated severity criteria for that disease. On the other hand, other factors tend to lead to over-estimation, *e.g.* the failure to identify recurrence of a disease as a result of the patient moving house.

Medical cause of death

France, like other European countries, exhaustively registers all deaths that occur throughout its territory. For every death, a medical certificate must be filled in by a physician recording all the relevant details (notably the main and immediate causes of death, and any intercurrent conditions). These certificates are eventually sent to National Institute of Health and Medical Research (Inserm-CépiDc, *Institut national de la santé et de la recherche médicale*) for processing and the compilation of annual statistics on causes of death. Diseases are classified in accordance with Version Nine of the International Classification of Disease. The whole process is made possible by the close relationship maintained between Inserm and the National Institute of Statistics and Economic Surveys (Insee, *Institut national de la statistique et des études économiques*) which provides details on each of the subjects (sex, age, place of residence, and social and occupational status). These data make it possible to carry out mortality analyses on the basis of important social and demographic parameters, as well as geographical considerations. International comparisons and temporal analyses are also possible. The most commonly used indicators are: overall number of deaths; the number of deaths due to each of the various causes; raw mortality rates; specific rates; age-standardised rates (comparative rates with reference to the age breakdown of the French population for both sexes as it was in 1990); excess mortality indices (ratios of rates). Analyses are based on specific causes of death, which can be problematic when it comes to elderly subjects who often suffer from multiple diseases affecting more than one organ. Moreover, as a result of the failure of certain forensic institutions to supply information, the figures on violent death tend to be underestimated.

Young people of under 15 years of age

The under-15 age bracket includes children and adolescents, although of course, the demarcation is somewhat arbitrary given the continuous nature of the development process and the huge variation between different individuals with respect to the age of puberty.

The Census conducted in March 1999 registered nearly 10.5 million individuals of 14 or under living in mainland France. This figure is falling (from 11.2 million in 1982 through 10.8 in 1990) as is the proportion of the overall population in this bracket (from nearly 21% in 1982 through 19% in 1990 to 18% in 1999).

This trend is mainly due to a reduced birth rate although this parameter appears to have been on the increase following a minimum seen in 1993 and 1994 (with a total of 779,000 births registered in 2000).

Infancy and adolescence represents a period of both physical and psychological growth, a time of cultural and academic apprenticeship, and integration into society and social life. It is also a key period of experimentation with different habits and life styles, some of which – if they become ingrained – can either predispose to or reduce the likelihood of the later occurrence of specific diseases. Family life which is such a key factor in this development process has seen major changes in recent decades with single parenthood, working mothers and parental divorce and remarriage far more common these days.

Declared morbidity

In general, children are healthy between the ages of 0 and 14. Parents are rarely brought to declaring any disease affecting their child – on average, less than one problem per child with most of these being benign. The most common complaints fall into three categories (figure 1): respiratory disease (22% of all children); dental problems (20%); and eye problems (17%).

Acute upper airways infections, rhinopharyngitis, sore throat and laryngitis are among the most common complaints (11%), fol-

Part one Data about health status

Figure 1 **Main declared conditions among boys and girls of under 15 years of age. 1998**
(percentage suffering from at least one disease of health problem)

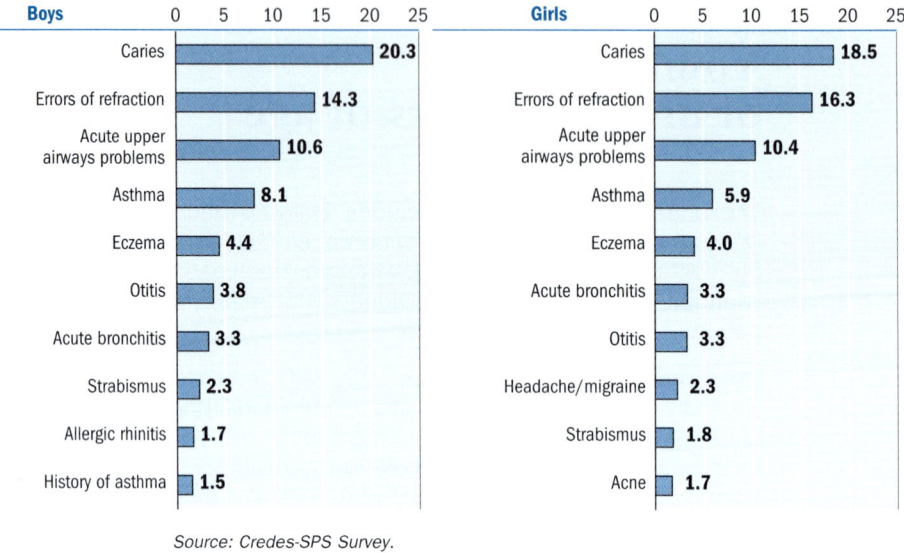

Source: Credes-SPS Survey.

lowed by asthma and pre-asthmatic conditions (8%), and acute bronchitis (3%). Asthma and allergic rhinitis are more common in boys.

The most common dental complaint is caries, whether they are treated or not (19% of all children).

Errors of refraction (myopia, hyperopia and astigmatism) and strabismus account for almost all declared ophthalmologic problems, and are slightly more common in girls.

No other problem is nearly as common. Skin diseases affect 6% of children, with 4% of these suffering from eczema; acne vulgaris is relatively rare at this age; 4.4% experience ear problems, mostly otitis (4%) with deafness and hypoacusis affecting less than 1%. Finally, 4% of children complain of various other symptoms, including headaches and insomnia.

Reasons for consulting an independent physician

Every year, children of under 15 account for 67 million consultations with a doctor in independent practice (either a General Practitioner or a specialist). The average number of reasons per visit in 1998 has remained stable at 1.3 since 1992.

The most common single reason is upper airways disease (figure 2) which accounted for 4 out of 10 visits in 1998. Acute infections such as rhinopharyngitis, sore throat, laryngitis and bronchitis are the most common, accounting for fully one-third of all consultations.

The second category is "Other reasons for solicitation of health care services" (22% of all consultations) which covers obligatory examinations for newborns and children (10%) and immunisation procedures (6%).

Lower down are infectious diseases, including parasitic infections (10%). Nearly half of these correspond to intestinal infections with diarrhoea being the immediate reason in 5% of cases.

One consultation in ten falls into the category of "Poorly defined symptoms or disease", the most common of such symptoms being coughing and fever.

Figure 2 **Main reasons for consultation with an independent practitioner among boys and girls of under 15 years of age. 1992. 1998** (percentage of consultations)

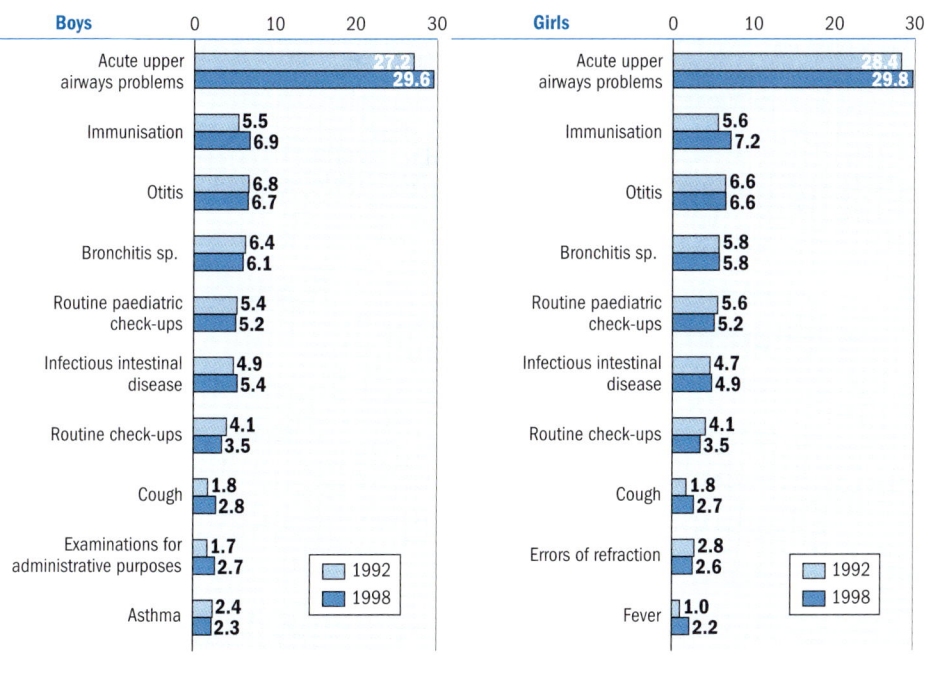

Source: Credes. Data: EPPM Survey 1992-1998. IMS-Health.

Part one Data about health status

Ear problems – basically otitis – account for 8% of consultations and, finally, skin and eye problems (notably eczema and errors of refraction or conjunctivitis) each constitute the reason for taking the child to see an independent practitioner in 5% of all cases.

Overall, if one takes the respiratory problems (mostly infectious) together with some infections of the ear and other organs, it is clear that most of the problems in this age group which lead to consultation with an independent physician have an infectious etiology.

There was little change in the reasons for such visits between 1992 and 1998, although there was a clear increase in the number of consultations for poorly defined symptoms, and a slight fall-off with respect to infectious problems.

Figure 3 **Main diseases of boys and girls of under 15 years of age treated in short-stay hospital departments. 1998**
(per 100,000 inhabitants)

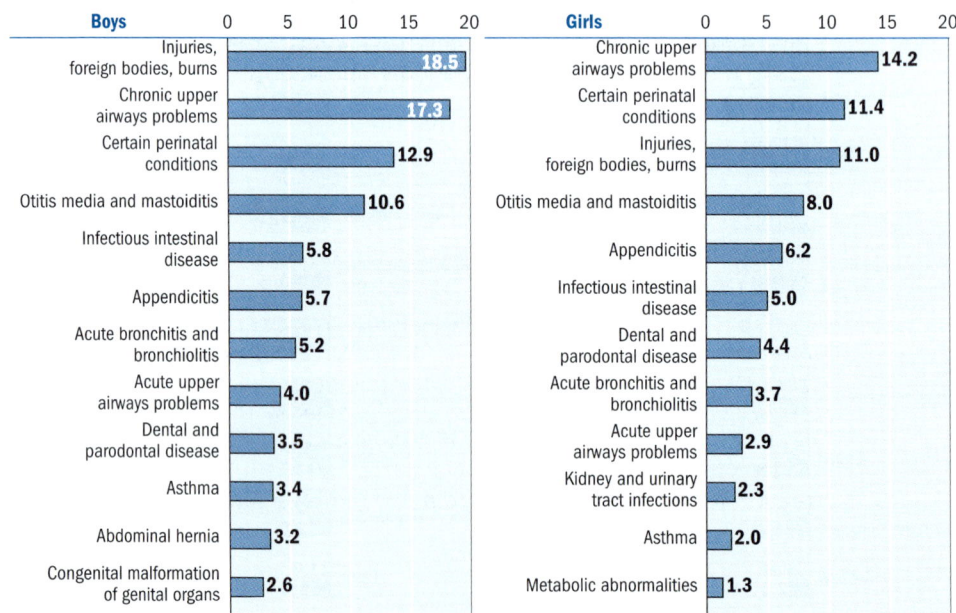

Source: PMSI. Ministry of Employment and Solidarity. Drees.

Reasons for admission into hospital-based medicine, surgery and obstetrics services

Hospital admission patterns are very varied within the 0-14 age bracket, with babies of under 12 months being admitted almost as often as the elderly, while the rate of admission of children of between 5 and 14 is well below the average for the population as a whole.

A clear difference is observed between the sexes, with boys being admitted more often. This may be due to specific diseases or greater male susceptibility to certain problems as well as the fact that boys engage in more high-risk behaviour. Another factor may be that the readiness of parents to take their children to hospital depends on the child's gender. This tendency was revealed in 1991-1992 in the household-based survey of health and health care conducted every ten years: boys of under 15 were taken to the doctor more often than girls for all reasons (disease, prophylactic treatment, accidents, etc.).

The most common reason for admitting a child of either sex of under 15 years of age into hospital is airways disease, be it acute or chronic (about 1 admission in 5), with traumatic injury, poisoning, and gastrointestinal problems, each accounting for about 1 in 10 admissions.

Minor surgery – often carried out in an outpatient context – is the reason for many admissions related to chronic conditions, including those affecting the upper airways (tonsilectomy and adenoidectomy), otitis media and mastoiditis (tympanostomy), and dental and periodontal disease (tooth extraction).

Both sexes are also admitted for other forms of respiratory disease, notably acute airways problems and asthma.

Physical injury is responsible for 19 hospital admissions per 1,000 in boys, and 11 per 1,000 in girls. The most common traumas are fractures of the arm and cranial injury in both sexes.

Appendicitis is another common reason for admission (6 per 1,000), as is intestinal infections (due to dehydration risk-related complications).

Naturally, in babies of under 12 months of age, perinatal problems (premature birth, hypotrophy and maternal complications secondary to pregnancy, delivery or postpartum) predominate, accounting for fully one-third of all admissions. This is followed by respiratory problems (15% of admissions), with acute bronchitis or bronchiolitis representing the second most important reason for the hospitalisation of babies in their first year of life.

Part one — Data about health status

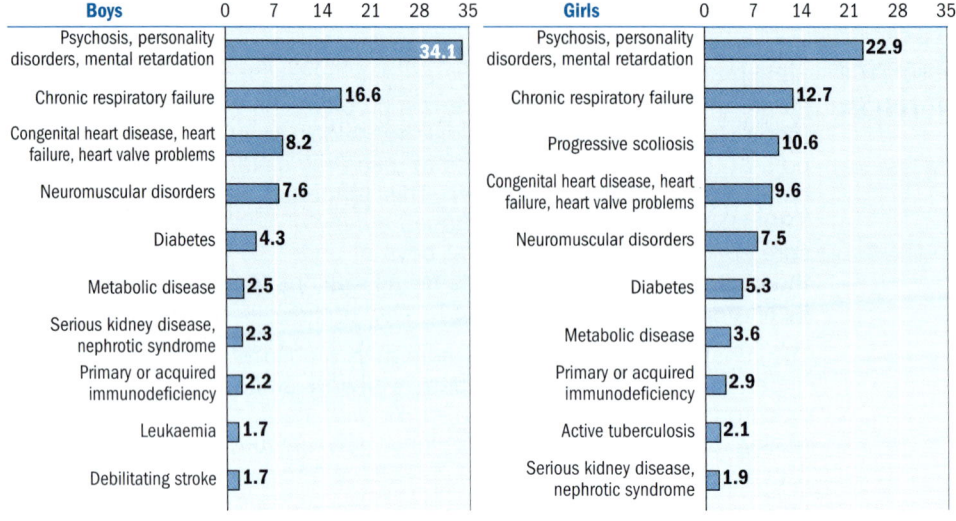

Figure 4 **Main long-term conditions in boys and girls of under 15 years of age covered by the health insurance system. 1998**
(percentage of reasons for recognition)

Source: Cnamts. National Medical Service Level.

Long-term conditions

Nearly 26,000 children of under 15 with national health insurance coverage (which covers more than 80% of all the population) were recognised as suffering from a long-term condition (LTC) in 1998. This represents about 4% of all LTCs recognised in that year and a frequency of 258 per 100,000 insurees.

As is true for all forms of disease, LTCs are more common in the very first few years of life: 44% of new LTCs concern children of under 4 as against just 29% of between 5 and 9, and 27% of between 10 and 14.

Before the age of 15, mental health problems are by far the single most important kind of LTC (29%). The most common is retardation (more than 2,000 new cases registered in 1998), and two other particularly severe forms can be singled out, namely major developmental problems which account for 1,300 cases (including 500 LTC admissions for autism) and Down syndrome (460 LTC admissions). Other common LTCs are serious chronic respiratory insufficiency (15 %) – mainly severe asthma – and congenital heart diseases and cardiovascular disorders (11%). Among girls, progressive structural scoliosis requiring orthopaedic or surgical correction accounts for about 11% of LTC admissions (compared with just 1% among boys).

Young people of under 15 years of age

Slightly less common among young children are severe neuromuscular diseases (8%), malignancies (6%) and insulin-dependent diabetes (5%).

Medical causes of death

The current annual number of deaths among children of under 15 in France is 5,000 which corresponds to 50 per 100,000, a relatively low figure compared with other European countries. It is important to make the distinction between the infant mortality rate and the mortality among children of between 1 and 14 years of age because both the rates and reasons for death are very different in these two sub-populations.

Under 12 months: annual mortality is 3,400 which corresponds to 473 deaths per 100,000 births. Half of these occur in the first week of life, and more boys than girls die throughout the first year of life (a boy is 30% more likely to die before 1 year of age than is a girl).

Sudden Infant Death Syndrome accounts for 10% of these deaths with markedly more boys dying thus (+ 50%). Other common causes are congenital heart diseases and problems associated with delivery (including hemorrhage and premature birth).

Between 1990 and 1997, infant mortality dropped dramatically (by nearly one half). The most marked reduction was seen for children of over 1 month although neonatal mortality also decreased; in particular, the incidence of Sudden Infant Death Syndrome fell by a remarkable factor of four, an impressive decrease which is largely due to changes related to sleep position. Death due to birth defects and violent deaths both decreased significantly in this period, although the study of death causes confirm the slight decrease in perinatal problems.

Figure 5 **Main causes of death in boys and girls of between 1 and 15 years of age. 1997**
(age-normalised rates per 100,000 inhabitants)

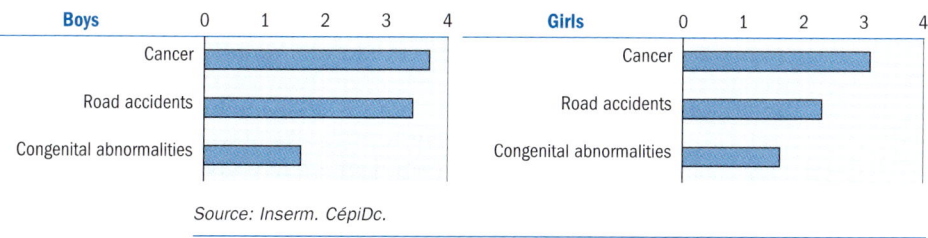

Source: Inserm. CépiDc.

Part one Data about health status

Between 1 and 14: in 1997, 1,900 children in this age range died (800 girls and 1,100 boys, *i.e.* a mortality rate 30% higher among boys than girls). Two causes predominate: violent death (40%), half in road accidents, and tumours to a less extent (20%).

The overall death rate amongst children of 1 to 14 years of age of both sexes is dropping sharply (by a factor of 25% between 1990 and 1997) with a similar trend seen for most causes of death, *e.g.* – 29% for accidents, – 26% for tumours, and – 31% for birth defects, etc.).

Main health-related issues in children of under 15 years of age

A significantly improved picture of health in the early years of life, largely due to the efficacy of measures to prevent Sudden Infant Death Syndrome

During pregnancy and the months immediately following birth, mother and child are now closely monitored and cared for by a specialist team of professional health care providers who are ready to implement both prophylactic and curative measures. The key health care providers here are General Practitioners and specialist physicians together with the Mother and Child Protection Service (PMI, *Services de protection maternelle et infantile*), and hospital neonatal and paediatric departments.

In the sub-population of babies of under 12 months of age, both the number of consultations with independent practitioners and the rate of hospital admissions are close to those of the elderly. Above and beyond the legally required check-ups (at 8 days, and 9 and 24 months), many children are taken to see their doctor on a regular basis for purely preventive purposes. The increased presence and enhanced efficacy of this care network over recent decades has led to a major reduction in infant mortality: this figure which had already halved between 1970 and 1990, was divided by almost 2 between 1990 and 1997 as a result of the implementation of an effective strategy to prevent Sudden Infant Death Syndrome. Today, the infant mortality rate in France is one of the lowest in the world at just 5 per 1,000 births.

This spectacular improvement is not always accorded its true import. Between 1980 and 1997, the number of babies dying before 1 year of age dropped from 9,000 to 3,400, corresponding to the saving of more than 5,000 lives every year. However, if one considers a hypothetical town with 10,000 inhabitants representative of France, this decrease means that instead of the one baby out of the 125 born in 1980 dying, now only one dies every two years. Thus, infant death – although traumatic for the parents – was always a rare event for the community as a whole, which is why this great step forward is not obvious in everyday life.

The available data provide only a limited picture of the health of the very young and cannot be used to make any very precise predictions about their future health. Advances in neonatal medicine entail questions about the future for children born well before term with a current total of 9,000 babies per annum being delivered before 33 weeks of term as it is estimated that 30% of all cases of major psychomotor and sensory handicap occurring during early childhood are due to prematurity sequelae. The question is not simply how to monitor these children for epidemiological purposes (see box below), but also involves ethical questions concerning which the National Ethics Committee recently published a report.

Moreover, although a great deal of work has shown the fundamental importance of both a child's emotional environment in very early life and the parent-child bond which is constructed during this period, it is by no means sure that adequate attention is paid to these factors when it comes to health policy because the consequences – which can take many years to become apparent – are so difficult to document. By way of example, little is known about the non-medical consequences of the reduction in the average time spent in a maternity ward following childbirth (a decrease of 0.8 days between 1989 and 1998). Similarly, there is little discussion of the fact that breast-feeding is far less common in France than in other countries despite overwhelming evidence of its beneficial effects. In this context, recent legislation on paternity leave represents a step forward.

RATIONALISING PERINATAL CARE: AN EPIDEMIOLOGIST'S POINT OF VIEW

According to a recent Expert Committee report on maternal death in childbirth in France, the rate is no longer going down, having remained stable at about 10 per 100,000 births for the last ten years (a rate which is about twice as high as that in some Scandinavian countries). However, even if the rate appears stable, this does not mean that it cannot be decreased. Reviews of medical records suggest that 30% of maternal deaths could be prevented. Comparison with data from Britain and other European countries shows that the excess mortality in France is due to an increased incidence of fatal haemorrhage, a problem which French experts believe can be overcome by improved perinatal management. A survey recently conducted in different regions indicates that the logistics of the health care system are a major factor in outcomes in this respect.

As regards the babies, various studies on post-natal care have clearly shown that perinatal management is a primordial factor when it comes to the subsequent development of babies born very prematurely, and in the risk of their developing long-term disability. Despite improvements in this field, the absolute number of handicapped children is not falling because more children are being born prematurely, and premature children are surviving for longer.

From these observations, it is clear that, in high-risk situations, the quality of care is a key factor in outcome. As a result, it is crucial that the health care system be organised in such a way as to guar-

Part one Data about health status

antee access to appropriate, high-quality care for all mothers and children who need it.

Although the need for intensive care in high-risk situations is recognised by all, the topic of low-risk pregnancy engenders more controversy. Intrusive monitoring can have an iatrogenic effect that outweighs any potential benefit. Two recent articles and an editorial in the *Lancet* show that prenatal surveillance can be reduced in terms of the procedures performed, and that a permanent specialist supervision is unnecessary.

Therefore, the current data indicate that the way forward is to do more and do it better in high-risk situations, and do less (still doing it better) otherwise. This is an issue which will have to be addressed in years to come not only in the area of perinatal care but in a whole range of other medical disciplines as well.

No definitive conclusions can be drawn about the relative efficacy of the logistics of different health care systems from the data available from randomised studies and general surveys. This is partly because, in many of those countries with particularly impressive perinatal outcomes, health care systems are organised in very different ways, *e.g.* in Holland, 30% of deliveries are performed at home whereas in Finland, nearly all are performed in very big establishments.

The absence of any clear indication as to the advantages of a certain mode of organisation is not a justification for failure to develop a consistent policy, the absence of which would be more detrimental than any specific form of organisation.

Because institutions and learned bodies cannot formulate decisions and recommendations only on the basis of scientifically validated data, developing instruments to evaluate any measures implemented is an essential step. In this context, it is vital to accept the idea that decisions taken in the past might not have been the best in the circumstances, and that they might have to be "rethought".

For the establishment of such instruments, a consistent perinatal monitoring system will have to be put in place, and this system will have to be extended to monitor two extra kinds of indicator:
– long-term outcomes in the children,
– long-term outcomes in the mothers.

In conclusion, in the absence of any concrete data as to the advantages or disadvantages of any particular mode of organisation of the health care system, any recommendations will have to be issued with care. This does not mean avoiding the making of decisions, but will entail the establishment of a rigorous evaluation system.

Gérard Bréart, Inserm U149

References: [3, 7, 39].

Accidents are the most important immediate danger to the health of children, and the situation in France is worse than in many other European countries

Between 1 and 14, admission into hospital and death are far rarer events than in any other age bracket. However, accidents and their consequences are common, being the reason for 40% of the deaths and 12% of hospital stays. This makes accidents the most serious short-term risk for children's health. Boys are at greater risk with a death rate due to accident 30% higher than that of girls, and a hospital admission rate for physical injury twice as high.

Traffic accidents are responsible for half of the 800 deaths in accidents per annum, and also for many injuries: 2,400 serious injuries (necessitating a hospital stay of over 6 days), and 12,000 less serious, according to figures for 1999 compiled by the police and the gendarmerie. Of the children dying following traffic accidents, 25% are on foot and 23% on bicycles or scooters.

Ordinary accidents are very common among children, although rarely serious. However, every year, dozens of children die from drowning, falling or burns, and other accidents can have very serious consequences.

European research – referred to in a recent report on accidents amongst children in France [42] – has revealed a link between socio-economic level and accident-related pathology: underprivileged children are more likely to die in an accident. The same report draws attention to the paucity of reliable information on the consequences of accidents (resultant functional impairment, disability and handicap) and presents the results of two French studies on outcomes in the cases of hospitalised children. Serious sequelae are experienced in 6 to 7% of cases, with no difference between the sexes but with prevalence increasing with the age of the children. Every year, a number of accidents associated with sport and leisure activities would be likely to have long term consequences.

The major decrease in the number of accidental deaths among children of under 15 in recent years is evidence of the efficacy of preventive policies implemented in the context of both road and ordinary accidents. However, this decrease has been less rapid than elsewhere and, in Europe, France has one of the highest accidental death rates (in particular for children of between 1 and 4), nearly twice as high as in Northern European countries. This inferiority – particularly when it comes to sporting and traffic accidents – is also evident from the results of the HBSC survey conducted in 1993-1994 (under the auspices of the WHO) on children of 11, 13 and 15 years old in 24 European countries.

Many factors can be invoked to account for this situation, perhaps principally a lack of awareness on the part of the French population. Thus, taking again the example of the hypothetical town with 10,000 inhabitants, one of the 1,800 children of under 15 will die as a result of an accident every three or four years. Since only one in four young victims of road accidents is a pedestrian, this means that a child on foot will only be killed once in every twenty

Part one Data about health status

to thirty years. It is difficult to mobilise a community to tackle such a rare problem, although particularly dramatic accidents or attention-focusing events can change this.

Serious disease is relatively rare in childhood; the most common serious problems are mental disease, cancer and asthma

Serious disease is relatively rare in childhood. The 26,000 children (with national health insurance coverage) suffering from a LTC admitted into hospital every year represent only 4% of all LTC recognitions while this age bracket contains 18% of the population.

Serious mental problems, notably mental retardation and major developmental problems (*e.g.* autism), account for 29% of LTC recognitions in children under 15 years of age.

Serious, chronic respiratory failure (15% of admissions) is usually associated with severe asthma which is itself a common complaint in children (8%) and constitutes the reason for 2% of all consultations with independent physicians. The real figures are probably somewhat higher because asthma is under-diagnosed. Asthma is a potentially serious disease which leads to more than 30,000 admissions into hospital and about twenty deaths every year among children of under 15.

Numerous studies have indicated that the prevalence of asthma is on the increase, along with that of all other forms of allergic disease (see box below). This increase in prevalence is not paralleled by changes in either the reasons for consultation with an independent physician between 1992 and 1998. Neither did the number of resultant deaths rise in the period 1990 to 1997; this suggests that improvements have been made in diagnosis and/or management of the asthma.

Malignancy, leukaemia and central nervous system tumours account for a moderate proportion of LTC recognitions (6%) but a disproportionate number of deaths (20%) in children of between 1 and 14. Nevertheless, therapeutic progress has significantly reduced cancer mortality, especially from leukaemia.

These figures on children suffering from serious diseases justifying LTC recognition can be considered in the light of those on children with major deficiencies compiled by Inserm Unit 149 and the Isère RHEOP Registry. The prevalence of such serious deficiencies is about 9 per 1,000 at 8 years of age indicating that between 6,000 and 7,000 children in each generation are affected. The most common deficiencies affect the motor system (39%, cerebral palsy being the most common), intellectual function (34%, notably Down syndrome) or are psychiatric in nature (25% for autism or psychosis). Less common are auditory (10%) and visual (7%) deficiencies.

PAEDIATRIC ALLERGY

In recent years, the incidence of allergic disease has been rising to the point that allergy is now a massive public health problem. In France, approximately 25% of all children have some form of allergy, three-quarters of these manifesting respiratory symptoms.

The frequency of asthma has risen by 50% every ten years over the last two decades. According to the ISAAC survey, 9% of all children and 12% of all adolescents in France suffer from asthma, and 3% of hospital stays are associated to this disease, with a total of 2,000 deaths from this disease per annum (counting all ages). In parallel, the frequency of rhinitis and conjunctivitis has tripled in twenty years so that now 7% of children and 15% of adolescents suffer. Finally, 5% of those of under 8 years of age have some form of food allergy.

Three different mechanisms are involved in the pathogenesis of allergy:

Immediate hypersensitivity (Type I hypersensitivity in the Gell and Coombs classification system) involves IgE (the class of antibodies which causes most allergies) directed against environmental (often airborne or occurring in certain types of food) allergens such as house dust mites, pollen, animals, fungi, etc. Symptoms occur very rapidly after exposure (within minutes or hours). Immediate hypersensitivity is most common in children of under 15.

Type III hypersensitivity is mediated by immune complexes and symptoms only develop six to twelve hours after exposure to the allergen.

Delayed-type hypersensitivity (Type IV) is mediated by T lymphocytes and the symptoms do not develop for 48 to 72 hours following exposure.

Allergic symptoms can appear at very young age, *e.g.* atopic dermatitis commonly manifests in the first few months of life. Most asthmatics have symptoms before they reach 5 years of age.

Asthma is often the most severe symptom of allergy in children. According to the WHO, there are 200 million asthma sufferers in the world. The severity of the disease seemed to increase up until the mid-1990's, as indicated by WHO mortality figures which attributed 150,000 deaths to this cause in 1998. However, in countries in which national recommendations on how to manage the disease have been implemented, its impact seems to be waning.

Asthma has major repercussions on quality of life, and results in significant absenteeism from school (or work). Apart from indirect costs, asthma is a major and growing financial burden, accounting for 1.5% of all health care expenditure in the developed world.

According to a 1998 International Consensus Position (Third International Paediatric Consensus: Asthma Management in Children), asthma in childhood can be classified on the basis of three different grades:
- Grade I, occasional intermittent asthma,
- Grade II, frequent intermittent asthma,
- Grade III, chronic asthma.

Allergic rhino-conjunctivitis has traditionally been divided into seasonal and non-seasonal (perennial) forms, although because of changing exposure conditions and increasing allergenic loads, the

current tendency is to ignore this distinction and use a classification based on:
– intermittent rhinitis: fewer than four days a week and less than four episode a year,
– persistent rhinitis: more than four days a week or more than four episodes a year.
In babies, food allergy tends to manifest as gastrointestinal upset although in older children, symptoms may also be systemic, cutaneous or respiratory. The main allergen for babies is cow's milk protein; after 3 years of age, the most common is peanuts which, together with cow's milk protein, eggs, fish and mustard account for 78% of all cases of food allergy.
Predisposition to allergic disease is governed by numerous factors. Heredity is clearly involved although the increase in the incidence of the disease in recent years must be due to changing environmental factors given the improbability of mass genotypic change. Interactions may occur between mother and foetus *in utero* which affect the child's predisposition to allergy, especially in pregnant women who smoke. Recent work on immune system maturation in early childhood points to a protective role for respiratory infections, and exposure to bacteria, fungi and endotoxin in general. It is believed that an environment laden with diverse antigenic stimuli (*e.g.* the countryside) pushes the maturing lymphocyte system towards a protective (Th1-type) response, whereas the absence of daily stimulation predisposes to allergy (*i.e.* Th2-type responsiveness). Certain factors related to domestic conditions may predispose to allergy, including overheating or humidity, poor ventilation, pets, pot plants, passive smoking, and volatile organic compounds or nitrogen dioxide released into the air from unvented gas or petroleum stoves. Finally, atmospheric pollution plays an indirect role in triggering attacks in certain regions and in certain climatic conditions.
Reducing the frequency and severity of allergic reactions involves cutting down exposure to the guilty allergens (by eliminating them from the sufferer's environment as far as is possible), symptomatic treatment with antihistamines, cromolyns and local (or even oral) corticosteroids, and specific immunotherapy (desensitisation). The final point to be made is to draw attention to the strong protective effect of breast feeding vis-à-vis allergy; preventing allergic disease in this way is an investment in the future.

Jean Bousquet, Inserm U454
Emmanuelle Fleurence, Intercommunal Hospital Centre, Créteil

Close inspection of the figures reveals that these children with severe deficiency only represent one half of all the children covered by Departmental Commissions of Special Education, the other half suffering from problems of undefined character and etiology.

Therefore, seriously ill children are relatively few. Most of them will have to live for a long time – possibly their whole life – with their disease, and the relative rarity of their problems often compromises the extent to which their special needs are catered for in the society in which they live. Thus, once more taking the hypothetical town with a population of 10,000 inhabitants, about 5 children will be admitted into hospital for a LTC every year, including one with mental disease and 1 with asthma. Assuming that these diseases are persistent but not life-threatening at this age, the total number of children of between 0 and 14 who are seriously ill and consuming health care resources in this town will be about 70, but there will be no more than ten with any one, specific type of problem: it is difficult to justify special services for such a small population in need. Thus, any specific measures will have to be implemented at a larger scale.

Benign infectious diseases (notably respiratory and ENT conditions) consume significant resources but little is done to prevent them

During the first years of life, the immune system is maturing and still learning to recognise common pathogens, so a number of commonplace infections – mostly involving the airways – are inevitable. Respiratory and ENT infections account for over 40% of the 67 million annual consultations with independent practitioners, and more than 20% of hospital admissions. In babies of under 12 months, these problems represent the second reason for admission into hospital. They are also responsible for various forms of surgical intervention (mainly in an outpatient context), e.g. tympanostomy, adenoidectomy and tonsilectomy. Moreover, they can have a significant impact on the social and professional lives of parents.

The attitude to these problems is largely a fatalistic one and the primary response from the authorities to these mainly viral infections is often a call to restrict the prescription of antibiotics, for both financial reasons and ecological ones (given the adverse effect of the widespread taking of unnecessary antibiotics on bacterial resistance).

However, various factors which potentiate the risk of contracting many of these problems have been identified, including passive smoking (40% of women of between 25 and 40 years of age smoke), atmospheric and domestic pollution, and close contact with other children. Although breast milk has been demonstrated to be protective against such infections, only 45% of French mothers are feeding their baby naturally even when still in the maternity ward (according to a 1998 perinatal survey). Finally, the prophylactic value of keeping one's hands clean and nose clear is often under-estimated, in which respect parents and others who come into regular contact with children have a key educational role to play.

So far, a few locally based preventive initiatives have been undertaken, mainly under the auspices of the PMI, but, despite the significant financial and social costs incurred as a result of these problems (many of which are probably avoidable), no global programme has ever been implemented to bring together everyone who might be concerned, both from within the health care system and outside of it.

Immunisation, dental care, glasses, and minor surgery: the value of routine procedures is often inadequately recognised

Many professionals – General Practitioners, specialists, dentists and orthodontists, and PMI and school health service personnel – are involved in screening and caring for a number of common childhood health problems, and in prevention.

The most common problem is still dental caries, be they treated or not (declared for 19% of children of under 15) although numerous studies have shown significant improvement in this matter in recent decades. Between 1987 and 1993, the percentage of children of 12 years of age with an intact set of permanent teeth rose from 12 to 35%.

Similarly, routine screening for auditory and visual deficits (mainly conducted by the PMI and school health service) has led to the identification of most children with such problems (nearly 20% of children wear glasses). This is all the more relevant when the importance of these senses in learning, and therefore school integration, is taken into account.

More generally, routine examinations, immunisations, and check-ups conducted with a view to the signing of a certificate account for 20% of consultations with independent or hospital practitioners. Some minor surgical procedures are also classified as prophylactic measures, *e.g.* the extraction of wisdom teeth, the correction of abdominal hernias, etc.

Performance in this area is far from perfect and certain specific deficiencies could be singled out: the inadequacy of the resources attributed to school health services; gaps in vaccine coverage; and the lack of efficiency of the system caused by poor co-ordination between the various different professionals involved in children's health care. Nevertheless, this form of provision – which is accorded little glory or medical recognition – is undoubtedly making a significant contribution to the health of today's children, and therefore to their current and future quality of life, although the exact extent of the benefit is difficult to gauge, particularly with respect to long term impact.

Behavioural and mental health problems are difficult to quantify

The last WHO Report on health across the planet drew attention to the high incidence of behavioural and mental health problems among children and adolescents (with between 10 and 20% of all children of under 15 affected, depending on the study) and the fact that insufficient heed is paid to this issue.

The various information sources used for this report do not constitute an effective instrument for constructing an accurate description of these problems in France. In practice, behavioural and mental health problems are not always recognised by the family and, if they are recognised, they are often not declared. Moreover, they are often not diagnosed by health care providers unless specialised care is indicated. Thus the desire to avoid branding the child as handicapped is superimposed on the difficulty in diagnosing conditions which are so often progressive and polymorphic. Our review of these problems will therefore have to be based on an analysis of the prevalence in the sub-population as a whole of certain symptoms (tiredness, headaches, insomnia, etc.), behaviour patterns (addiction, violence, high-risk behaviour), developmental problems, learning difficulties, emotional problems, the inability to adapt to new situations, and most significantly, evidence of the superimposition of any combinations of these features.

Very little information is available on very young children since no relevant data are collected during the regular check-ups organised by the PMI or school health services, apart from a few details on learning difficulties. These indicate that 8% of the children attending nursery school suffer from delayed language acquisition and 15% abnormal fine motor function. A three-yearly survey recently commissioned by the Ministries of Education and Health together with the Institute for Public Health Surveillance (InVS, *Institut de veille sanitaire*) focusing on 6-year-old, fifth and ninth grade children should provide extremely useful data in the future on both somatic and mental problems.

Far more data is available on pre-adolescents because numerous studies on large scale have been conducted to investigate the attitudes and behaviour patterns of young people from the age of 11 or 12 up (Baromètre santé 2000, ESPAD 1999, HBSC 1994 and 1998, etc.).

All of these studies show that boys tend to express their difficulties in the form of antisocial behaviour (violence, risk-taking, abuse of psycho-active substances, etc.) whereas girls tend to verbalise them or express them in a more introspective form (attempted suicide, functional and mood disorders, eating disorders, etc.).

According to the Baromètre santé 2000 survey, nearly 1% of boys and 3.5% of girls of between 12 and 14 claim to have already made an attempt at suicide. Boys are more often the authors and the victims of violence: 13% confess to having struck someone in

Part one   Data about health status

the preceding 12 months, and 12% say that they themselves have been struck (compared with 3.5% and 3% of girls, respectively). The same male predominance is seen in alcohol consumption (see box below).

THE YOUNG AND HEALTH: IMAGES, FEARS AND EXPECTATIONS

Health is not a daily concern among the young who feel that in this respect their stock is inexhaustible and can be threatened by nothing. When asked to define what health means to them, their image is a very positive one, associating it with pleasure, seduction, freedom, independence, well-being and rapport with other people. In contrast, being in poor health means feeling bad, being cut off from other people and not getting any pleasure out of life.

Major differences emerge between boys and girls. Girls construct a health universe at a younger age, and they situate themselves from the outset in a time frame. Very young girls already see themselves as mothers, and are conscious of their internal bodies (and can use words to describe them). At all ages, girls are more open to ideas about prevention and are therefore precious intermediaries when it comes to disseminating information on this subject. In contrast, boys have less of a structured idea of health – they live more for the moment, interested in action and improving their performance, and their perception of health and body is far more functionally conditioned.

In the course of adolescence, action takes priority for many boys and both sexes begin to become conscious of their bodies. From 12 onwards, boys perceive their bodies in a different way from girls, especially with respect to faults and negative aspects. Girls assess their quality of life – on both the somatic and psychological fronts – lower than do boys, and this persists throughout life. From the same age onwards, boys differ from girls in the degree of high-risk behaviour that they engage in, the first evidence of the male tendency to externalise rather than internalise suffering.

Girls experience more depression and anxiety, have more fears for themselves, and generally worry more about road accidents, cancer, heart disease, AIDS, suicide and depression. As is well known, they are extremely sensitive about their appearance although the gap with respect to boys in this regard is narrowing rapidly.

These generalisations about health in the young need to be interpreted carefully and the idea of coping behaviour – personal strategies implemented to deal with stressful events and challenges – can be very helpful. This idea developed in the USA makes it possible to pinpoint differences in reactions to identical situations which are dependent on the readiness to seek help from without.

Differences exist between boys and girls in this respect too. Girls are far more likely to exploit social resources and seek information in the event of difficulty. They accept advice and are far more willing to verbalise their problems. Somatic and psychosomatic complaints are often in effect calls for help.

Boys are more often in denial of stressful realities in their lives. They often delay dealing with a problem until action becomes unavoidable, and they are more ready to adopt a flight strategy or embark on a pattern of high-risk (or "experimental") behaviour. They are probably less able to express themselves at a linguistic level which allows them some distance from their emotions.

Given the complexity of the relationship between the young and health, we need to pay close attention to the programmes proposed to help in this field.

There is no place for moralistic rhetoric or propaganda if the message is to be heard by those at whom it is aimed. The message must address the anxieties of adolescents, and take into account their long-term commitment and need for freedom and independence.

Christiane Dressen, CFES, Vanves

References: [1, 4, 9, 33].

DRINKING IN THE YOUNG

The Europe-wide *Health Behavior in School-Aged Children* (HBSC) survey conducted in 1994 and again in 1998 on a representative sample of schools in 28 countries (under the auspices of the WHO Regional Office in Copenhagen) gives figures on drinking among children of between 11 and 15 years of age.

The situation in France is relatively "good":

– France is near the top of the list for the fraction of children who have never touched alcohol: 50% of 11-year-olds, 32% of 13-year-olds and 14% of 15-year-olds; for comparison, the corresponding figures for Britain are 23%, 6% and 4%, and those for Italy are 30%, 13% and 5%. Before the age of 13, boys are slightly more likely to "experiment" than girls in all countries (about 5 boys for every 3 to 4 girls) but this difference disappears later.

– France is around the middle of the list when it comes to regular drinking (*i.e.* at least once a week): 9th place at 11 (6% of boys and 3% of girls), and 14th place by 15 (31% of boys and 15% of girls).

– France is also relatively well situated in terms of the fraction of students who admit to having been intoxicated on least two occasions: under 1% at 11, and by the age of 15, only 20% of girls and 29% of boys. In Britain, 3% of girls and 9% of boys have already been drunk by the age of 11, and 50% of both sexes have been so by 15.

– Between 1994 and 1998, regular drinking (at least once a week) among 15-year-olds diminished to the greatest extent in France: down by 9% among boys and by 3% among girls. In contrast, the number of episodes of intoxication increased over this period (up by 5% among boys and by 7% among girls), a trend that was observed in all countries.

Thus, starting from a situation that was probably worse than elsewhere, there is now less drinking amongst French children of under 15 years of age than in most other European countries. However, it should not be forgotten that this is largely due to, on the one hand deterioration in other countries, and on the other hand a change in drinking habits from regular low-level consumption to binge drinking.

Source: [34].

Part one Data about health status

Interpreting such data is a complex endeavour, as outlined in the HCPH Report on "Psychological disturbances in adolescents and young adults" *(La souffrance psychique des jeunes adultes)* [14]. Although psychological disturbance may express itself in the form of various types of behaviour and problem, these parameters cannot in themselves be treated as a reliable measure of the underlying problem because so many social and environmental factors predispose to or inhibit their expression. Moreover, different problems and behaviour patterns are associated with different forms of psychological disturbance. Nevertheless, the fact that psychological parameters are difficult to analyse should not result in a failure to recognise and attempt to tackle the resultant problems which can have a terrible impact on the child's current state, as well as repercussions throughout his or her life.

Widespread excess weight and obesity: a worrying tendency due to overeating coupled with reduced physical activity

Infantile obesity is another problem which is difficult to gauge on the basis of the information available from the sources used for this report. However, in contrast to the situation with behavioural and mental health problems (with which obesity can be grouped in many respects), this parameter is easy to quantify. A recent study conducted by the Nutrition Unit of the Institute for Public Health Surveillance on a representative sample of children of between 7 and 9 years of age showed that 14% of boys and 18% of girls are overweight or obese. This high prevalence and the ongoing upward trend are extremely worrying: apart from the adverse social and psychological impact at the time, childhood obesity is a risk factor for obesity in adulthood and therefore for a whole range of associated diseases, including diabetes, cardiovascular diseases, certain forms of cancer, respiratory problems, joint diseases, etc.

The two key factors in this deteriorating situation are changes in eating habits (increased snacking and the consumption of foodstuffs containing large amounts of sugar) and a reduction in the overall level of physical activity (largely due to television and video games).

Obesity is still not seen as a health problem (it does not figure either on the list of declared diseases or as a reason for consulting an independent physician) and is therefore not being addressed as such. The recent establishment of the National Health and Nutrition Programme *(Programme national nutrition santé)* is nevertheless evidence of an increased awareness of the importance of preventive measures in this area.

People of between 15 and 44 years of age

According to the 1999 Census, there are 25 million people of between 15 and 44 living in mainland France. The numbers of men and women are equal since the higher male death rate has by this time compensated for the imbalance seen in children.

After a slight increase between 1982 and 1990, the proportion of the population in this age bracket has since dropped off fairly sharply to just 42% in 1999.

This is the age at which people enter into active life, and this applies these days as much to women as to men. It is also the age of procreation. The mean age of mothers giving birth has been steadily increasing by about 0.1 year per year to reach 29.3 in 1998. Childbirth before the age of 20 has become extremely rare (just 0.7 children per 100 women of under 20) and the frequency of childbirth between the ages of 20 and 24 halved in fifteen years to 5.2 children per 100 women. Fertility is now more or less identical in the 20-24 and the 35-39 age groups, and is not very different in the 25-29 and the 30-34 groups.

Declared morbidity

As for the other age brackets, the problems most commonly declared by people of between 15 and 44 years of age are dental caries and errors of refraction (myopia, hyperopia and presbyopia). Three in four people declare caries, be they treated or not, and this figure can be associated with the 4% of this population (with no difference between the sexes) who carry dental prostheses. More women experience errors of refraction (40% of women compared with 30% of men). In the vast majority of cases, neither caries nor refractive problems lead to major disability although both can cause pain and necessitate significant expenditure on treatment: although routine dental care is well reimbursed by the insurance system, dental prostheses and spectacles are not.

Back pain is also very common in this age bracket with 1 person in 10 declaring it as a problem.

Colds, sinusitis, sore throats, etc.: many young adults still have acute upper airways infections with 1 person in 10 declaring such involvement, *i.e.* almost the same incidence as in children of between 0 and 14.

Part one — Data about health status

Although headache and migraine are often considered as exclusively "female" problems (declared by 18% of women), men are not entirely immune (6%).

Varicose veins and circulatory problems affecting the lower limbs are far more common in women than men (10% *versus* 2%).

Difficulties associated with menstruation are experienced by 6% of all women in this age group and this constitutes one of the most commonly mentioned problems.

Much research conducted both in France and elsewhere has drawn attention to the current increase in the incidence and severity of asthma. According to the Health and Social Coverage *(Santé protection sociale)* survey, 6% of 15-44 year-olds declare themselves as currently suffering from asthma, and 3% declare having a history of the disease.

Although entirely benign, acne vulgaris can be unsightly and can have a significant psychological impact. This condition is now declared by 5% of women and 3% of men: the availability of more effective treatment modalities and the intense promotion of certain products to a young target audience are both undoubtedly factors in the increase in frequency with which this problem is being declared.

Figure 6 **Main declared conditions among men and women of between 15 and 44 years of age. 1998**
(percentage suffering from at least one disease or health problem)

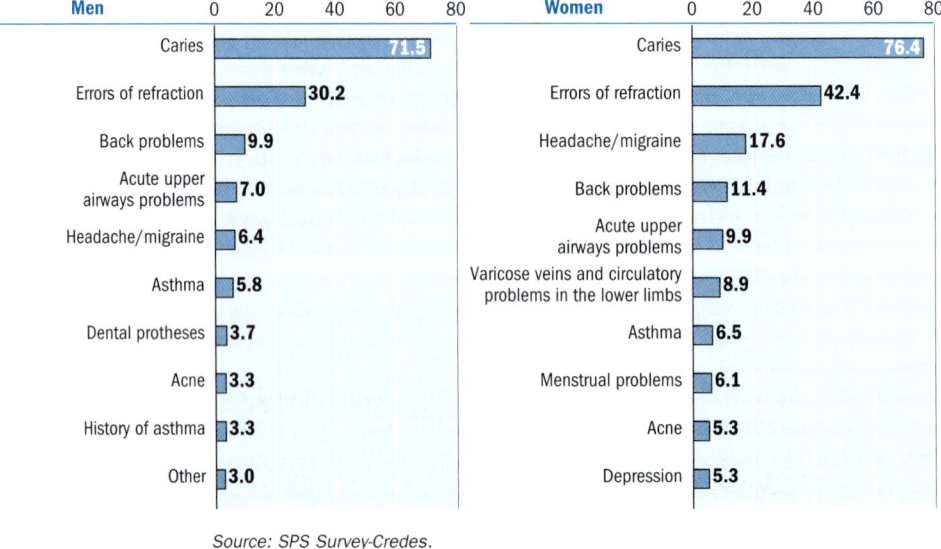

Source: SPS Survey-Credes.

People of between 15 and 44 years of age

Finally, depression is declared by 5% of women and 2% of men in this age bracket.

Between 15 and 44 years of age, men and women tend to declare the same types of disease although in all cases, more women are affected. Three problems in particular are declared far more often by women, namely headache and migraine, varicose veins, and depression.

Reasons for consulting an independent physician

In 1998, the population of people between 15 and 44 years of age accounted for 126 million consultations with an independent physician (either a General Practitioner or a specialist).

Consultations for reasons associated with sexual activity or genital problems were particularly common amongst women in this age bracket: contraception (12% of consultations), prenatal

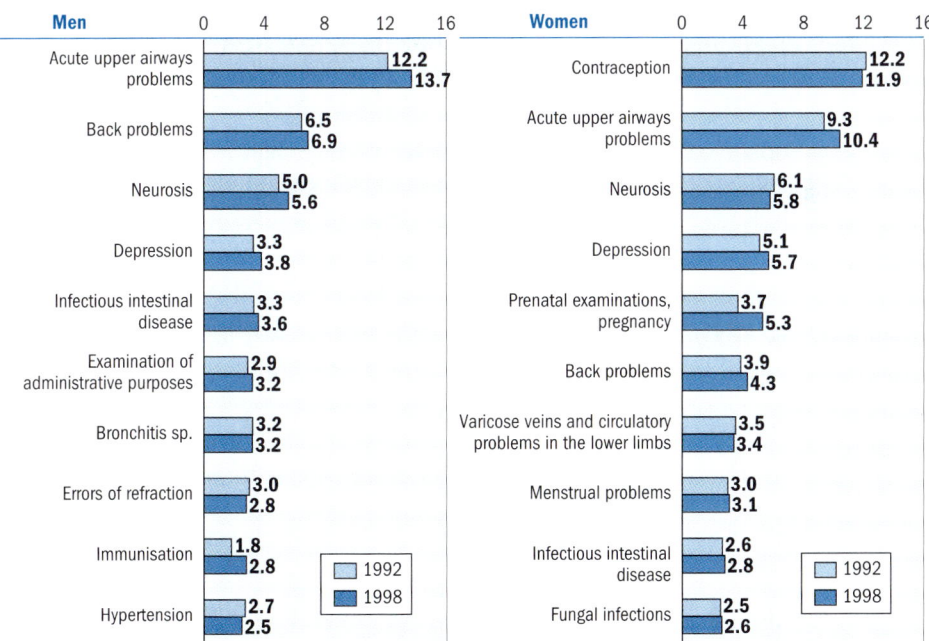

Figure 7 **Main reasons for consultation with an independent practitioner among men and women of between 15 and 44 years of age. 1992. 1998**
(percentage of consultations)

Source: Credes. Data: EPPM Survey 1992-1998. IMS-Health.

Health in France / February 2002

examinations and monitoring of pregnancy (5%), menstrual problems (3%), and pregnancy-related complications (2%).

A high proportion of consultations followed directly from morbidity that had been perceived and was declared, including acute upper airways problems, back pain, errors of refraction and, particularly in the case of women, depression, varicose veins and menstrual problems.

Mental health problems figure significantly in this age range with neurotic symptoms mentioned in 5% of consultations (without any differential between the sexes) and depression in 5% of consultations with men and 3% with women (although depression is more often declared by women). The 1% of consultations for male "tiredness" or "malaise" could also reasonably be included in this category.

Other common reasons include infectious intestinal disease (3% for both sexes), bronchitis in men (3%) and fungal infections in women (3%).

Finally, men in particular often see an independent physician for immunisations (3%) and examinations conducted for administrative purposes (3%), the latter probably related to the fact that sport is seriously practised by many men of this age.

Thus, analysis of the reasons for making an appointment with an independent practitioner shows that most concern relatively minor problems, although the number of such consultations is high and therefore they warrant a response in terms of public health.

No significant changes in the reasons for consultations were observed during the 1990's, apart from a slight increase in the incidence of acute upper airways infections (although this may be entirely due to an epidemic in 1998).

Reasons for admission into hospital-based medicine, surgery and obstetrics services

In 1998, the 15-44 age bracket accounted for a total of 4,850,000 admissions into hospital, *i.e.* 190 admissions per 1,000 inhabitants. Sixty per cent of these admissions were of women.

For men in this age bracket, the leading reason for hospitalisation was physical injury (295,000 instances, *i.e.* 17% of all admissions). The corresponding rate in women was three times lower.

Among the women in this age bracket, 40% of admissions were directly related to fertility or pregnancy. For 750,000 births, there was a total of 930,000 admissions, either during pregnancy, for delivery or post-partum (30% of all stays). To these figures have

People of between 15 and 44 years of age

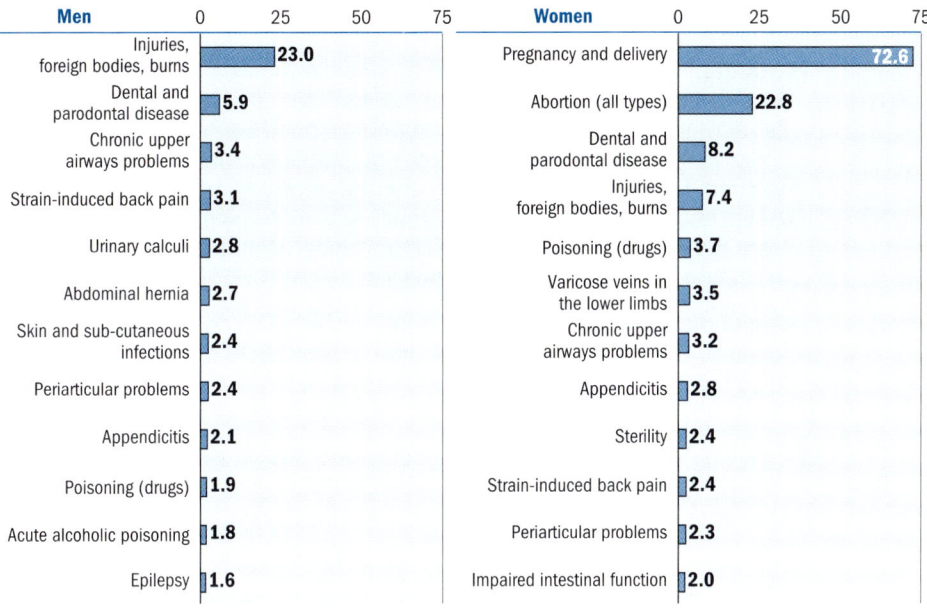

Figure 8 **Main diseases of men and women of between 15 and 44 years of age treated in short-stay hospital departments. 1998**
(per 1,000 inhabitants)

Source: PMSI. Ministry of Employment and Solidarity. Drees.

to be added those for the monitoring of normal and high-risk pregnancies, and for prenatal screening (a total of 124,000 admissions).

Abortion is the second reason for admission in women (292,000). The reason for the discrepancy of one third between this figure and the number of legally declared elective abortions is due to spontaneous and therapeutic interruptions of pregnancy, and also to the tendency of health care establishments to fail to declare all abortions.

Finally, 30,000 admissions per annum are for the treatment of sterility.

Dental and parodontal diseases represent the second cause for hospitalisation in men (76,000 admissions per annum, *i.e.* 6 per 1,000) and the third in women (100,000, *i.e.* a rate of 8 per 1,000). The great majority of these admissions are for the extraction of wisdom teeth (140,000 interventions per annum for both sexes).

Chronic upper airways problems account for 40,000 admissions per annum (without any gender differential), mainly for tonsilectomy and adenoidectomy – both of which procedures are still commonly practised in France in, among others, young adults despite the fact that their utility is questioned.

Back problems account for more stays among men than among women (40,000 *versus* 30,000).

Current PMSI data do not make it possible to put a reliable figure to the annual number of attempted suicides, but roughly 90% of all admissions for drug poisoning correspond to such attempts. Drug poisoning is the fifth cause of admission into hospital in women (47,300 admissions), and the tenth in men (24,900). Since the PMSI figures do not cover psychiatric institutions, it is very difficult to gauge the true importance of mental disease as a reason for admission into hospital.

Appendicitis accounts for a total of 62,000 admissions per annum, 3 per 1,000 in women, and 2 per 1,000 in men.

Other common causes for hospitalisation are:
– in men, urinary calculi, abdominal hernias, skin and subcutaneous tissue infections, joint problems, and acute alcohol poisoning (23,000 admissions per annum);
– and in women, varicose veins in the lower limbs.

Overall, the hospital admission rates for men and women in the 15-44 age bracket are similar if maternity-related hospitalisation is discounted. This is because the high rate of admission of men for physical injury is cancelled out by the higher number of admissions of women for problems involving the genital organs (including cancer) and the digestive tract (dental problems, appendicitis, etc.).

Long-term conditions

A total of 131,000 individuals of between 15 and 44 years of age and covered by the national health insurance system (which covers over 80% of the population as a whole) were recognised as suffering from a LTC in 1998. This bracket accounts for only 18% of all LTCs recognised despite the fact that it includes fully 42% of the total population, which serves to illustrate the low level of morbidity in this sub-population.

The psychiatric condition of 44,000 of these patients is such that the victim is exempted from the patient-payable portion. This corresponds to schizophrenia and delusional states (14,000), severe personality disorders (14,000), severe depression or neurosis (8,000), bipolar disorder (2,000), and alcohol-induced mental problems (1,000). These represent one-third of all recognised LTCs in this age bracket, so mental disease represents the main type of heavily incapacitating chronic disease in young

Figure 9 **Main long-term conditions in men and women of between 15 and 44 years of age covered by the health insurance system. 1998**
(percentage of reasons for recognition)

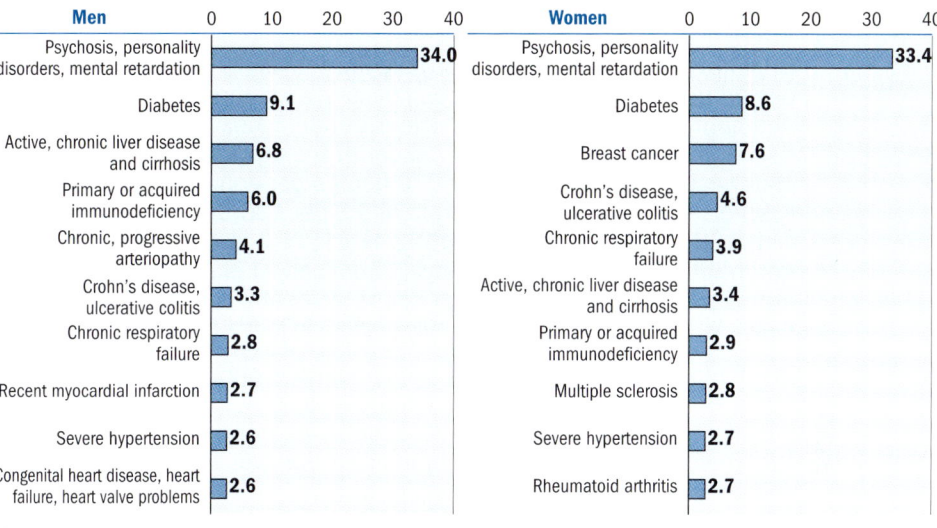

Source: Cnamts. National Medical Service Level.

adults. Two-thirds of schizophrenics are male whereas two-thirds of all depressives are female.

Three other pathologies which are under-represented in the data from the other sources used to compile this report also constitute a common reason for recognition of a long-term condition: diabetes, with 12,000 people of between 15 and 44 years of age admitted per annum; chronic liver disease with 5,000 cases of chronic viral hepatitis and 1,000 cases of alcoholic cirrhosis; and inflammatory bowel diseases with 5,000 patients suffering from ulcerative colitis or Crohn's disease.

Medical causes of death

The overall death rate between 15 and 44 years of age is low: 111 deaths per 100,000 inhabitants in 1997. There is a major discrepancy between the death rate in men (158 per 100,000) and women (64 per 100,000), a differential which has not changed since 1990.

Violent death is the primary cause of death in the 15-44 age bracket both for men (1 in 2) and women (1 in 3). Among these, the most common among men is road accidents with a total of three times more men dying in this way (although this is still the

Part one Data about health status

second most important cause of death among women). The main cause of death in women and the second in men is suicide with 4,400 deaths in 1998, with a risk multiplied by four in men.

Despite the efficacy of tritherapy and a significant reduction in mortality, AIDS remains a major cause of death among young men.

Drinking and smoking are already significant killers of men in this age group (although not nearly as ravaging as in the older groups) and come a close second to violent death. Smoking is a major risk factor for lung cancer and cancer of the bronchi and the trachea which are responsible for 670 deaths per annum in this age bracket. This corresponds to a rate of 5.3 per 100,000 (compared with 168 per 100,000 in the 45-74 bracket). It is worth pointing out that the number of women dying from cancer is rising sharply, representing today the seventh cause of death in women (210 per year) whereas it was practically negligible just a few years ago.

In addition to smoking, alcohol consumption is another important factor in the 460 deaths per annum due to cancer of the upper airways and digestive tract. Alcohol is directly implicated in 900 male deaths each year (cirrhosis of the liver, alcoholic psychosis and alcoholism).

Figure 10 **Main causes of death among men and women of between 15 and 44 years of age. 1997**
(age-normalised rates per 100,000 inhabitants)

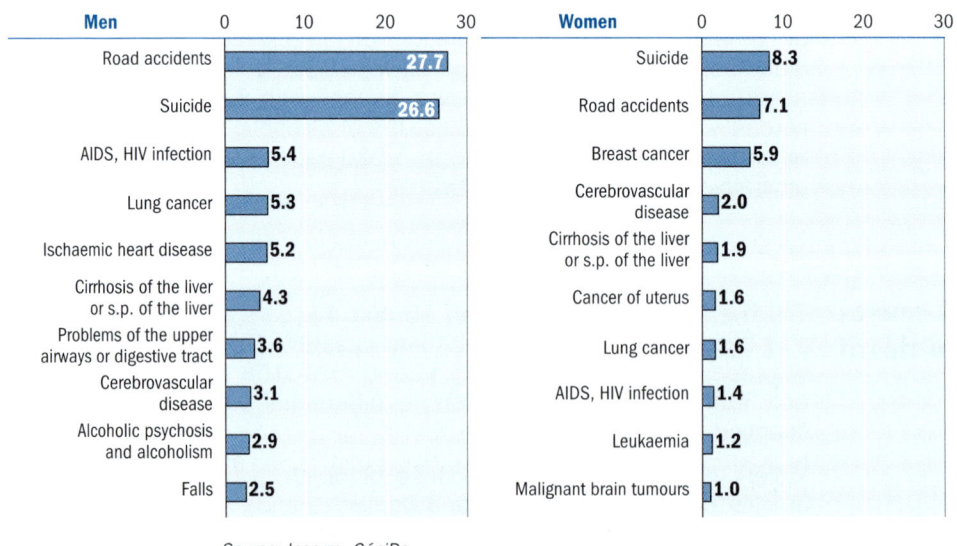

Source: Inserm. CépiDc.

Cardiovascular disease is already beginning to kill significant numbers of both men and women in this age bracket, although 3 times more men die of heart disease, and 1.5 times more of stroke.

Finally, gynaecological cancers are a common cause of death in women, notably breast cancer (450 deaths) and cancer of uterus (210).

Main health-related issues in people of between 15 and 44 years of age

Physical injuries and violent deaths – often linked to heavy drinking – are key factors in male health in this age bracket

Violent death takes a particularly heavy toll in this age group with France occupying third place among European countries (together with Spain and behind Portugal and Finland) in this respect.

External causes of injuries and poisonings actually constitute the leading cause of both death and admission into hospital, with traffic accidents and suicides being the main culprits. These two alone account for most excess mortality in young adults and in young men in particular. The magnitude of this differential is particular to France and the current rate of reduction in the annual number of deaths on the road remains quite inadequate to give any prospect of reaching the levels seen in countries like the United Kingdom where the corresponding rate is less than half that in France.

A similar observation could be made when it comes to deaths as a result of accidents in the workplace, the number of which still remains unacceptably high despite regular reductions over recent years. Comparing the French situation with that in England and Wales [26] gives an idea of the progress which could be made in avoiding avoidable deaths: in France, the overall mortality rate between 25 and 44 years of age is 234 per 100,000, whereas the corresponding figure in England is 128 per 100,000, a differential which is largely due to violent death.

Excessive drinking underlies many physical injuries and violent deaths. In 1993, 30% of all those assumed to be responsible for mortal traffic accidents were over the legal blood alcohol limit. Alcohol is also known to play a role in suicide, not only immediately prior to the actual act but also in terms of its deleterious effects on family and social life.

Otherwise, acute alcoholism accounts for 23,000 admissions of men into hospital per annum, and is a common reason for use of the emergency services.

Already among the men in this age bracket, heavy drinking leads to a significant number of deaths through chronic disease (900 in 1998 due to cirrhosis, alcoholic psychosis or alcoholism). Combined drinking and smoking also causes deaths (460 deaths due to cancers of the upper airways or digestive tract). Among those of between 15 and 44 years of age covered by national health insurance, there are 1,000 LTC admissions for alcohol-induced mental problems and another 1,000 for alcoholic cirrhosis.

Although the average consumption of alcohol is certainly on the decrease, French society is nevertheless still over-tolerant of excessive drinking and the efforts made by the authorities to correct this situation remain ineffective. Contributory factors include the difficulty in applying the legislation pertaining to the advertising of alcoholic beverages, the power of the producers' lobby group, and the lack of any recent publicity campaign against alcohol abuse. However, it can be hoped that the extension of the remit of the Interdepartmental Mission for the Fight against Drugs and Drugs Addiction (Mildt) to cover alcohol and tobacco represents the first step in a change of public policy.

Certain forms of cancer are appearing at a younger age, particularly in women

The frequency of cancer rises sharply with age but this is not to say that young people are unaffected since 24,000 new cases (*i.e.* 10% of all new cases) develop every year in those aged between 15 and 44.

Of these, 14,000 occur in women. More than half involve the breast, cervix, uterus or ovaries, and regular gynaecological examinations help identify disease at an early stage, especially in the case of cervical cancer for which the screening of women from the age of 25 is now recommended (with a national screening program due to be launched in 2003). In contrast, systematic screening for breast cancer has not been shown to be of any value in this age bracket, largely because the mammary radiographs of young women are often difficult to interpret. The priority therefore is to provide women with effective treatment modalities – and conservative ones, whenever possible. Significant progress has been made in this respect in recent years, although questions arise about disparities between different groups in terms of access to treatment, especially reconstructive surgery. Because of the possible adverse effect on the patient's perception of herself, the treatment of breast cancer – probably to a greater extent than the treatment of other forms of cancer – needs to be informed by a full exchange with the care providers, leading to the definition of a consensual strategy. A White Paper published by the National Anti-Cancer League in 1999 indicates that much remains to be done.

The special case of women with a high family risk of breast cancer warrants specific mention. Half of these women carry a mutation in one of the genes associated with breast cancer *(brcA1* or *brcA2)* which means that there is a 90% chance that they will develop breast cancer at some point in life. A genetic test now exists to identify carriers of these mutations. Once identified, the prophylactic options for carriers consist of either bilateral mastectomy and ovariectomy (because these mutations also predispose to ovarian cancer), or regular mammography starting at the age of 30. So far, only the first of these two options has been shown to have any effect on mortality: it is obvious that such a radical preventive measure justifies in-depth consideration and discussion on the part of care providers and, more importantly, the patient herself.

Attention must be drawn to the emergence of lung cancer in women in whom it was hitherto practically non-existent. In 1997, 210 women of between 15 and 44 died of this disease, representing a 72% increase since 1990. The results of Baromètre santé 2000 show that almost a half of all men and women of 18 now smoke on a regular basis, an average of 10 cigarettes a day for women and 8 for men. This suggests that female lung cancer figures will explode in the next twenty years.

In men of this age, cancer takes more diverse forms, although cancer of the lung, lips, mouth and pharynx are most common (accounting for 1,120 cases per annum including 765 among people between 40 and 44 years of age), all largely consequences of smoking and drinking. Thus, against a background of sharply decreasing overall cancer-related mortality, the number of people dying of lung cancer is remaining stable (nearly 700 per annum).

Controlling fertility and preventing sexually transmitted disease (notably AIDS) are priorities among young adults

The number of new cases of AIDS stopped falling in 1998 and this disease remains a major concern for the sub-population of between 15 and 44 years of age. Apart from the risk of premature death, the possibility of HIV infection has had a major effect on sexual life, in particular that of young adults. Whereas the advent of effective means of female contraception (the pill and the IUD) had reduced the risk of unwanted pregnancy in previous years, the AIDS epidemic introduced the spectre of death into sexual relations, and necessitated the unwelcome use of condoms.

Certain regions are more touched than others by this disease, with two-thirds of all cases recently declared being in just four regions, namely Île-de-France, Provence-Alpes-Côte-d'Azur, Aquitaine and Antilles-Guyane.

A total of 850 cases were diagnosed in men in this age bracket during the year 2000. Of these, the virus was transmitted in the course of homosexual relations in 38%, heterosexual relations in

29%, and intravenous drug use in 22%. In the same year, 358 women were diagnosed with the disease, most of whom were infected during sexual relations with a man. The fraction of women being infected has risen over time (sex ratio of 5 in 1990 and of 2.5 in 2000).

The introduction of new, more effective therapeutic modalities for HIV-positive patients in the mid-1990's led to significant decreases in both the number of new cases and the corresponding mortality rate. However, in 2000, 4 out of 10 people of between 15 and 44 years of age with full-blown AIDS only discovered that they were infected with HIV at the time of diagnosis. The proportion who had not been tested for infection prior to the appearance of full-blown disease depended on the transmission mode: 53% for heterosexual transmission, 39% for homosexual transmission, and 14% for intravenous drug abusers. Half of all those young adults who had been aware of their HIV status prior to the diagnosis of AIDS had not previously received any form of antiviral treatment.

Thus, most new cases of AIDS involve people who have either not been screened and not received any antiretroviral treatment, or who know that they are infected but have still not been given any antiretroviral treatment. These findings draw attention to the importance of campaigns to disseminate information and publicise the importance of prevention.

Another sexually transmitted infection, genital herpes, is extremely widespread and its incidence is on the increase. However, the seriousness of this health problem is under-estimated as was highlighted by the results of the 1996 Herpimax study which were presented at a recent French Consensus Conference: the prevalence of infection with herpes simplex virus 2 (HSV2, the form which causes most cases of genital herpes) is 18% in women and 14% in men, although only 20% of all those infected are ever diagnosed. Because of the widespread nature of this viral infection together with the fact that genital herpes can promote the transmission of HIV, obtaining better epidemiological data on HSV2 infection is a priority, and structures need to be put in place to improve prevention, diagnosis and treatment.

Finally, available means of contraception have not in any way precluded the problem of unwanted pregnancy, especially amongst poor young women (see box below).

In conclusion, the strategies in this area to be focused on by the authorities and institutions involved in health must be primarily preventive ones focusing on sexual life and habits.

CONTRACEPTION, ABORTION AND PUBLIC HEALTH

Although the use of medical means of contraception has steadily increased in France since the 1970's (over 80% of women of between 18 and 44 years of age now depend on either oral contraceptives or an intra-uterine device [IUD]), the number of cases in which contraception fails has remained relatively stable. The percentage of unwanted pregnancies significantly decreased between 1970 and 1985 but the number of elective abortion has remained fairly constant over the last twenty years, and a slight increase has even been observed recently among women of under 25. It is estimated that more than 200,000 elective abortions are performed every year, *i.e.* 15 per 1,000 women of between 15 and 49, which is close to the average rate in European countries. It could be true that today, women may be more ready to request an abortion in the event of contraception failing, but this "contraceptive paradox" also raises questions about the accessibility of different means of contraception and about the accessibility of elective abortion.

Contraception failures are not confined to women or couples who do not use any means of contraception at all. In practice, the number of women who do not wish to have a child and yet do not use any means of contraception is very low (under 3%), and about 10% of first experiences of sexual intercourse today are unprotected [19]. The real problem stems from a failure to use effective contraception systematically.

Access to contraception

Differences in behaviour between different social classes and geographical areas were recorded in the 1970's, but these had disappeared by the time of the Ined survey in 1994 which addressed the use of oral contraceptives and IUDs by adult women. In a very recent survey however on sexuality among young men and women of between 15 and 18 years of age, differences were detected in contraception practices according to educational history [19]. At the time of their first sexual intercourse, more of those in vocational training used an oral contraceptive, whereas more high school students used condoms. However, it is difficult to draw any conclusions about specific links with educational profile because the age of sexual initiation itself depends on class, with children of the lower classes tending to begin sexual activity at a younger age. This prefigures general behavioural differences vis-à-vis the risks associated with sex. Nevertheless, data on pregnancy and elective abortion rates suggest that some degree of social selection does indeed exist with respect to access to contraception, *e.g.* pregnancy is more common in poor girls. The attitude to motherhood is certainly different in different social classes, and pregnancy during adolescence might not inevitably be classified as "unwanted" by everyone. In fact, for many adolescents, pregnancy is wished for and motherhood represents a way of acquiring an identity and social status. Nevertheless, elective abortion is still more common among poorer young girls: 8% of girls in vocational training declare having already had at least one abortion, compared with just 1% among those following a conventional, academic curriculum.

Therefore, in terms of prevention policy, reducing social inequality with respect to access to contraception represents a priority. This will entail designing and implementing special, targeted programmes which will have to take into account the fact that, while the data presented here indicate that socially conditioned disparities in access to contraception are an important factor, there is another important question to be tackled, namely that of the inability of certain women (of all ages) in a socially vulnerable situation to control their lives in the way that is prerequisite for the rational use of contraception.

When contraception "fails"

Social inequalities should not be thought of merely in terms of association with some particular set of socio-economic groups. Other factors would seem to be at play in some contraception failures according to recent data collected in an Inserm survey. Suitably targeted preventive policy might be able to cut down high-risk behaviour in this area. Thus, incompatibility between the means of contraception used and the woman's living conditions, and emotional and sexual situation can lead to failure. Above and beyond improving the awareness of doctors, it is the very nature of the doctor-patient relationship which is at issue here, notably with respect to empowering women to choose the most suitable means of contraception for themselves. Lack of information (which mainly affects younger women) is rarely the only factor. Apart from structural reasons (e.g. the inaccessibility of institutions in a position to give them the relevant information), the fact that women lead sexual lives that they themselves perceive as socially unacceptable represents a fundamental obstacle when it comes to raising their consciousness about effective means of contraception. Although inhibitions on talking about sexuality and contraception within the family have been lifted to some extent, there are nevertheless many young women who are reluctant to or cannot talk about intimate subjects with their parents. This is why different types of centre where young men and women can go to talk about their problems and get advice need to be established (or maintained, in the case of those already in existence). Such centres should be set up so as to genuinely respond to the needs of young people.

Finally, any measure intended to enhance the independence and status of women – by indirectly contributing to changing social attitudes to sexuality – will tend to promote the rational, effective use of contraception by women.

Availability of elective abortion

In the event of the failure of contraception, one woman in two today resorts to elective abortion. Two recent reports [13, 30] review the health care system and draw attention to ways in which it is not functioning well, in particular the inability of the public sector to perform all requested elective abortions. This is due to budget limitations, disapproval of the procedure, and low staff status, and leads to inequality, particularly with respect to those women living in a precarious situation. Some women are obliged to go abroad for the operation. Recent research on access to abortion [29] revealed that lack of information about establishments offering the procedure was a source of inequality, and that women who consulted their General

Practitioner from the outset were not ultimately dealt with as well as those who consulted elsewhere. It is also important to draw attention to the fact that access to RU486 (the "morning after pill") remains limited with only 28% of the 40% of eligible women actually obtaining it in 2000.

Focus on prevention

People living in an insecure or vulnerable situation are at greater risk for problems related to sex, be it the need for abortion, or sexually transmitted disease (the incidence of which has been on the rise again in recent years), including HIV infection. Access to means of prevention needs to be further improved, not only from the point of view of the dissemination of information but also-and more importantly-at the level of the social and financial accessibility of various means of contraception and prevention. As stated by Calvez [5], *"risk-taking is not the result of human weakness but of a type of social experience which does not allow people to make the association between sexual risks and their current situation, and which fails to give them a context in which to organise their preventive behaviour"*. This is why we need to review the concepts underlying our preventive policy and the methods used to implement it, notably the extent of consultation between researchers and those responsible for public policy as well as players on the ground. Major innovations have already been introduced in this respect in the field of HIV infection, and these should be extended to cover other risks associated with sexual activity, notably elective abortion and other sexually transmitted diseases.

Nathalie Bajos, Henri Leridon, Inserm U292

References: [2, 5, 13, 19, 21, 29, 30].

Mental suffering – which affects men and women alike – is poorly accounted for

The magnitude of the mental health problem is difficult to gauge from the available data but it is nevertheless great with 5% of women and 2% of men claiming to suffer from depression. It is by means of analysing drug use and treatment patterns that the real picture emerges: 10% of all outpatient consultations are for neurotic symptoms or depression among women, and nearly 9% in men. In 1998, among people of between 15 and 44 years of age with National Health Insurance coverage, 8,000 were recognised as suffering from a long-term condition (LTC) in the form of either depression or neurosis, a figure which represents 6% of all admissions in this group. A survey conducted by the Credes on a representative sample of the French population revealed even higher age-specific prevalences with 4% of males of between 16 and 19 years of age suffering from depression, rising to 10% by the age of 30 and remaining stable thereafter. Among women, the situation was even worse with fully 14% of under-20 year-olds being depressive, rising to 20% thereafter. Therefore, several million people of between 15 and 44 suffer from depression with only a minority receiving any specific treatment. Depression is often difficult to diagnose for an independent practitioner, at least in the early stages when the symptoms are not perceived as debilitating by the victim. A priority area for action is General Practitioners' awareness and knowledge of this problem. The above-mentioned apparent under-treatment of depression, especially by the prescription of anti-depressant drugs, remains to be reconciled with the paradoxical observation that the level of psychotropic drug consumption is particularly high in France.

In this age group, by far the most common reasons for LTC recognition are psychosis and severe personality disorders which together account for one-third of all such admissions, *i.e.* more than 40,000 per annum among those with national health insurance coverage alone (without any differential between the sexes). An age breakdown shows the peaks to be located in the 25-29 sub-population of men, and between 40 and 44 for women.

Finally, death by suicide is an obvious manifestation of extreme psychological suffering, and this represents the second cause of death amongst both men and women (3,500 and 1,000 deaths per annum respectively). This cause of mortality is not decreasing unlike those of other causes. Hospital admissions following suicide attempts (corresponding to about three-quarters of all such attempts) are steadily increasing amongst those of between both 15 and 24 (300 admissions per 10,000 inhabitants) and 35 and 44 (360 per 100,000).

Headache, migraine, back pain and circulatory problems affecting the lower limbs: problems which cause suffering and lead to massive consumption of health care resources

At this age, certain diseases are already in evidence which, although by no means life-threatening nevertheless entail significant pain and disability, and lead to massive consumption of health care resources. Thus women declare in a large proportion headaches and migraine, back pain and circulatory problems affecting the lower limbs. Headaches and migraines as well as back pains are found in men but at lower frequency. Back pain represents the leading occupational problem and the leading reason for disability leave. In 2000, 4% of all the employees of EDF-GDF (the French national gas and electricity utility) took time off work for a back problem (acute or chronic spinal arthrosis, sciatica or disk lesions). More women take time off work for this reason, and the problem rises steadily with age (from 1% at 25 to 5% at 45).

Changes in lifestyle underlie the trend towards increasing body weight

Living and eating habits have considerably evolved in recent years. Broadly speaking, calorie intake has decreased somewhat but physical activity has decreased disproportionately as a result of easier working conditions, generally lower energy expenditure in daily life (*e.g.* driving instead of walking), and the increase in time spent watching television. Over the same period, the food processing industry has taken over a large part of the diet with products that are rich in sugar and animal fat. As a result, the French – following their counterparts in the USA – are getting fatter, a worrying trend given the causal role of excess body weight in the development of serious health problems such as diabetes and cardiovascular disease.

The ObEpi survey based on data volunteered by the subjects themselves (in which weight figures are probably therefore under-estimated) shows that the number of French people that are overweight or frankly obese increased in just four years. According to this survey, in the year 2000, 40% of the French population were overweight (with 10% falling into the clinical category of obesity). The prevalence of excess body weight rises sharply between the age brackets of 15-24 and 35-44: from 11 to 29% in women, and from 12 to 46% in men. Meeting the targets set by the National Nutrition and Health Plan is becoming an ever more urgent priority in this country.

Nevertheless, a period characterised by generally good physical health

Despite all these various health problems, the period of life between 15 and 44 years of age is generally characterised by good physical health.

The overall death rate is low – of the order of 1.6 per 1,000 for men, and 0.6 per 1,000 for women – and falling steadily. Admission to hospital is relatively rare, barely any higher than that between 1 and 14 at 140 admissions per 1,000 for both sexes alike if hospital stays related to pregnancy and childbirth are discounted.

It is not therefore very surprising that at this age health is perceived very positively by nearly three people in ten, and judged satisfactory by more than 60% of them (according to the 1997 Credoc survey).

However, it is important to put this into context with respect to differences between the sexes, in particular between the ages of 15 and 19. In fact, according to the Baromètre santé 2000, women across the board perceive their general state of health (associating physical and mental health, and social well being) as significantly lower, especially young women of between 15 and 19 years of age. This is because of high levels of anxiety and depression.

Part one — Data about health status

ROAD ACCIDENTS

Road accidents have a considerable impact on overall health. Every day, 22 people are killed, and 74 seriously injured on French roads, and in 2000, the number of people who died within 30 days* of a road accident reached 8,079 [31]. Table 1 gives a breakdown of the 7,241 reported deaths broken down according to age and type of road-user.

The number injured is far higher: according to the National Ministerial Road Safety Watchdog (Onisr, *Observatoire national interministériel de sécurité routière*), the 2000 total was 161,681, of which 26,971 (17%) were classified as "serious" injuries**. Data from the National Institute for Research on Transport and Safety (Inrets, *Institut national de recherche sur les transports et leur sécurité*) clinical database for the Rhone region paint an even more alarming picture with a total number of victims nearly double that of the Onisr [20]. The Inrets figures document eight times more cyclists injured than do the Onisr statistics.

The number of victims per 1,000 inhabitants is dependent on age and sex. The 2000 figures show a national level of 8.6 victims per 1,000 young people of between 15 and 24 compared with just 3.5 victims per 1,000 adults of 25 to 44. In the former age bracket, there were two male victims for every female one [31].

These data on death and injury represent the tip of the iceberg when it comes to the impact of road accidents on overall health because most of the associated problems only emerge after the accident. Outcomes among those of 15 to 24 who had been injured in a road accident were investigated in a study conducted in the Franche-Comté region [32], from which some results are presented below.

The young are most affected. Most of the injuries correspond to cranial trauma which can have repercussions for many years, *e.g.* pain, physical and psychological sequelae, and adverse effects on social life.

Table 1 **Number of deaths on the roads in 2000**

	Pedestrians	Cyclists	Motor cyclists	Car drivers	Total
0-14 years	78	31	42	180	331
	23.6%	9.4%	12.7%	54.4%	100%
15-24 years	59	31	452	1,390	1,932
	3.1%	1.6%	23.4%	71.9%	100%
25-44 years	153	48	631	1,574	2,406
	6.4%	2.0%	26.2%	65.4%	100%
45-64 years	169	62	141	960	1,332
	12.7%	4.7%	10.6%	72.1%	100%
65 years and over	324	79	35	802	1,240
	26.1%	6.4%	2.8%	64.7%	100%
Total	783	251	1,301	4,906	7,241
	10.8%	**3.5%**	**18.0%**	**67.8**	**100%**

* The number of dead within 30 days is estimated by multiplying the number of dead reported immediately after the accident by a factor of 1.06.
** An injury is considered as "serious" if it entails a hospital stay of longer than 6 days.

People of between 15 and 44 years of age

Outcomes of injuries sustained by those of between 15 and 24 years of age*

Five years after the accident:
Pain 68% are still taking pain killers
Sequelae experienced in 54% of those who suffered cranial injury
Psychological repercussions 38% have some form of psychological sequela, and 13% experience psychological distress
Social life 52% report adverse effects vis-à-vis their career

Details on the accidents-such as the Onisr figures presented in Table 2 which relate health impact to place and day of the week-may give clues about how to implement effective measures.

For example, these figures show that two deaths out of three occur on isolated country roads whereas two injuries in three result from accidents in town. Fatal accidents are 40% more common on Saturdays and Sundays.

Table 2

Accidents broken down according to level of urbanisation and day of the week

	Fatal	Involving injury
Number of accidents		
In town	2,137	80,729
On country roads	5,506	40,494
Mean per day		
Saturday	27	356
Sunday	26	291
Other days	19	334

Data from different countries

In 1999, the death rate on French roads was one of the highest in Europe [20].

Number of deaths within 30 days of the accident per million inhabitants

	1990	1994	1999
United Kingdom	94	65	60
Germany	126	121	95
France	199	156	143
Spain	232	144	146

Key determinants

Areas in which action could be taken are summarised below. Driving at a speed suitable to road and traffic conditions depends on driver behaviour, and the condition of both the vehicle and the road.

---

* Results of a survey carried out on a sample of serious injuries: 80% had suffered cranial trauma [32].

Part one Data about health status

Dangerous driving is particularly common among young men, a fact which is reflected in the annual mortality figures. Tiredness, alcohol, and the use of recreational drugs and psychotropic medications all affect a driver's ability to react – the increased incidence of accidents on Saturdays and Sundays may be linked to this problem.

Controlling vehicular performance at the design and manufacture stage represents a key factor if appropriate speeds are to be ensured. Finally, the condition of both the roads and the vehicles on them deserves constant, close vigilance.

Main causes of road accidents

1. Drivers' behaviour
    Dangerous driving
    Alcohol and psychotropic drug use
2. Poor state of roads
3. Factors related to vehicles
    Built-in performance
    Maintenance

Regional programmes to address these factors can create a suitable framework in which appropriate measures can be designed and co-ordinated to involve all concerned in improving the situation.

Bernard Junod, National School of Public Health, (Égéries department), Rennes

People of between 45 and 74 years of age

The 1999 Census recorded 19 million people of between 45 and 74 years of age living in France. After having remained fairly stable between 1982 and 1990, this figure rose by nearly three million in the ensuing nine years. This is because, by the 1990's, the generation which was decimated by the First World War had largely passed, and those born in the population explosion following the Second World War (the "baby-boomers") were beginning to enter the group. As a result, the overall proportion of 45-74 year-olds rose by 4%, from 28% to 32%. Projecting to 2020, the ageing of the baby-boom generation coupled with their increased life expectancy is expected to give rise to a significant increase in the number of people in this age bracket up to a total of about 23.5 million, representing 37% of the population as a whole.

The fact that more men die before their time (premature death being conventionally defined as death before the age of 65, see the box on page 112) leads to an imbalance of the sexes in this group which contains 9,800,000 women as against just 9,100,000 men.

Declared morbidity

The period between 45 and 74 years of age represents a time of change during which multiple health problems frequently appear, from commonplace ailments entailing more or less inconvenience or pain to serious, life-threatening diseases. It is also during this period that serious attention needs to be paid to risk factors.

The most common problems involve the eyes (94% of this subpopulation), and mouth and teeth (82%).

Most of the eye problems are errors of refraction (myopia, hyperopia and presbyopia) which are slightly more common among women, although the differential is far less marked than in the preceding age bracket and is probably mainly due to an overall difference in age.

Mouth and tooth problems boil down to caries and the need for prostheses. Two-thirds complain of caries, be they treated or not, and one-third have dental prostheses (crowns, bridges or removable denture), compared with just 4% of those of between 15 and 44.

Ear problems correspond to loss of hearing function which is declared by 9% of women and 16% of men.

Part one Data about health status

Circulatory and joint problems are declared by more than 40% of people of between 45 and 74 years of age, a clear change since these problems only affect 9 and 16% respectively of those falling into the 15-44 age bracket.

Although the total prevalence of these two problems is the same in both sexes (44%), this masks major gender-related differences.

Circulatory disorders are far more common in women (52% *versus* 35%), with varicose veins and other venous deficiencies involving the lower limbs being declared by 1 in 3 women compared with 1 in 10 men. In contrast, the same number of each sex declares high blood pressure.

With respect to bone and joint problems (declared by 37% of the men in this age group and 50% of the women), back pain and osteoarthritis are more common in women (respectively 30% and 18% in women *versus* 23% and 10% in men).

Among the diseases most frequently declared, disorders affecting lipid metabolism (hypercholesterol-aemia and combined hyperlipidemia) affect equal numbers of both sexes (16%).

Figure 11 **Main declared conditions among men and women of between 45 and 74 years of age. 1998**
(in percentage suffering from at least one disease or health problem)

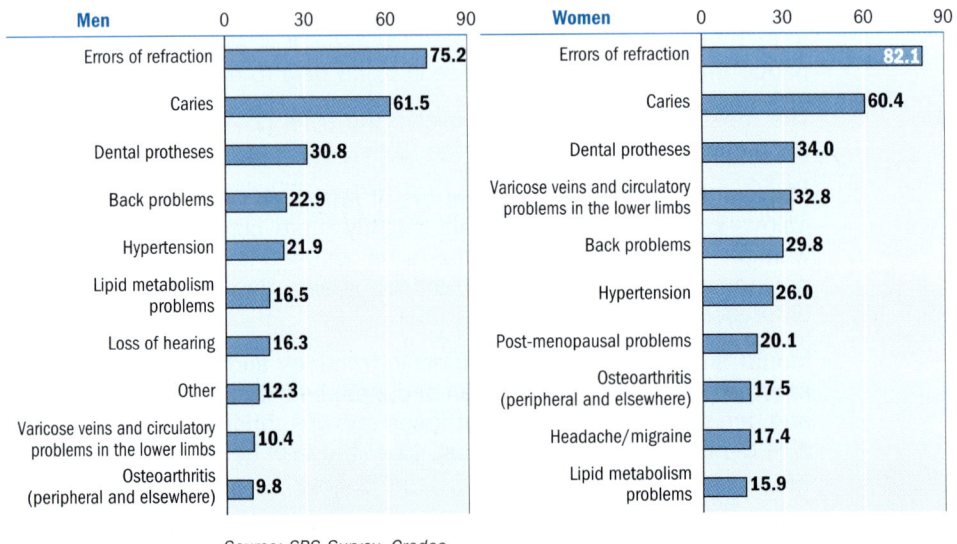

Source: SPS Survey. Credes.

Taking the broad view, of the ten most commonly declared problems, eight are experienced by both men and women. The exceptions are deafness (7th place among men and 15th place among women) and headaches and migraine (17% of women compared with just 7% of men).

Problems associated with menopause are declared by 20% of all women.

Reasons for consulting an independent physician

People aged between 45 and 74 had as many consultations with independent physicians as those in the 15-44 age bracket (125 million, in total) although they constitute a smaller fraction of the population.

Cardiovascular disease – practically absent in the younger group of subjects – is one of the major reasons for such consultations, accounting for 3 in every 10. Both sexes experience cardiovascular problems but more women seek the advice of an independent practitioner.

Hypertension is the reason for 21% of male consultations, and 18% of female ones, but more men are seen for ischaemic heart disease (6% of consultations), arteritis (3%) and arrhythmia (3%). One in ten female consultations are for varicose veins or circulatory problems involving the lower limbs.

At this age, metabolic problems become a major reason for consulting an independent physician, notably problems with lipid metabolism, especially hypercholesterolaemia, which account for 10% of all consultations. Diabetes is another common disorder in this group, responsible for 6% of visits by men and 4% by women.

Otherwise, 7% of female consultations are for problems associated with menopause. Management of these diverse disorders at an early stage is essential if the appearance of serious health problems is to be prevented or delayed, problems which figure prominently among the reasons for admission into hospital.

Mental problems are another reason for consultations with an independent physician, particularly by women: one in six female consultations are for psychological problems – mainly depression or neurotic symptoms – compared with just one in ten among men.

Consistently with the declared morbidity findings, joint and bone disorders are another common reason for consultation, with back problems being the third most important reason among men (7% of all consultations), and the sixth among women (6%).

Respiratory disease is mentioned in one consultation in seven although acute upper airways infections – the leading reason for

Part one Data about health status

Figure 12   **Main reasons for consultation with an independent practitioner among men and women of between 45 and 74 years of age. 1992. 1998**
(percentage of consultations)

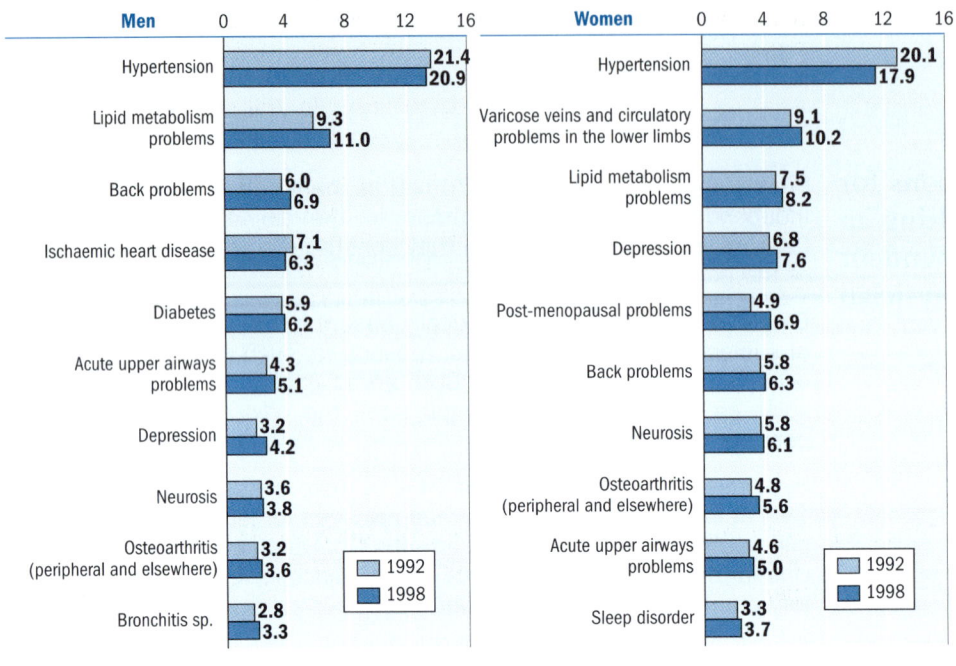

Source: Credes. Data: EPPM Survey 1992-1998. IMS-Health.

consultation in both of the younger age brackets – only incites 5% of visits. In men, however, bronchitis is relatively common.

Finally, although far less common than in the oldest age bracket, sleeping disorders are the reason for nearly 4% of all consultations of 45-74 year-old patients with independent physicians.

Reasons for admission into hospital-based medicine, surgery and obstetrics services

The age of 45 largely corresponds to the end of the period of female fertility which was associated with 40% of all hospital stays of women of between 15 and 44. In parallel, the rate of admission of men of between 45 and 74 increases to exceed that of women. In this age range, the reasons for admission are at their most diverse, with the ten leading reasons accounting for only one quarter of the total (compared with one-third in the oldest age bracket and one-half for younger patients). This is due to the fact that it is during this period of life that chronic conditions affecting multiple organs begin to be superimposed on all the other possible reasons for admission into hospital.

Physical injury is the leading reason for admission in women, and the second in men. Traumas are more diverse in both nature and location in men (including dislocations and strains, cranial injuries and broken limbs) than in women (in whom fractures of the limbs are predominant). This is because men are at significant risk of a variety of accidents (domestic, work-related and road accidents) whereas most accidents in women are falls (the consequences of which are often exacerbated by nascent osteoporosis).

Ischaemic heart disease is the leading reason for admission of men into hospital, underlying one stay in twenty. This disorder is also one of the main reasons for the admission of women but the absolute number of associated admissions is four times lower. Other cardiovascular problems are represented, *e.g.* varicose veins involving the lower limbs is the third reason for admission of women into hospital, and arrhythmia and impaired conduction are among the ten leading reasons for men.

Figure 13 **Main diseases of men and women of between 45 and 74 years of age treated in short-stay hospital departments. 1998**
(per 1,000 inhabitants)

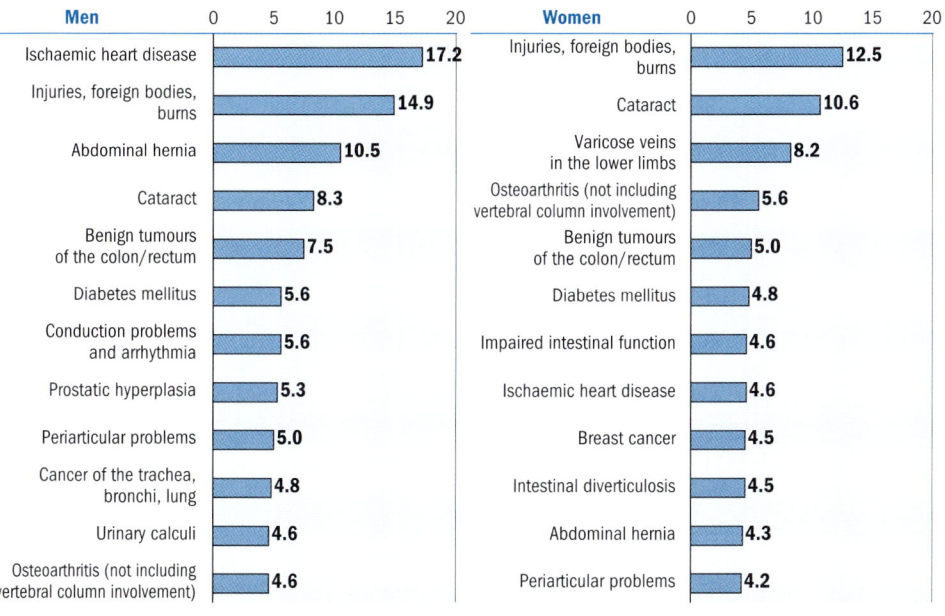

Source: PMSI. Ministry of Employment and Solidarity. Drees.

Major differences between the sexes are seen when it comes to admission into hospital for gastrointestinal disorders: in men, abdominal hernia is the most common (accounting for 11% of all hospital stays) whereas women are more often admitted for intestinal functional disorders (5%) and diverticular disease of the colon (5%).

Two types of tumour figure among the ten leading reasons for admission of each sex: benign tumours of the colon and rectum (both sexes) and lung cancer (men) or breast cancer (women).

Diseases involving the joints or bones are also common, especially periarticular conditions and osteoarthritis of the hip and the knee. Most hospitalisations in this context are for total joint replacement procedures. The admission rate for total hip replacement rises between the ages of 50 and 80, before dropping off thereafter. This procedure tends to be tackled at a younger age in men whose admission rate is higher up to the age of 75 (whereas the admission rate of women is higher after this age). Similarly, the frequency of total knee replacement surgery increases up to the age of 80 and then falls off; this operation is twice as common in women.

Diabetes represents the sixth most common reason for hospital admission in both men and women, although the way in which PMSI data are collected means that the real incidence of this disease is under-estimated. This is because, if the reason for admission is diabetic damage to an organ which is resulting in a specific, classifiable clinical problem, the reason recorded is the latter rather than diabetes. Thus, diabetic retinopathy is counted as a "disease of the eye or its appendages" rather than as an "endocrine, nutritional or metabolic disease".

Prostatic hyperplasia is already a fairly common reason for hospitalisation in this age group, although it is really after 75 years of age that this reason becomes major.

Finally, cataract is the third most important reason (after trauma and maternity) for admission into hospital, taking all ages across the board. This problem really begins to appear frequently between 45 and 74 years of age, constituting the fourth most important reason for the admission of men in this age bracket (1 in every 40 admissions), and the second most important for women (1 in 25).

Long-term conditions

In 1998, 400,000 people of between 45 and 74 years of age with National Health Insurance coverage (which covers over 80% of the entire population) were recognised as suffering from a LTC

People of between 45 and 74 years of age

Figure 14 **Main long-term conditions in men and women of between 45 and 74 years of age covered by the health insurance system. 1998** (percentage of reasons for recognition)

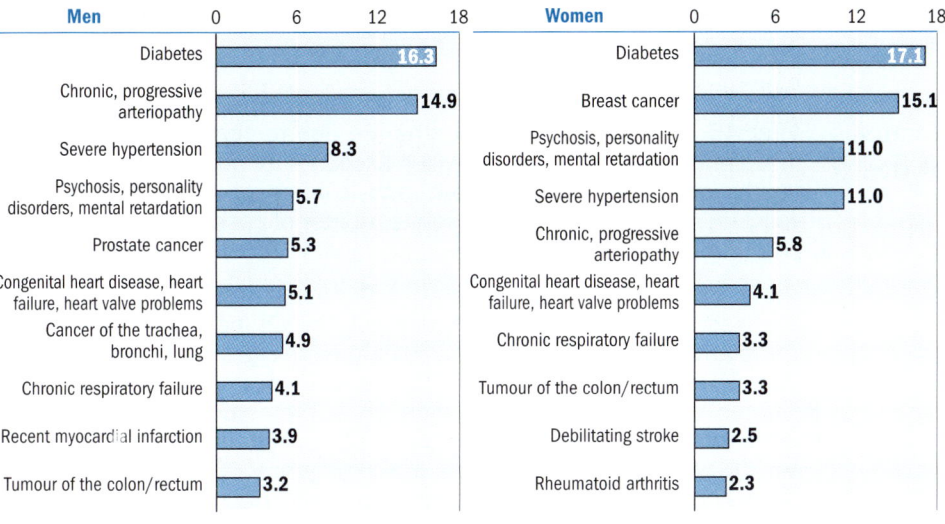

Source: Cnamts. National Medical Service Level.

in 1998. This corresponds to 55% of all admissions for just 32% of the overall population.

Cancer and cardiovascular disease each underlie 30% of these cases, cardiovascular disease being predominant in men (80,000 LTC admissions *versus* 43,000 for women) whereas cancer is the most common reason in women (57,000) although the absolute number of men recognised as having cancer is actually greater (66,000).

Ischaemic heart disease, infarction and severe high blood pressure are the most common cardiovascular complaints, followed by heart failure.

Among the various forms of cancer, prostate cancer is the most common reason for LTC recognition of men (12,000 cases per annum), followed by malignancies involving the upper airways or digestive tract (11,500 cases) and lung cancer (11,000 cases). In women, breast cancer alone accounts for 46% of all LTCs recognised in patients suffering from cancer (with 26,000 new cases in 1998).

Other common LTCs admission include diabetes – the third most important frequently recognised between the ages of 45 and 74 accounting for 37,000 men and 30,000 women. Mental disease

Part one — Data about health status

(depression, neurosis, serious personality disorders, dementia and psychosis) is no longer the leading motive of LTC admission, as was the case for both of the younger age brackets, although 19,000 women and 13,000 men in this age group are recognised as suffering from this kind of condition.

Medical causes of death

After 45 years of age, most deaths are due to common chronic diseases, in particular cancer which accounts for nearly half of all deaths of both men and women, and to a lesser extent cardio-vascular disease which arises in one quarter of cases in men and one fifth in women.

The pattern in France compared with that in other countries changes with age. Between 45 and 60, French mortality figures are relatively high (which is also true before the age of 45) whereas after 60, they are relatively low. This is so for both sexes but the differential is more marked for men. Thus, premature death (conventionally defined as death at under 65) is high in France (221 per 100,000), a fact which the major progress made in recent years should not be allowed to obscure (the corresponding figure was 300 per 100,000 in 1982) (see box below).

Figure 15 **Main causes of death among men and women of between 45 and 74 years of age. 1997**
(age-normalised rates per 100,000 inhabitants)

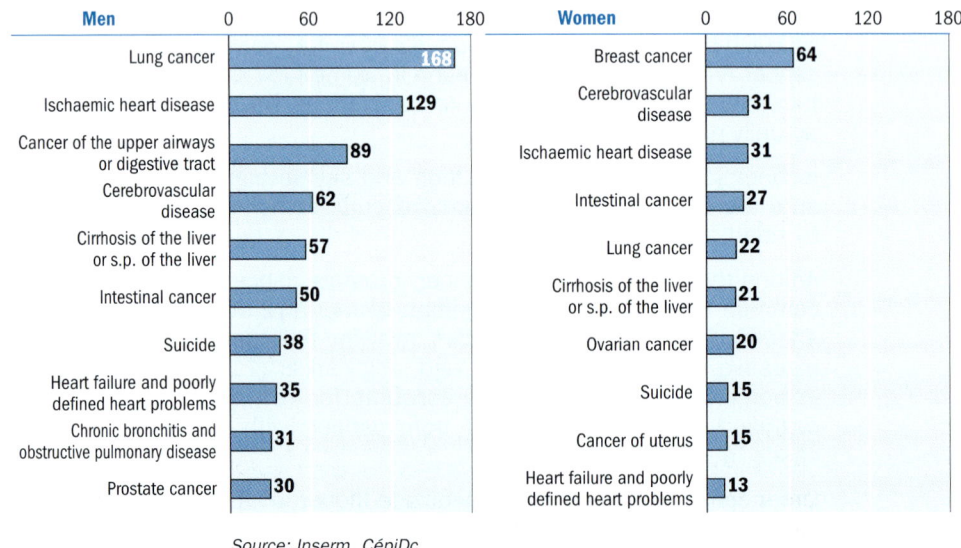

Source: Inserm. CépiDc.

Between 1990 and 1997, death rates fell by 10% (although the absolute number of deaths rose over this period as a result of the increased number of people in the relevant age bracket), but not at a rate any faster than that in the most elderly sub-population. This reduction in mortality in both sexes was due to across-the-board decreases for all major diseases apart from respiratory and skin diseases, and deaths due to congenital anomaly.

While the profile of causes of death in men has not significantly changed, the fraction of deaths secondary to circulatory problems has fallen in women. It is worth noting that, although mortality due to respiratory disease is relatively low (5%), the overall situation is deteriorating with no change in the number of men dying, and more women dying from this type of condition.

Analysis of death from malignancy reveals a highly dynamic picture. Lung cancer causes the death of one of eight male deaths and is a rising cause of mortality among women (having increased by a factor of 40% in terms of absolute numbers, and by 25% in terms of percentage): this is a foretaste of the terrible public health consequences of women smoking which are largely yet to come. In contrast, tumours of the upper airways and digestive tract constitute the cause of death which has seen the most positive change in men (a reduction of 25%) due to reduced excessive drinking: similar effects are seen in other alcohol-related causes of death. In women, death due to breast cancer is not decreasing at all and this disease is still responsible for 1 in 9 deaths of women of between 45 and 74. Mortality associated with both prostate and cervical cancer has decreased, and that associated with ovarian cancer is unchanged. Intestinal tumours tend to kill fewer people, a trend which is more obvious in women.

The numbers dying as a result of the two major cardiovascular causes of death have significantly diminished since 1990: in the case of ischaemic heart disease, by a factor of 20% in men and by 30% in women; and in the case of cerebrovascular disease, by 20% in men and 25% in women. A third group of cardiovascular diseases (covering heart failure and poorly defined heart conditions) also figures in the top ten causes of death and is also causing fewer deaths.

The number of deaths due to cirrhosis is continuing to fall in both sexes, following the same trend as for other alcohol-induced problems. Fewer people are dying by suicide, although it is in this age group that the suicide rate is highest.

Respiratory diseases (bronchitis and obstructive pulmonary disease) are unchanged or on the increase (30% of men and 40% of women are suffering from pneumonia and bronchopneumonia). Since this trend is observed in older people, it is a public health issue which warrants analysis and close monitoring.

Part one Data about health status

PREMATURE DEATH WHICH CAN BE AVOIDED IN FRANCE

If one compares death rates in various countries of a similar level of economic development, one observes that France is in a generally positive situation, especially its women who have the lowest death rates in the entire European Union. This overall situation is due to low death rates among older people in France. However, if the spotlight is turned on "premature" death (*i.e.* death before 65), France is not so high and indeed, for men, it is near the bottom of the list.

Therefore, addressing the problem of premature death is a priority area for action in French public health policy. Death before 65 accounts for one-fifth of all deaths, equivalent to 110,000 deaths per annum (77,000 men and 33,000 women). A man is 2.5 times as likely to die before 65 as a woman. Cancer is the cause of the greatest proportion of these deaths (more than one-third in men and nearly one half in women), lung cancer being the most common in men and breast cancer in women. Cancer is followed by violent death (which accounts for about one-fifth of the total). The premature death rate steadily fell from 1990 on, but this trend was bucked in 1998 when this death rate rose slightly in both sexes.

As was done in the two previous reports, it is useful to focus on two particular indicators associated with premature mortality:
– "deaths which could be avoided by cutting down high-risk behaviour": *i.e.* smoking, drinking, dangerous driving, etc. These corresponding causes of death include lung cancer and cancer of the upper airways and digestive tract, cirrhosis, road accidents, falls, suicide and AIDS;
– "deaths which could be avoided by improving health care": deaths from causes which could be cut down by improving the care system (including screening programmes), possibly combined with changes in individual behaviour patterns. These causes include ischaemic heart disease, cerebrovascular disease, breast cancer, cancer of uterus, testicular cancer, Hodgkin's disease, leukaemia, asthma, ulcers, appendicitis, hernia, influenza, and maternal mortality...

In men, mortality which is due to "high-risk behaviour" and avoidable has 3 times as much weight as that associated with the care system. In women, the opposite is true: it is the mortality which is related to the care system and avoidable which is the more frequent (mainly due to cancer of the breast and uterus). Between 1990 and 1997, the number of deaths due to both of these groups of causes fell in both sexes, although the overall drop in men was greater. However, the figures for lung cancer in men remained more or less constant (and even increased a little in 1998), and the number of women of under 65 dying of this form of cancer in general is rising significantly.

With respect to "deaths which could be avoided by cutting down high-risk behaviour", France occupies a relatively poor position in the European Community so that, despite steady improvement over recent years, it is at the same level as Germany and Denmark – for alcohol-related deaths (among both men and women). Similarly, the highest number of deaths below 65 due to lung cancer is seen in France (and Belgium). Finally, France is among a group of countries where the suicide rate is higher than elsewhere.

Main health-related issues in people of between 45 and 74 years of age

The period between 45 and 74 years of age is the time when morbidity first becomes important as risk factors (obesity and high blood pressure) accumulate and commonplace ailments (eye and teeth problems, varicose veins, sleeping disorders, etc.) begin to appear together with, in some cases, more serious diseases. Risk factors, especially for cardiovascular disease, figure prominently in declared morbidity and among the reasons for consultations with independent practitioners. In a certain fraction of cases, these lead to disease with a resultant effect on hospital activity. This is illustrated by the disproportionate number of all LTC recognitions (55%) involving patients in this bracket (which amounts to just 32% of the overall population).

The two major groups of chronic pathology which will become predominant towards the end of life really begin to appear between the ages of 45 and 74, namely cancer and cardiovascular disease. Cardiovascular disease is more frequent and leads to the consumption of more health care resources, but cancer kills more people.

Death, from being a rare event, often due to some external cause (*e.g.* an accident), becomes far more familiar in this intermediate age group. Mortality rates increase precipitately, more or less doubling every ten years. One person in 100 dies at around 60. Many of these early deaths (which are more common in men) are due to long-standing behavioural patterns or environmental factors (*e.g.* smoking, drinking, occupational exposure, etc.).

More than 60% of malignancies appear between 45 and 74 years of age

Of the 240,000 new cases of cancer per annum (according to figures from the Francim network), 150,000, *i.e.* over 60%, affect people of between 45 and 74 years of age; of these, 90,000 are in men and 60,000 in women. The incidence rate in males rises sharply with seven times more cases appearing between 70 and 74 than appeared between 45 and 49; the corresponding ratio in women (in whom rates were already higher at younger ages) is only two.

The high incidence of malignancy is reflected in the hospital-based figures with 275,000 admissions of men and 173,000 admissions of women (not counting repeat sessions for chemotherapy and radiotherapy).

Lung cancer dominates the picture because of its poor prognosis (with just 7% survival after five years) and high incidence which make it the biggest killer of all the cancers in this age bracket. In 1995, there were an estimated 15,000 new cases in men, and 2,000 in women, most of whom died.

Part one Data about health status

Most cases of cancer of the upper airways and digestive tract occur in men: 15,000 new cases a year in men compared with just 1,700 in women in this age bracket. Both the incidence of these cancers and the corresponding mortality rate is dropping due to reduced drinking, although these tumours which are also associated with smoking remain a major cause of early death.

Malignant breast tumours are common in women with 23,000 new cases per annum, representing nearly 40% of all new cases of cancer in the women of this age bracket. This type of cancer becomes increasingly common from 35 up, reaching a maximum incidence at 60. Nevertheless, the low corresponding mortality (6,100 in 1997) is evidence of its relatively fair prognosis in the short term although this form of cancer remains the main cause of female death in this age bracket.

Between 45 and 74 years of age, colorectal cancer develops in 20,000 people per annum (according to the 1995 figures), 12,000 men and 8,000 women.

Two other forms of cancer are relatively common: prostate cancer in men, the prevalence of which becomes very high in the elderly but which nevertheless affects a significant number of men from the age of 55 on (with 14,500 new cases per annum appearing in the 45-74 age bracket); and cancer of cervix and uterus in women (with 5,000 new cases per annum).

Cancer incidence and mortality figures point up the importance of primary prevention and screening strategies.

Primary prevention of risk factors constitutes the first priority area for action.

Smoking is the main cause of avoidable death, as is tragically highlighted by the increasing incidence of lung cancer and mortality from this disease among women in recent years.

Similarly, although alcohol consumption has been regularly dropping over recent decades with corresponding decreases in related mortality, it remains significantly higher than in many economically comparable countries. The need for action to limit alcohol abuse is also occasioned by the role drink is known to play in accidents and acts of violence.

The arrival of middle age together with the appearance of the first symptoms of ageing is often an ideal moment for behavioural changes. The benefit of quitting smoking at any age is well characterised although of course, the earlier this step is taken, the better (with never beginning in the first place being the ideal strategy).

Nutrition is also a key factor which is now known to play a central role in the occurrence of many diseases. People need to be encouraged to eat a healthy diet (*e.g.* one containing plenty of fruit and vegetables) by appropriate, sustained educational measures, and possibly by improvement of the supply side. This is the objective and job of the National Health and Nutrition Programme.

Occupational exposure constitutes another area in which preventive policies need to be consolidated. For example, asbestos is not only the main risk factor of mesothelioma, but it is also involved in certain forms of lung cancer.

The second major area for action in the matter of cancer prevention is in screening. For certain forms of cancer (notably breast, cancer of cervix and uterus), how to conduct useful mass screening programmes is now well understood and it remains only to summon the will, mobilise the resources and establish the appropriate monitoring modalities to ensure efficient diagnosis of these treatable conditions. In addition studies and assessments should be commissioned so that rapid progress can be made on other forms of cancer for which an ideal screening protocol has not yet been definitively identified (notably colorectal and prostate cancer).

OCCUPATIONAL HAZARDS: FACTORS WHICH REMAIN SIGNIFICANTLY UNDER-ESTIMATED

The international scientific literature demonstrates that occupational factors are a very significant determinant of public health. Notably, it is clear that approximately one-third of the socially-based differential in the number of deaths due to cancer in industrialized countries is due to occupational exposure to carcinogens, and that this fraction rises to about 50% in the cases of lung and bladder cancer. Apart from cancer (which has been extensively researched), many other health problems have a largely or partially occupational etiology, *e.g.* muscle and joint problems (at least 30% of adult males experience back pain, mostly work-related, and in recent years, in all the countries which record the relevant data, it is obvious that there has been a genuine epidemic of periarticular disorders), impaired hearing, sterility, non-malignant respiratory disease, dermatological conditions, neuro-psychiatric disorders, cardiovascular disease, etc. Above and beyond exposure to toxic physico-chemical and biological agents, work-related psycho-social factors also have major effects, not only on psychological well-being but also on somatic health.

The French system for compensating workers for occupational diseases is based on "Tables" which stipulate criteria for the recognition of various diseases and hazardous forms of exposure. This system is controversial in that it results in a global under-estimation of the true incidence of occupational disease, and because the likelihood that an occupational disease will be recognised as such varies enormously between different parts of the country. This under-estimation probably affects all occupational diseases for which there exists a table providing for their treatment and is usually difficult to quantify. But the partial data available in the field of cancer and musculo-skeletal disorders give a measure of the magnitude of this problem.

About 500 cases of cancer were recognised as occupational in etiology in France in 1999 whereas projections based on the international scientific literature would put the true figure at several thousand. The example of cancer due to exposure to asbestos-which is actually a particularly well recognised occupational exposure factor-is striking: in 1998, 413 cases of cancer were officially attributed to occupational exposure to asbestos whereas a "low" 1996 estimate attributed about 1,950 deaths to asbestos in that year.

A similar situation is observed with periarticular disorders, particularly carpal tunnel syndrome, for which disease an occupational etiology is well established. A recent study conducted in Montreal – the results of which are readily extrapolated to France – showed that carpal tunnel syndrome had been induced by work in a large fraction of manual workers presenting for surgery to correct the problem (76% of the men and 55% of the women). However, in France, despite 130,000 annual interventions being performed for this indication alone, only about 2,000 cases of any type of periarticular disorder are recognised as occupational in origin. Even if only a fraction of these interventions were performed in manual workers, it is clear that the occupational etiology of this disease is being seriously under-estimated. And this is true of a disease for which – unlike cancer – the symptoms appear soon after exposure, usually while the person is still working and therefore still being monitored by the occupational health system.

One consequence of the under-estimation of the causality of occupational factors is that inadequate attention is paid to prevention in the workplace. The French system of compensating occupational disease was designed as a financial sanction for businesses to oblige them to take adequate preventive precautions and improve working conditions. The major under-estimation of the importance of the problem in general is highly prejudicial to the efforts made in the fields of information and prevention, both of which are key when it comes to cutting down the incidence of avoidable, occupational diseases.

Moreover, in the absence of any reliable, specific domestic data, we are obliged to estimate the incidence of such problems on the basis of international statistics in the literature. The first disadvantage of this situation is that it leads to generally invalid estimates because the fraction of the incidence of any disease due to occupational exposure is highly dependent on the specific characteristics of the exposed population. But most important of all, it leads to under-estimation of the incidence of occupational disease, a problem which always appears more serious when it is measured on the basis of domestic figures compiled in a co-operative initiative on the part of a large number of different collaborators, rather than on the basis of foreign data, the dissemination of which is limited to a few specialists in the field.

Marcel Goldberg, Inserm U88

References: [15, 18, 22, 24, 38].

Cardiovascular disease represents a gamut of seriousness, from everyday ailments through risk factors (which are now often manageable) to life-threatening crises

Similarly to cancer, 3 in 10 women and 1 in 10 men suffer from varicose veins or circulatory problems affecting the lower limbs, problems which sometimes cause severe pain and account for 10% of the reasons for consultation with a physician.

High blood pressure – which is at once a risk factor and a disease in its own right – is declared by one-quarter of all people of both sexes and requires attentive management by an independent practitioner (accounting for 1 consultation in 5). The same is true for problems with lipid metabolism, another risk factor for cardiovascular disease which is declared by 1 person in 6 and mentioned in 1 in 10 consultations with an independent practitioner.

Although risk factor management by independent physicians is not always perfect (as shown in recent Cnamts work on high blood pressure), such care is probably one of the main factors underlying the recent rapid decrease in cardiovascular mortality rates, specifically mortality due to ischaemic heart disease, strokes, arrhythmia and conduction problems. Nevertheless, ischaemic heart disease still represents the leading reason for the admission of men into hospital and the second cause of death in men of between 45 and 74 years of age; in women it is the third most important cause of death.

Cardiovascular disease – mainly ischaemic problems – is also the most common reason for early retirement due to ill health in men of between 50 and 60 (accounting for 23% of all pensions granted to men of this age group in 1998).

Two other major risk factors for cardiovascular disease, diabetes and obesity, are also particularly common in this age bracket. Diabetes is declared by 6% of people, constitutes a common reason for consultation, and accounted for 414 LTC admissions per 100,000 people covered in 1998. According to the ObEpi survey conducted in the year 2000, nearly 14% of men and 12% of women of between 45 and 64 were obese.

Again like cancer, preventing cardiovascular disease involves a dual approach: combating behavioural risk factors such as smoking, inadequate physical activity and poor eating habits; and improving the screening for and management of risk factors.

Part one Data about health status

CARDIO-VASCULAR MORTALITY IN FRANCE

The reduction in the death rate due to cardiovascular disease in France since 1970 is all the more spectacular given that it has occurred in a southern European country where, despite differences between regions, cardiovascular mortality is far lower than in Finland or Scotland, or in the United States. It is not known to what extent differences between different countries are genetically determined or environmental in origin, and nor is it known whether the decrease in cardiovascular mortality in Europe and the United States is due to a decrease in the incidence of new cases or improved care. This has been a controversial topic ever since the first evidence of the regression of the "epidemic" was observed in the United States in the 1960's. Various interpretations have been proposed, particularly in the context of the results of the Monica study. However, for the time being, the most pragmatic approach to this multifactorial form of disease would seem to be a systematically holistic one.

The two central tenets of public health policy are to reduce the extent to which the population as a whole is exposed to cardiovascular risk factors, and to enhance how those who are at risk or are already ill are being managed. In this way, it is hoped to reduce cardiovascular mortality in France by a factor of 20% every ten years. Between 45 and 75 years of age it is vital to avoid the trap of seeking, on the one hand to concentrate exclusively on screening for cardiovascular risk factors and treating them with drugs, and on the other hand massively increasing radiological, surgical and pharmaceutical treatment beyond the age of 75. This traditional interventionist approach favoured by the medical community – which is very profitable for the health care industry – is immediately appealing to the man in the street but it is fraught with danger at the individual level and entails huge cost at the national level. Thus, what is the benefit to risk ratio of intensive treatment to lower cholesterol if this strategy puts the patient at risk for cancer or depression (neither of which is a stated possible adverse reaction at this point in time)? Or if aggressive anti-hypertensive treatment is compromising quality of life? Although the results of randomised clinical trials have pointed to significant benefit, both from drugs (lipid-lowering, anti-hypertensive and anti-platelet drugs) and surgical modalities (*e.g.* coronary stenting and carotid surgery in the elderly), the spread of these therapeutic modalities entails a major iatrogenic risk, a risk which is all the more unacceptable if the true benefit is limited. In order to maximise benefit-to-risk and benefit-to-cost ratios on the care provision side of public cardiovascular health policy, professional health care providers now need to consider a more holistic approach based on across-the-board improvement.

This means improving the accuracy and reliability of blood pressure measurement and medical testing, and instigating regular physical examinations and tests to orient the care strategy. It also means improving monitoring over the months and years following any kind of procedure in order to reduce associated mortality and morbidity.

The question of behaviour is at least as important as that of which medical procedure is the most suitable. This includes modifying eating habits, increasing the level of physical activity, reducing alcohol consumption and convincing people to quit smoking, which in turn means formulating positive incitements – for the various different age groups – to promote healthy behaviour patterns. Encouraging behaviour to prevent cardiovascular disease at the level of the family from pregnancy onwards will necessitate not only a wide range of different paramedical care providers (midwives, dieticians, etc.) but other professionals, *e.g.* school meal planners, teachers of children and students of all ages and all types (*e.g.* both academic and vocational), the food processing industry, advertisers, sports organisers, etc. The benefits to be obtained by reducing the dietary intake of salt, calories and unsaturated fat are scientifically demonstrated so all efforts should now be directed towards implementing appropriate measures at all ages, in all cultures, everywhere, and matched to all social circumstances.

Therefore, the first priority of cardiovascular health policy should be aimed at those at risk and those already sick, *i.e.* improving screening and the management of disease and risk factors. Measures should focus on quality with a view to cutting down adverse reactions and cost. This alone could furnish the 20% decline in the death rate from cardiovascular disease at all ages targeted for the next ten years. The second objective – if it is effectively applied and if the French people goes along with it wholeheartedly – could result in the almost total abolition of death from cardiovascular disease before 75 years of age by the year 2050. The minimum is to avoid a recrudescence of cardiovascular mortality around the year 2020 when factors like smoking amongst the young, lack of exercise, and excess weight (as a result of over-eating or compulsive eating) will compound one another resulting in an increased incidence of metabolic disease which might last several decades.

With the objectives and methods thus set at the beginning of the 21st Century, future successes can be expected which will make failure-which is possible in certain areas-seem only the more unacceptable.

Joël Ménard, UFR Broussais-Hôtel-Dieu, Paris

Mental disease, an underestimated problem in this age bracket

In children, and to an even greater extent adolescents and young adults, the good physical health of the vast majority means that the spotlight tends to be focused on psychological problems. And in the elderly, the high level of dementia and cognitive deficiency is increasingly recognised these days. However, in the 45-74 age bracket, the widespread emergence of physical problems of variable severity can lead to psychological and psychiatric problems and diseases being relegated into the background.

Nonetheless, this period of life is characterised by a number of destabilising changes, such as retirement, the departure of children from the family home, and menopause for women. All these factors can help to induce or exacerbate psychological disturbance.

Thus, in this age bracket, there are 5,000 successful suicide attempts per annum, 3,500 of which are by men. This is a significant fraction of the total of 11,000 across all ages. And the number of unsuccessful suicide attempts which finish in some form of contact with the care system is estimated at 40,000.

The findings of the HID survey suggest that 4% of people suffer from some form of mood disorder or depression, and that 5% are afflicted with some other mental problem. Mental problems are also at the root of massive care consumption with depression and neurotic symptoms among the ten leading reasons for consultation with a physician.

In 1998, 13,000 men and 19,000 women were recognised as suffering from some psychiatric long-term condition, either depression, personality disorders, dementia or psychosis. Among women of between 50 and 60 (and all other age groups, in fact), psychiatric problems represent the leading reason for the granting of disability leave by the national health insurance system. In men in this age range, such problems rank in third place (accounting for 16% of admissions) after cardiovascular disease (discussed above) and joint and bone conditions.

Therefore, in this age bracket, mental disease represents an important public health issue which requires redoubled effort to improve prevention, diagnosis (particularly the identification of the various problems and the helping of subjects with suicidal tendencies) and care.

MENTAL HEALTH: REALITIES AND ISSUES

When trying to evaluate psychiatric morbidity, one is immediately confronted – to a greater extent than in other fields of health – with questions of definition. Apart from schizophrenia and perhaps dementia, there is a lack of consensus – in both France and in the world in general – concerning the major groups of psychiatric disorder, including among others mood problems, anxiety, personality disorders and addiction [35].

Even when epidemiological surveys are conducted using standardised instruments, all data on general populations show that cultural determinants, specific to the concerned society, are vital in the definition of what exactly constitutes pathological; this applies to affect (*e.g.* sadness), behaviour (*e.g.* isolation) and symptoms (*e.g.* compulsive disorder), although understanding the importance and significance of all these entirely depends on establishing where the frontier lies between the normal and the pathological. In France, ideas of mental health and mental distress going well beyond the confines of the field of psychiatry are gaining ground [37]. This is leading to the focus being placed on social and behavioural phenomena which are associated with psychological status.

Nevertheless, the major broad groups of mental problem can be listed:
– Depression, the lifetime prevalence of which is between 17% and 20% for the entire population, and the simple prevalence around 5%. Because patients suffering from this type of problem rarely see themselves as sick, depression is rarely the explicit reason for seeking

medical help. As a result, it is under-diagnosed and insufficiently managed [36]. Progress in both of these areas must be considered as a priority.
- Suicide, the rate of which in France is above that in comparable Western countries. Since health care system deficiency is not at issue in this area, most of this excess mortality can be ascribed to cultural and social factors, to which primary prevention is most relevant.
- Addiction which, for this age group, mainly corresponds to alcoholism. Heavy drinking is a somatic risk factor but it is also a major co-morbidity factor in various psychiatric disorders (including depression and anxiety) as well as in high-risk behaviour and the actual act of suicide. Although alcoholism has decreased in recent years, it still constitutes a major social problem which cannot be ignored.
- Chronic psychosis which affects about 2% of the population. This type of disease entails major social problems and serious loss of quality of life for the patients and their families. Although most cases of chronic psychosis are diagnosed in France, therapy and psycho-social rehabilitation are under-developed, and the segregation of the social services and the health care system means that patients' daily needs are often poorly provided for. Social support for these patients should be divorced from the logistics of the health care system [43].
- Personality disorders and anxiety: there is little consensus on either the epidemiology or the best way to treat these problems, but fuller consideration is urgent.
All these psychiatric problems entail – for patients, their families and society – serious consequences, both economic and social. Therefore, managing them better represents a priority, despite the fact that access to this type of care is associated with certain specific problems:
- Recognising that a problem exists, both on the part of the patient and the professional. Better popular understanding of mental disease would lead to improved realisation of the need for treatment in victims.
- Social representations [16] are still heavy with received ideas, fearful projections, and misconceptions based on abnormality and incurability. A resolute effort to combat the stigmatisation of psychiatric disease is indicated.
- Without specific action, the number of practising psychiatrists is going to decrease over the coming years [28]. Therefore, it will be necessary to establish a network system in which specialists can operate in the context of the primary care system, although this is not guaranteed to resolve the entire problem.

Denis Leguay, Mental Health Centre, Angers

References: [16, 43].

Menopause presents a serious health problem for women in this age bracket, both with respect to the symptoms with which it is associated and the osteoporosis that it induces

Women undergo menopause at the age of about 50 and commonly experience various kinds of functional symptoms (including hot flushes, depression, insomnia, asthenia, reduced libido, weight changes, etc.) which can have a significantly deleterious impact on the quality of their life. Menopause is also accompanied by an increased cardiovascular risk and reduced bone mass, the latter possibly leading to spontaneous or easy fracturing of certain bones.

One woman in five of between 45 and 74 years of age declares problems associated with menopause. Apart from the actual symptoms experienced and a degree of heightened awareness as a result of high-profile publicity campaigns concerning this subject, this high frequency may be partly due to the fact that medical treatment modalities are available for the management of both the symptoms and the risk of osteoporosis, notably hormone replacement therapy. Menopausal problems are the reason for 1 consultation in 13 with an independent physician among women in this age bracket.

However, the management of osteoporosis is far from perfect, as shown by the high number of women of between 45 and 74 admitted into hospital each year for the treatment of fractures (36,000 fractures of the upper limb, 11,000 fractures of the neck of the femur, and 20,000 other fractures of the lower limb) although, of course, not all fractures are associated with osteoporosis. Guidelines on strategies for the prevention of osteoporosis and its consequences were formulated in 1996 by a group of experts working under the auspices of Inserm. Apart from certain recommendations concerning research, these guidelines make suggestions on measures to be implemented in early decades of life (making sure that calcium and vitamin D intake is sufficient) as well as during menopause (actively compensate for oestrogen deficiency, possibly by undertaking hormone replacement therapy) and after the age of 60 (regular screening, and large-scale curative and prophylactic treatment).

Commonplace problems can become seriously incapacitating but may be treatable

The vast majority of people of between 45 and 74 declare conditions which can be broadly qualified as "commonplace problems". These are mainly mild forms of sensory organ impairment, dental problems, disorders involving the venous system, joint and bone conditions, back pain and osteoarthritis, or symptoms like sleeping disorders.

Neither the data on declared diseases nor those on reasons for consultation with physicians give any indication of the degree of inconvenience entailed by these various problems although back problems in particular can cause enormous pain: it is extremely widespread with one third of all women in this age group and one-quarter of the men declaring, and it is also a common reason

People of between 45 and 74 years of age

for sick leave. For example, at EDF-GDF (the French national gas and electricity utility) where a record is kept of reasons for sick leave, 5% of employees aged between 45 and 54 took time off work at least once for this reason in the course of the year 2000. Joint and bone problems – mainly conditions affecting the spine and peripheral joint involvement – give rise to a significant fraction of all early retirements (with a pension paid by the National Health Insurance System) for disability among both men (21%) and women (23%).

These diseases cannot be considered as serious in the sense that they are in no way life-threatening but they can cause significant disability, and some respond to surgery, thereby enhancing the patient's quality of life. Taking eye problems as an example: apart from routine errors of refraction (which can be corrected using spectacles or contact lenses), nearly 180,000 cataract operations are performed each year. And to treat osteoarthritis – declared by 1 woman in 5 and by 1 man in 10 – 40,000 first-time total hip replacement procedures and 18,000 first-time total knee replacement procedures were performed in 1998, mostly on patients of over 65 years of age. In the context of common operations, mention could also be made of surgery performed to correct carpal tunnel syndrome.

Those of 75 and over

The demographic importance of the sub-population of 75 years of age and over is rising fast, both in absolute numbers and in terms of the fraction of the entire population it represents. Between 1990 and 1999, the number in this group rose from 4 to 4.5 million, an increase of 10%, and, as a percentage of the population as a whole, this group has gone from 7.1% in 1990 to 7.7% (the most recent figure). This has been accompanied by a general ageing within this population: the number of people of over 85 years of age in France rose from 740,000 in 1982 to 1.4 million in 1999.

These trends are common to all developed countries and are going to continue through the coming decades. According to Insee demographic projections, by 2020, the number of people of 75 and over in France will have reached 6 million, representing 9.6% of the population as a whole. The number of people of over 85 years of age is going to drop off up until 2005 (because of the low birth rate between 1915 and 1919), after which it will start to rise, reaching 2.1 million by 2020.

These changes mainly result from a significant decrease in overall mortality at advanced age. In 2000, a 75-year-old man could expect to live for an average of another ten years (compared with eight years in 1970), and a woman thirteen years (compared with ten years in 1970). The sustained differential between male and female life expectancy is why women predominate in older age groups, accounting for two-thirds of all those of over 75, and three-quarters of all those above 85.

As well as being longer, the lives of the elderly have changed in many other ways in the last few decades as a result of various factors. Among these, economic factors are very important, with advanced age no longer going hand in hand with poverty, as was often the case in previous generations. The average standard of living of retired people is now equivalent to that of those in work, and the number living in poverty has fallen five-fold since 1970. In parallel, their state of health has improved, as measured by the parameter of disability-free life expectancy (historical figures for which are available for the 1980's and 1991) with today's 65-year-old men and women being able to expect to live significantly longer without any kind of major disability than their parents.

Most old people (90% of those of over 75) still live in their own home although, unsurprisingly, the rate of institutionalisation is higher among the very old (15% of those of over 80 were living in a retirement home or a long-term care unit in 1999, compared with 14.3% in 1990).

This picture probably goes a long way to explaining why subjective impressions of health have been rising amongst the elderly over the last few decades. According to the results of the regular Credoc survey of people living in their own homes, the percentage of people that judged their own state of health as relatively good for their age rose between 1980 and 1998. This trend was observed at all ages although the increase was far more marked among those of over 60, rising from 76 to 89% in the 60-69 age bracket, and from 78 to 85% among those of 70 and over.

Declared morbidity

Declared morbidity figures from the SPS survey only deal with people still living at home, excluding those in institutions (whose average state of heath is poorer) who represent 10% of this entire age bracket, and 15% of those of over 80.

The frequency of most diseases increases with age, so it is not surprising that most elderly people declare multiple pathological states. The mean number of declared problems per person rises from three in the general population to over seven after the age of 75.

Sensory impairment, mainly ocular and auditory, is particularly common in the elderly. As in all the other age brackets, most of the ophthalmologic problems are errors of refraction (presbyopia, myopia or hyperopia) which affect 70% of this sub-population. Most of these problems are corrected and 80% of elderly subjects declare that they use spectacles. Cataract is another common problem and, in contrast to errors of refraction, this is more specific to this age group affecting 25% of the men and 32% of the women. It is impossible to stipulate whether these figures apply to surgically corrected or un-operated cataract on the basis of the data from this survey. Some degree of auditory impairment is indicated by 31% in this sub-population although only 8% declare using a hearing aid.

The accumulation of problems associated with the mouth and the teeth is illustrated by the high numbers in this age group carrying dental prostheses, either fixed (crowns or bridges) or removable (prosthesis): two-thirds of this population declare at least one dental prosthesis. Caries, be they treated or not, are also widespread with a declared prevalence of over 30%.

Cardiovascular disease is a major issue with nearly three-quarters of elderly subjects declaring some form of cardiovascular involvement. The most common condition is high blood pressure (44%). Vein problems involving the lower limbs are commonly declared by women (31%) but by far fewer men (14%). Problems with lipid metabolism – which represent an important risk factor for cardiovascular disease – are declared by 16% of men and 19% of women.

More than half of this age group declare bone and joint problems, although they are more common amongst women (63% *versus* 43%). Most common are osteoarthritis and back problems.

Prostate disease is widespread in men with 19% of men of over 75 years of age declaring having undergone surgery and 13% declaring prostatic hyperplasia.

The rate of declaration of insomnia rises steadily with age to a level of 17% after the age of 75. As in all other age brackets, this problem affects more women (21% *versus* 12%). These figures could be compared with those for depression which affects 10% of women of over 75.

Figure 16 **Main declared conditions among men and women of 75 and over. 1998**
(in percentage suffering from at least one disease or health problem)

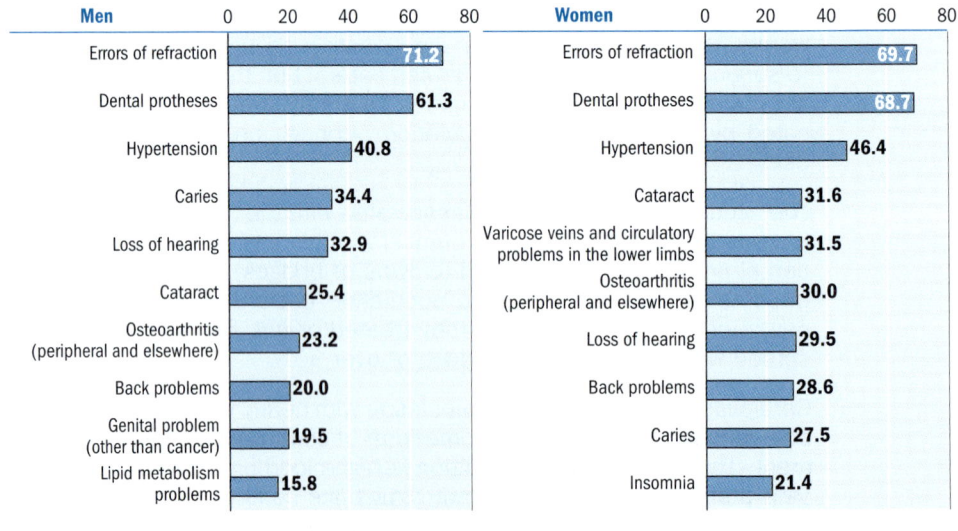

Source: SPS Survey-Credes.

Reasons for consulting an independent physician

The regularity with which elderly people consult independent physicians has sharply risen in the last few decades so that now, this group – whose previous level of care consumption was clearly lower than what it ought to be if the only factors involved were age and state of health – has now caught up with the others. General Practitioners are central care providers for this population with the number of consultations per patient per annum equal to 8 for those of between 70 and 79, and 10 for those of 80 and over (according to the 1991-1992 Ten-yearly Health Survey).

By far the most common reason for consultation is circulatory problems which account for more than 50% of visits by both men and women in this group, an even greater proportion than in the 45-74 bracket.

The most common cardiovascular problem in both sexes is high blood pressure (30% of consultations) followed by ischaemic heart disease, arrhythmia, heart failure and cerebrovascular problems. In addition, arteritis is a fairly common problem among men, and circulatory problems involving the lower limbs among women. As in the 45-74 age bracket, the fraction of consultations for cardio-vascular disease has dropped off somewhat since 1992 (from 55 to 52%), mainly because of decreases associated with ischaemic heart disease and cerebrovascular problems.

Endocrine and metabolic diseases account for 14% of independent consultations in both men and women of this age group, notably diabetes (5%) and lipid metabolism disorders (6%), mainly hypercholesterolaemia and combined hyperlipidemia.

Bone and joint problems incite more consultations by women (22% *versus* 14%), and, overall, the number of consultations for this type of problem has risen since 1992. For both sexes, osteoarthritis is the most common reason, followed by back problems.

Genito-urinary infections are more common in men because of the high incidence of prostatic hyperplasia which underlies fully 7% of consultations (up from 5% in 1992).

The proportion of consultations for mental problems is significantly greater for women (14% of all consultations) than for men (8%), although the reasons are similar in both sexes, mainly depression and neurotic problems.

Finally, symptoms which are not clearly associated with any specific pathology (*e.g.* dizziness, sleeping disorders, constipation, tiredness, malaise, etc.) are a particularly common reason for consultation with an independent practitioner among old people, accounting for 20% of all visits by both sexes, a figure which seems to be on the increase.

Part one   Data about health status

Figure 17   **Main reasons for consultation with an independent practitioner among men and women of 75 and over. 1992. 1998**
(percentage of consultations)

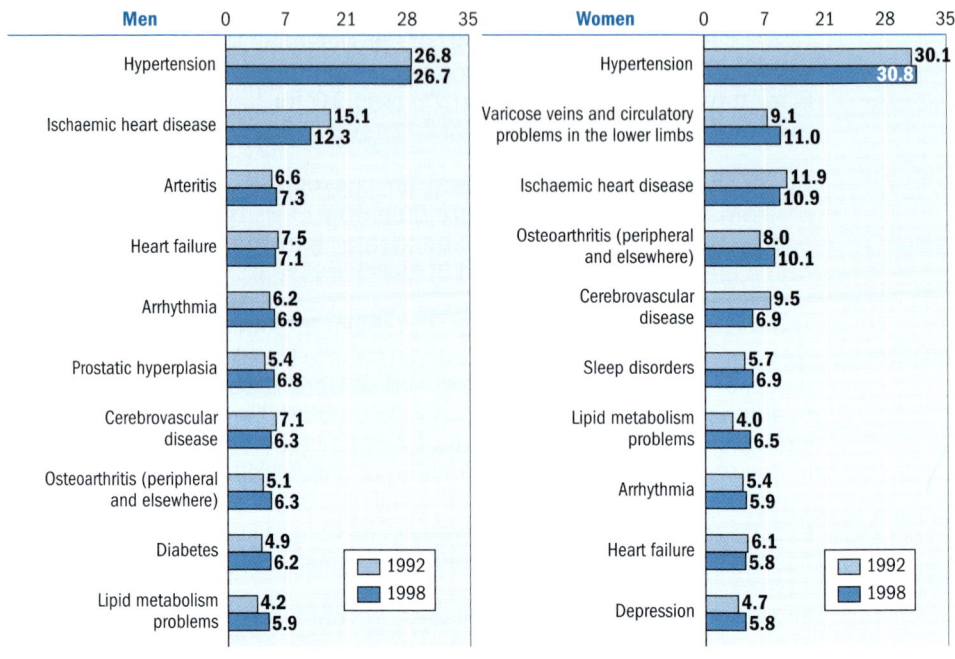

Source: Credes. Data: EPPM Survey 1992-1998. IMS-Health.

Reasons for admission into hospital-based medicine and surgery services

Hospital admission is a regular event in the population of people of over 75 years of age: just counting short stays and discounting psychiatric establishments, there are 682 admissions per 1,000 men in this group, and 520 admissions per 1,000 women per annum. This corresponds to a total of 2.3 million admissions, i.e. 16% of the total of 14.7 million annual admissions into both public and private sector units providing short-term care.

As it is for consultations with independent practitioners, circulatory system disease is the leading reason for admission into hospital in this age bracket, accounting for almost 1 stay in 5. Heart failure, ischaemic heart disease, arrhythmia and cerebrovascular diseases are the main specific complaints, for each of which, the admission rate for men is 1.5 to 2 times higher than that for women.

Four other groups of diseases follow, each responsible for about 10% of all admissions. These are diseases of the eye or its appendages, tumours, gastrointestinal disease, and physical injuries and poisoning. In men specifically, respiratory disease accounts for approximately another 10% of all admissions.

The high frequency of ophthalmologic problems is due to the high number of admissions for cataract (9% of all admissions in this age group, 20% of which are in an outpatient context), a condition in which the lens of the eye becomes opaque but which can easily be corrected by surgery. The procedure can be scheduled well in advance and outcomes are now extremely good, explaining the three-fold growth in the number of admissions for this indication between 1986 and 1998.

Tumours constitute the main pathology in 13% of stays by men and 8% by women. Locations are diverse with prostate cancer being particularly common in men, and colorectal tumours (either benign or malignant) relatively common in both men and women.

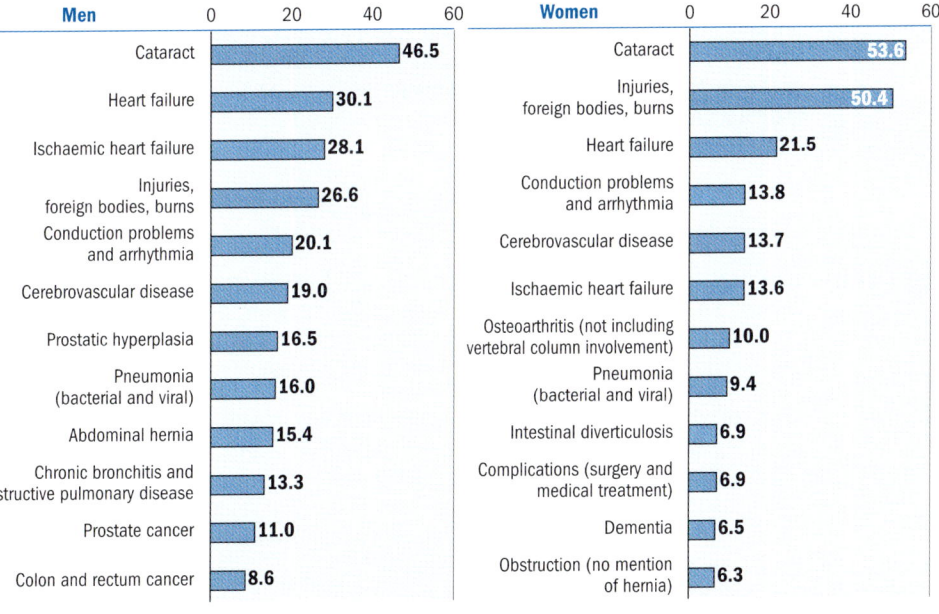

Figure 18 **Main diseases of men and women of 75 years and over treated in short-stay hospital departments. 1998**
(per 1,000 inhabitants)

Source: PMSI. Ministry of Employment and Solidarity. Drees.

Part one Data about health status

The conditions involving the digestive tract which necessitate the highest number of admissions of old people into hospital are hernias (inguinal hernias account for about 2% of all men's stays), intestinal diverticulosis (both with and without complications), and intestinal obstruction.

Most admissions for trauma are associated with falls, and in this group – in contrast to the picture in the other age brackets – the vast majority of such admissions (80%) are of women. The most common fracture is of the neck of the femur in both sexes, although this injury is 2.5 times more common in women. Next are fractures of the upper limb in women, and head injuries in men.

The admission rate for fractures of both the femur and the upper limb has not significantly changed in recent years.

Bacterial and viral pneumonia underlie 2% of admissions, with a slightly higher frequency in men (bringing this reason close in importance to chronic bronchitis and other obstructive pulmonary diseases).

Osteoarthritis (mainly involving the hip or the knee) accounts for 10% of admissions of women.

The admission rate for prostatic hyperplasia (half of which included transurethral prostatectomy) fell by 20% between 1986 and 1998.

Finally, although dementia is an extremely common problem in this age bracket, it does not lead to many admissions into medicine or surgery services in hospitals (7 per 1,000 women, and 6 per 1,000 men) since it is usually managed in psychiatric units, long-term care facilities, or at home.

Long-term conditions

In the 80% of this sub-population covered by National Health Insurance, 163,000 were recognised as suffering from a LTC in 1998. Thus, this age group which represents only 7% of the population as a whole accounts for 23% of all such cases.

The most common category of LTC in both men and women in this age group is cardiovascular disease corresponding to 41,000 cases in women and 26,000 in men, representing about 40% of the total in both cases. The three most common forms are chronic, active arteriopathy (mainly ischaemic heart disease), heart failure and severe hypertension.

Cancer is the reason for about 43,000 LTCs recognised per annum: 22,000 men (*i.e.* 1 in 3 admissions) and 21,000 women

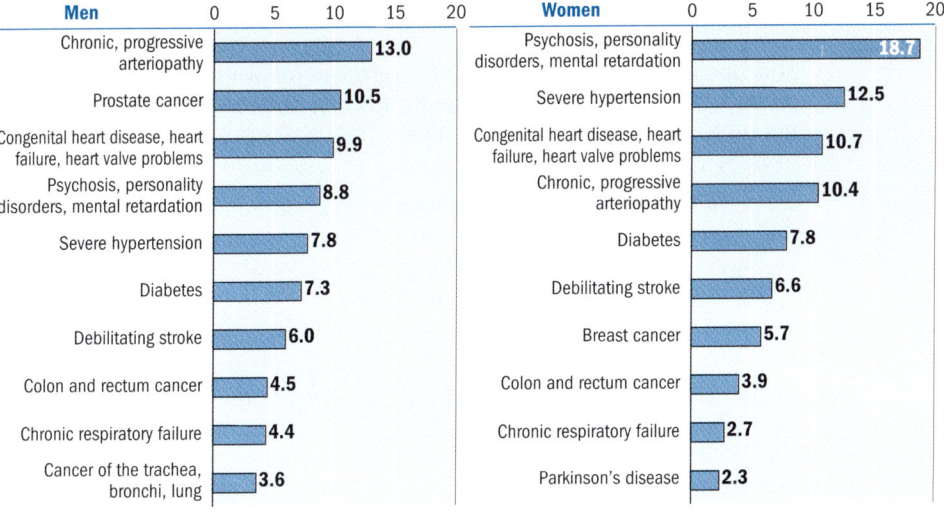

Figure 19 **Main long-term conditions in men and women of over 75 covered by the health insurance system. 1998**
(percentage of reasons for recognition)

Source: Cnamts. National Medical Service Level.

(1 in 5). The most common forms in women are breast and colorectal cancer, and the most common form in men is prostate cancer with colon, lung and bladder cancer far behind.

Mental problems – 85% cases of dementia in this age group – were recognised as a LTC in 18,000 women in 1998 (1 in 5 admissions), and nearly 6,000 men (1 in 10).

Diabetes accounted for 12,000 admissions, severe chronic respiratory failure 5,000, and incapacitating Parkinson's disease a further 4,000.

Medical causes of death

Although mortality is fairly high in young French adults, that in the elderly is much lower than in other countries of the European Union, especially in women.

Moreover, death rates are still falling rapidly. Thus, between 1990 and 1997, the death rate in people of over 75 years of age fell by about 10%, with no difference between the sexes. Decreases were seen for all major diseases but particularly spectacular drops were observed for trauma and other forms of violent death, cardiovascular disease and gastrointestinal conditions. Only deaths due to pathologies involving the nervous system and sensory organs rose (by 10% in men and 25% in women), rises largely explained by an increase in the number of deaths from Alzheimer's disease and Parkinson's disease (an increase which is at least partially due to increased recognition and diagnosis of these conditions).

The absolute number of deaths is greater for women (191,000 *versus* 132,000) but this is due to the fact that women are more numerous in this age bracket; in fact, the death rate is 50% higher in men.

As in the 45-74 age bracket, cardiovascular disease and tumours are the two main causes of death although the order is reversed in those of over 75 with cardiovascular disease accounting for more deaths (40%) than tumours (20%). Third is respiratory disease (10%) followed by trauma and poisoning (5%).

The forms of cardiovascular disease which constitute the main killers are cerebrovascular disease, ischaemic heart disease and heart failure, each accounting for about 10% of all deaths. The mortality rates associated with all these conditions dropped significantly between 1990 and 1997, resulting in a global decrease in cardiovascular mortality over this period (down by 15%). Arrhythmia and hypertension also figure among the ten most common causes of death in this age group.

The most common mortal forms of cancer are lung and prostate cancer in men, breast cancer in women, and intestinal cancer in both sexes. Mortality decreased between 1990 and 1997 for most forms, but particularly marked reductions were seen in stomach cancer (both sexes), cancer of uterus (women) and malignancies involving the upper airways and digestive tract (men). The only areas in which the death rate rose were lung cancer in women (up by 20%) and cancer of the pancreas in both sexes.

The most common mortal respiratory diseases are pneumonia, bronchopneumonia, chronic bronchitis, and obstructive pulmonary disease. Between 1990 and 1997, the number of deaths due to bronchopneumonia rose (by 10% in men and 15% in women), as did the number of women dying from chronic obstructive pulmonary disease.

Physical injury and other forms of violent death account for a far lower proportion of deaths in people of over 75 years of age than in the younger age brackets. However, this is only because of the preponderance of other causes and it is among the elderly that both the absolute number of violent deaths (16,000 in 1997) and the associated mortality rate are at their highest. Nearly one half of all these deaths are associated with falls, although the corresponding mortality rate has dropped since 1990 (down by 30%). It is also among the elderly that the suicide rate is at its highest.

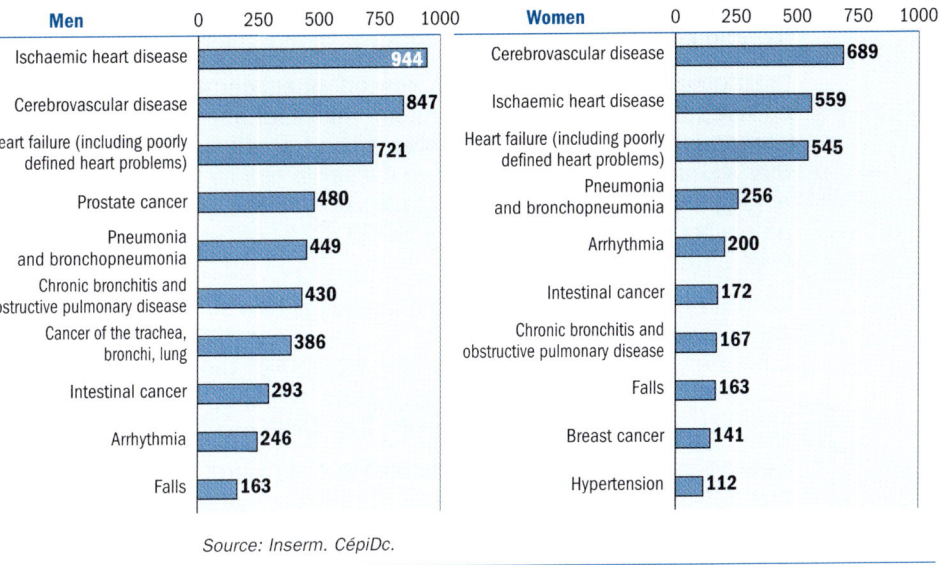

Figure 20 **Main causes of death among men and women of 75 and over. 1997**
(age-normalised rates per 100,000 inhabitants)

Source: Inserm. CépiDc.

Main health-related issues in people of 75 years of age and over

Cardiovascular disease is widespread, serious and entails massive care consumption

Cardiovascular disease is at the forefront of the health problems of people of 75 years of age and over, accounting for 44% of declared morbidity and 40% of deaths (although the latter figure should be interpreted with caution because of the difficulty often associated with defining a cause of death in the very old).

In parallel, the management of cardiovascular disease in elderly patients involves huge health care resources, these conditions being responsible for half of all consultations with independent physicians, 20% of hospital stays, and 22% of hospital days. It is therefore unsurprising that cardiovascular disease accounts for nearly 40% of LTCs in this age bracket.

More than one case of cancer in four appears after the age of 75

Cancer is a major killer of people of over 75 and is also responsible for significant care consumption, especially in the hospital context because of the expense of the relevant treatment modalities (surgery, radiotherapy and chemotherapy): cancer underlies 10% of hospital stays and 9% of days spent in the context of short term admissions. And the real figures are probably much higher given the fact that chemotherapy and radiotherapy sessions – of which there are many in a course of cancer treatment – are poorly evaluated by the information-gathering instruments used for this report. All this is consistent with the significant proportion of one in four recognised LTCs corresponding to some form of cancer.

Estimates made by the Francim network of cancer registries can be used to derive incidence figures. The resultant numbers will necessarily be minimum estimates since the registries are less than exhaustive when it comes to cancer in elderly patients but, among the total of 240,000 new cases of cancer in the population as a whole each year, at least 65,000 (27%) occur in people of over 75 years of age.

Of these, 35,000 are in women, the leading form being colorectal cancer (nearly 7,000) followed by breast cancer (5,000). In men, prostate cancer alone accounts for 12,000 of the cases, with colorectal cancer (3,000), lung cancer (2,600) and cancers involving the upper airways and digestive tract (2,200) far behind.

Despite cancer being so common in the elderly, it is often poorly managed due to a certain degree of reticence attached to the diagnosis and treatment of malignancy in old people, a pattern which is associated with a defeatist attitude on the part of both family and the medical community. Another factor is the absence of concrete data from prospective clinical trials specifically conducted to evaluate the efficacy and safety of the various therapeutic protocols in elderly patients.

Nearly one elderly person in five has some form of mental problem, mainly dementia

The figures for declared morbidity and short term hospital admissions do not give an accurate picture of the prevalence of mental problems in people of over 75 years of age, partly because of failure – conscious or unconscious – on the part of the sufferer to declare this type of problem, and partly because most of these patients are dealt with in psychiatric units or long term care establishments which are not covered in the PMSI figures used to compile this report.

Nevertheless, mental health is a major issue in the elderly, as highlighted by the results of the HID survey which estimate the prevalence of mental problems in this population at a level of 18% (*i.e.* affecting a total of about 800,000 individuals). The prevalence in people living in institutions is far higher (45%) than that in people still living at home (15%).

- Being both common and serious, dementia is far and away the most important single mental problem. The etiologies and pathophysiological mechanisms of these conditions which are organic in origin are many and various.

ALZHEIMER'S DISEASE

Alzheimer's disease was thought for a long time to represent an acute form of the normal ageing of the brain, an irreversible process which inevitably occurs towards the end of life and about which nothing can be done. However, in the course of the last decade, improved understanding of the disease has brought physicians, nurses, patients and patients' family members to realise that Alzheimer's disease is an entity like any other, serious but nevertheless one which can be mitigated by appropriate measures. Because this change in attitude only occurred very recently, and also because of the major increase in the incidence of the problem associated with the general ageing of the population, Alzheimer's disease sometimes seems like an emerging disease, and one that is emerging at a frightening rate.

Alzheimer's disease is by far the most common underlying cause of dementia, accounting for two-thirds of all such syndromes. Its clinical symptoms are progressive loss of cognitive function and memory loss, often associated with deterioration in language, attention, calculating, orientation in time and space, and higher functions such as those which govern planning, initiating and performing a series of tasks in an organised fashion. These symptoms are often accompanied by behavioural and mood problems. Cognitive degeneration has progressive impact on daily activities and independence: first affected are domestic activities (*e.g.* shopping, handling the household accounts, taking medications, driving, etc.) followed by the routine functions of daily life (washing, dressing, eating, and general mobility).

Alzheimer's disease is by far the commonest reason for profound dependence and institutionalisation of the elderly, and it is also the leading cause of death associated with the complications of either being bedridden or failure to take care of associated pathologies.

The disease can have a devastating impact on the patient's family, spouse and children especially, because of its relentless character, long-term progression and the general difficulty of behavioural problems. Apart from psychological and financial repercussions, the burden can affect the health of the intimate caregivers (among whom mortality is increased by more than 50%).

Above and beyond its frequency and the terrible disruption of the lives of patients and their families, other characteristics make Alzheimer's disease a huge public health problem.

Firstly, for simple demographic reasons, the frequency of dementia in general and Alzheimer's disease in particular is growing; if no progress is made on the prevention front, by 2010 there could be 800,000 patients with dementia, of whom 550,000 with Alzheimer's disease.

Alzheimer's disease is costly, with a mean annual per patient price (irrespective of severity) estimated at 18,294 euros in 1993 in France. This includes medical consumption, assistance by both paid and volunteer aids (accounting for 30% of the total) and institutionalisation. At the current prevalence of 430,000 cases, this comes to a total overall annual bill of 7.93 billion euros.

Alzheimer's disease is a neglected, under-treated disease. In 1990, only two out of every three cases of installed dementia had been diagnosed, and only one in three cases of nascent dementia.

Part one   Data about health status

> Although there has been progress, the therapeutic nihilism and the difficulties of treating dementia mean that early stage disease is often ignored. In many cases, the symptoms are simply tolerated by those close to the patient and medical advice is not sought until a relatively late stage. In other cases – especially among the upper classes – it remains a taboo area with the same result. Many doctors – both General Practitioners and specialists – do not consider that the limited potential benefit of centrally acting acetylcholinesterase inhibitors justifies a proactive attitude, and that, in the final analysis, ignoring the problem and providing reassurance is ultimately their best course of action. This option is no longer valid given the demonstrated efficacy of providing family caregivers with support and information, especially in the early stages of the disease. Under-treatment of dementia is not confined to France; it has been documented in Sweden, the United States and Canada.
>
> For all these reasons, Alzheimer's disease is associated with an inequal access to care: financially-based inequality linked to the inability to pay for psychological counselling, home help or nursing care; inequitable access to care because of socio-cultural factors, those that "ask the most" being those that "get the most"; and finally, inequality due to remoteness from specialised centres or to differences in the importance attached to dementia and its management by professional care providers. The Local Information and Co-ordination Centres for the Elderly (Clic, *Centres locaux d'information et de coordination pour les personnes âgées*) programme has been developed to address these problems.
>
> **Jean-François Dartigues, Inserm U330, Bordeaux**
>
> *References: [8, 10-12, 23, 41].*

Degenerative forms, notably Alzheimer's disease, are the most common.

Age-specific data on the incidence and prevalence of dementia were collected in a co-operative European study of eleven representative cohorts of people of 65 years of age and over. These figures can be used to estimate the number of people in France currently suffering from dementia at 660,000 (70% of whom are women, and two-thirds of whom are over 80), including about 430,000 patients with Alzheimer's disease.

There are an estimated 165,000 new cases of dementia arising every year, 70% in people of over 80 and more than 71.5% in women. Of these, about 110,000 are of Alzheimer's disease. The huge discrepancy between these estimates and the actual annual figures for LTC recognition for dementia (under 20,000 among those with national health insurance coverage) bears witness to the massive under-recognition of this condition (although caution is warranted when comparing figures in this way).

It should be noted that dementia and Parkinson's disease are the only causes of death among those of 75 and over for which the rate rose between 1990 and 1997.

- Suicide accounts for about 1,800 deaths per annum but, because of the high mortality for other reasons, this does not appear as one of the most important reasons for death even though it is in this sub-population that the suicide rate is at its highest (reaching 45 per 100,000, *i.e.* 3.5 times higher than in the 15-44 age bracket). As in all the other age brackets, the suicide rate is higher in men than in women (4 times higher in this sub-population).

- Depression is declared by 8% of elderly subjects still living at home, and this pathology accounts for 5% of reasons for consulting an independent practitioner. The latter, relatively low figure needs to be interpreted in the knowledge that depression is often difficult to recognise in the elderly for a number of reasons, notably physical degeneration with advancing age, complex interactions with somatic problems, depression, and even cultural prejudices which condition the opinion that sadness and withdrawal are normal in old people.

In the 1996-1997 Credes Annual Insurance Coverage and Health Survey in which depression was specifically addressed, its prevalence among women of 75 and over was estimated at 20%, and at 12% in men of the same age. The same study detected a generation effect with a significantly higher prevalence of depression among those born between 1920 and 1929, *i.e.* those who were of between 10 and 25 years of age during the Second World War.

Arthritis and fractures resulting from falls are responsible for many surgical procedures

- Globally, 27% of all those of 75 and over claim to suffer from osteoarthritis, and 25% from back problems (which are likewise often osteoarthritic in etiology). These incite respectively 9% and 3% of consultations with independent practitioners and their incidence is apparently on the rise.

In women, osteoarthritis accounts for 10% of all hospital admissions, mostly involving the hip or knee. Nearly one-half of all these 38,000 annual admissions of people in this age group are for surgery with, according to PMSI figures, a total of 10,000 total hip replacements (in the context of first-line, simple arthroplasty) and 6,800 knee replacements per annum.

This explains the relatively high proportion of elderly subjects who declare having such implants: nearly 8% with a hip replacement (360,000) and 3% with a knee replacement (140,000).

- Falls are very common events in the lives of elderly subjects.

Although only a small minority ever result in serious physical injury, falls nevertheless have a major impact on hospital admission and mortality figures: each year, 91,000 elderly subjects are admitted into hospital with a fracture of either the femur or the upper limb (the most common forms of injury), with 80% of these admissions involving some form of surgical intervention. About 7,600 deaths per annum are associated with a fall.

This death rate has dramatically decreased in recent years (a 33% drop between 1990 and 1997) although hospitalisation rates for fractures of the femur and the upper limb have remained stable.

Above and beyond any immediate physical repercussions, a fall can have significant long term impact in an elderly person, not only in terms of loss of function but also in the form of psychological consequences which are complex and difficult to identify. A bad fall can result in prolonged loss of mobility and impairment of physical capacities, and can induce in some people a profound fear of falling again which leads to a loss of self confidence. All these tend to result in the abandoning of normal, daily activities which itself can accelerate the loss of motor and cognitive function.

Despite the major resources dedicated to the management of motor deficit, fully half of all subjects of 75 years of age and over have some form of this type of problem according to the HID survey.

Sensory impairment is common and inadequately managed

Nine out of every ten elderly subjects still living at home declare an ophthalmologic problem, mainly errors of refraction (*e.g.* presbyopia) which may be age-related or may have been preexisting. The vast majority of such problems are managed with spectacles which are worn by 85% of people after the age of 75. However, certain progressive conditions can compromise visual function, cataract being the most widespread with 29% of all those of 75 or over declaring it as a personal problem. This condition responds excellently to surgery and, of the total of 400,000 annual admissions for this operation, 200,000 are of patients in the elderly bracket. The number of hospital admissions for this form of surgery tripled between 1986 and 1998, a period during which advances in surgical technique resulted in improvement of the benefit-to-risk ratio associated with the intervention, and therefore to an increase in the number of suitable candidates.

Nearly 1 elderly subject in 3 living at home claims some form of auditory impairment, the most common being simple, age-related presbycusis, a progressive, bilaterally symmetrical loss of hearing which, unlike visual problems, is often unperceived by the subject him or herself because it results in a decrease in the intelligibility of the spoken word rather than an evident reduction in volume.

VISION AND THE ELDERLY

Visual problems can occur at any age but it is at the extremes that people are most commonly affected, the very young and the old. Nowadays, although visual deficiency in children is on the decline due to progress in prevention, therapy and rehabilitation, in the elderly it is on the increase, and this is entailing some entirely novel problems. The incidence of eye disease rises with age, so in a climate of increased life expectancy, the number of old people suffering from visual deficiency is going to rise in the coming years, and moreover, those affected are going to have to learn to live with their deficiency for longer.

All the epidemiological data show that the prevalence of visual deficiency rises exponentially after the age of 50. Projections based on international data estimate the number of people in France of 75 and over who are partially sighted at just over 250,000. After the age of 85, between 10% and 15% of the population are affected, and this reaches 25% if only those living in institutions are considered.

The term visual deficiency describes not a single entity but rather a spectrum from full-blown blindness to partial sight. However, although blindness has been recognised since Antiquity, the idea of partial sightedness is far more younger and only emerged about twenty years ago. Visual deficiency may be selective for central or peripheral vision, or can involve both. It is clear then that the functional impact of visual deficiency varies enormously from one person to another. The loss of central vision can make it difficult to read, write, watch television and recognise faces (and can complicate the commission of everyday tasks). The loss of peripheral vision compromises the perception of space and movement and so makes it difficult for the subject to move around, especially in an unknown environment. The partially sighted in general tend to go outdoors at little as possible. In the elderly, the effects of losing visual function are often compounded with the consequences of other forms of impairment, notably auditory and cognitive, and they may be exacerbated by both a reduced capacity to compensate by using other senses and a generally fatalistic outlook. Although visual deficiency can be a major component in the pathway to dependence, it is often neglected by family members and professional care providers because it is so difficult to predict and understand.

Some of the causes of age-related visual deficiency cannot be avoided, but others respond to treatment:

– Cataract is progressive opacity of the lens of the eye which results in gradual loss of vision. Even before frank deficiency, this condition can significantly compromise quality of life, *e.g.* it can disallow driving which is particularly inconvenient for those living in the rural areas. The treatment is surgical ablation and outcomes are very good. Cataract is very common, affecting almost half of all people of between 75 and 85 years of age. Despite the efficacy of surgery, uncorrected cataract remains one of the leading reasons for partial sight in the industrialised world.

– Macular degeneration is the result of accumulated degenerative damage to the macula retinae and is responsible for visual deficiency in 30% of those of over 75. Its impact varies enormously from simple difficulty reading to major central vision deficit. No treatment exists which is known to be effective in the medium-term. Macular degeneration is the leading cause of blindness in industrialised countries,

Part one Data about health status

accounting for about half of all cases in the 75-84 age bracket, and more than two in three in people of over 85.
– Chronic glaucoma is a complex disease of the optic nerve which results in progressive, irreversible erosion of the field of vision. It is very disabling and causes serious disruption of everyday life. Its prevalence is between 2% and 5% among those of over 70 which makes it the third most important cause of visual deficiency in the elderly. It can be treated with both drugs and surgery, and it can be detected in the early stages by screening: being insidious and painless, medical advice is often not sought early enough so systematic screening would be the best means of preventing this problem. Improving how visual deficiency is managed in the elderly will involve measures, on the one hand to prevent avoidable deficit and, on the other hand to help those whose visual function is already seriously impaired. The first depends on screening for diseases like glaucoma and generalising the treatment of curable conditions like cataract (certain populations – particularly those living in institutions – seeming to be excluded from access to this type of treatment in which there has been such dramatic technical progress in recent years). For those with installed visual deficiency, management will involve consolidating rehabilitation resources and reinforcing support structures for the blind and the partially sighted. Rehabilitation consists of teaching subjects how to get more out of their residual visual capacities and how to compensate for lost visual function by using other senses. This involves various types of health professional and is usually offered in specialist units (either within or outside of a hospital). Despite the demonstrated efficacy of visual rehabilitation, it is prescribed in France less often than in other comparable countries for a number of reasons, including a lack of suitable, specialist units, under-awareness of the potential benefits on the part of both professionals and patients, and high cost (especially since visual rehabilitation for adults is not reimbursed by the health insurance system). Rehabilitation necessitates close co-operation from the subject and it is often not a viable option for the very old. As a result, for this last population, reorganising their living space may be the only practical measure to be taken.

Visual deficiency in the elderly represents a genuine public health problem and, because it has hitherto been underestimated, its real economic impact needs to be evaluated more thoroughly. The situation in this respect is unlikely to improve in the light of the projected reduction in ophthalmologic care provision.

Marie-Sylvie Sander and Xavier Zanlonghi, clinique Sourdille, Nantes

References: [6, 17, 25, 27, 40].

Personal relationships can suffer with the victim communicating with others less and less, resulting in social isolation which is too often accepted in a spirit of resignation.

Early screening could identify those who warrant in-depth investigation and, if necessary, treatment, either in the form of a hearing aid or rehabilitation. All this would involve significant resources, notably the attention of health care professionals during the necesary period of adaptation. The great discrepancy between the number of elderly people who complain of hearing loss (nearly 1 in 3) and the number who wear a hearing aid (8%) is convincing evidence that there is room for improvement in this area.

The frequency of auditory and visual problems coupled with the fact that they are often inadequately managed explains the high prevalence of these visual and auditory impairments which, according to the HID survey, respectively affect 22% and 38% of all those of 75 years of age and over.

Part one Data about health status

Annexe

Table 3 **Main causes of death for men and women** (1998 and 1991)

	Men 1998		Women 1998		Combined 1998		Combined 1991	
	Number	%	Number	%	Number	%	Number	%
Cardiovascular disease	76,653	28.0	89,646	34.5	166,299	31.1	175,681	33.5
Cancer	89,310	32.6	58,371	22.5	147,681	27.7	143,267	27.3
Violent death	26,388	9.6	17,720	6.8	44,108	8.3	47,206	9.0
Respiratory disease	22,031	8.0	21,283	8.2	43,314	8.1	36,015	6.9
Digestive disease	13,937	5.1	12,257	4.7	26,194	4.9	26,646	5.1
Other causes	45,880	16.7	60,527	23.3	106,407	19.9	95,897	18.3
Total	**274,199**	**100.0**	**259,804**	**100.0**	**534,003**	**100.0**	**524,712**	**100.0**

Source: Inserm. CépiDc.

Table 4 **Life expectancy at birth and at 60 years of age for men and women** (in years)

	Men	Women
Life expectancy at birth		
2000	75.2	82.7
1991	72.9	81.1
1981	70.4	78.5
Annual increase 1981-1991	0.25	0.26
Annual increase 1991-2000	0.25	0.18
Life expectancy at 60 years of age		
1998	20.0	25.1
1991	19.2	24.4
1981	17.3	22.3
Annual increase 1981-1991	0.19	0.21
Annual increase 1991-1998	0.11	0.10

Source: Insee.

PART TWO

Health inequalities and disparities in France

Composition of the Working Group

President Jacques Lebas, High Committee on Public Health

Rapporteur Gérard Salem, Space, Health and Territory Laboratory, Paris X

Co-rapporteurs Pierre Chauvin, Humanitarian Institute, Hôpital Rothschild, National Institute for Health and Medical Research U444
Annette Leclerc, National Institute for Health and Medical Research U88

Members Marianne Berthod-Wurmser, National AIDS Council, Ministry of Employment and Solidarity
Jean-François Bloch-Lainé, High Committee on Public Health
Chantal Cazes, Directorate of Research, Studies, Evaluation and Statistics, Ministry of Employment and Solidarity
Michel Grignon, Centre for Research and Documentation of the Economics of Health
Marie-Laure Kurzinger, Space, Health and Territory Laboratory, Paris X
Pierre Larcher, Social Action Directorate, Ministry of Employment and Solidarity
Andrée Mizrahi, Association for Socioeconomic Questions on Health
Arié Mizrahi, Association for Socioeconomic Questions on Health
Anne-Bénédicte de Montaigne, National Institute for Health and Medical Research U444
André Ochoa, National Federation of Regional Health Surveillance Centre
Stéphane Rican, Space, Health and Territory Laboratory, Paris X
Robert Simon, General Health Directorate, Ministry of Employment and Solidarity
Denis Zmirou, High Committee on Public Health

Co-ordination Marc Duriez, General Secretariat of the High Committee on Public Health

The Working Group wishes to thank for their contributions Pierre Bazely, Regional Division of Health and Social Affairs, French West Indies
Catherine Catteau, Regional Division of Health and Social Affairs, Réunion
Alain Grand, Toulouse University, National Institute for Health and Medical Research U558
Eric Jougla, National Institute for Health and Medical Research, CépiDc
Thierry Lang, Toulouse University, National Institute for Health and Medical Research U558
Jean-François Ravaud, Centre for Research into Medicine, Disease and Social Science, National Institute for Health and Medical Research U502
Anne Tursz, Centre for Research into Medicine, Disease and Social Science, National Institute for Health and Medical Research U502
Pierre-Jean Thumerelle, Sciences and Technology University of Lille

Introduction

Health in France is improving, as evidenced by the country's record rate of increase in life expectancy at birth. France is one the few countries in the world where the vast majority of the population has access to generally excellent, state-of-the-art health care. This has come about as a result of major government investment in a social protection system which covers virtually everyone in the country. These unarguably true facts are supported by the recent – although controversial – ranking of health care systems by the WHO [119, 121].

At the same time, the impact of the process of globalisation (of information, of commodities, of services and of people) on government policies and the lives of individuals is being felt in the field of health, as everywhere else. Today, inequality in this sphere is increasing between rich countries, emerging economies, developing countries and the poorest parts of the world, a trend which is evident from gaping differences in terms of access to effective treatment and modern health care technology. And other iniquitous forms of inequality co-exist in today's world, namely between different social groups living in the same country. The dimensions of the gap tend to depend on the degree of development of the country concerned but it is an unjust and unacceptable situation by any criteria, and one which is politically charged.

Social and geographical disparities are more marked in France than in most other European countries and, according to many health indicators, differentials are growing. Particularly worrying is the fact that among the areas in which deterioration is evident are some of those which have been earmarked for special attention and increased investment such as the health of new-born babies and, more recently, HIV infection.

A few statistics are revealing:
- life expectancy at birth varied by more than ten years between the North and South of France between 1988 and 1992;
- life expectancy at 35 years of age for a middle class man was 6.5 years greater than that of a working class man between 1982 and 1996;
- the risk of a worker becoming disabled (using a standard scale on which the average in France is 100) is 113 compared to 89 for an executive;
- between the least and the most educated women, there is a three-fold difference in the rate of premature birth (3.4% and 9.2% respectively in 1995) and a two-fold difference in the incidence of low birth weight (11.3% and 5.8%);
- at the moment of the diagnosis of full-blown AIDS, whereas only 21% of people of French nationality are unaware that they were infected with HIV, the corresponding figure for North Africans is 32%, and that for those from Sub-Saharan Africa 54%.

Thus, health is improving in France, mainly due to improved standards of living in recent years but also to some extent because some of most important killer pathologies are being managed and controlled more effectively. But against this background, the fact that many glaring instances of inequality persist or are even becoming more acute is a sign that progress is not being equitably distributed between different parts of the country and through the different social strata. This very important subject is unfortunately poorly documented in France (not as well, for example, as in other European countries), probably because hitherto there has always been an unquestioning presumption that our curative care-based system and the massive resources mobilised in its name are equitably distributed throughout a population, all of whose members have exactly the same kind of needs. Recent research [61, 102, 126] has gone some way to beginning to question this prejudice and establish a preliminary review of the real situation.

The objective of the Working Group assembled to compile this part of the report by the HCPH is not to go back over this review in an exhaustive way but rather to identify the most important issues (including areas of ignorance) by means of critical analysis and comparison with the situation in other European countries.

The first part is devoted to socially-based inequality in France with particular reference to mortality figures but also to other topics on which recent data are available, notably disability and accident rates. The second part addresses, and to a large extent draws attention to for the first time, geographical inequality, initially between regions and then at the level of larger towns and other concentrations of the population. In the third part, the limitations of present approaches are reviewed, and possible ways of improving the situation are considered, notably focusing on the kinds of concept and instrument used in other countries to investigate and mitigate inequality. Moreover, an attempt will be made to integrate data on inequality in health with data from sources on poverty and social exclusion with a view to understanding and remedying this area of injustice. Throughout these main parts, summary information on specific topics will be provided (in boxes) to illustrate the text or to expand on certain points of view. In conclusion, recommendations are presented as to possible directions that those in charge of both social and health policy could profitably adopt (including deeper integration of the two fields) with respect to all the various components of the policy-making process, namely research, the interpretation of results, and the design and implementation of concrete measures.

Above and beyond details about how to investigate and identify questions related to inequality in health, we are convinced that the issue is essentially a political one, and one which can only grow in urgency as good health becomes a fundamental part of the popular value system and comes to be seen as an inalienable right. It is also a political question because the issue of equitable health naturally goes beyond the bounds of the health care system to encroach on practically every area of public policy.

Socially-based inequality in health

Since the 1960's, accurate, integrated data have been compiled on mortality and socio-economic status in France for men of working age and, less comprehensively, for women of the same age. However, up until recently no other data were available to investigate the relationship between social status and health. Then, in 2000, Inserm published the results of a study undertaken to review the relationship between social status and state of health at different stages of life, and complementary data have become available more recently in the form of the preliminary results of the Handicap, Disability and Dependency (HID) survey which focused on health and functional impairment, and on how the disabled are managed.

In this part of the Report, the focus will be on how inequalities as evidenced by mortality figures have changed over time together with an analysis of mortality-related differences between France and other European countries. Then morbidity will be addressed with reference to three indicators, namely premature birth and low birth

Part two Health inequalities and disparities in France

weight, dental condition (children and adults), and traffic accidents. It is important to emphasise from the outset that data are not available in many areas, either because the necessary data are simply not collected or because the relevant analysis is not carried out. The examples taken here are going to illustrate how causality is difficult to determine with respect to inequalities in health, drawing attention to our failure to understand all aspects of a highly dynamic question. Thus, although income differentials (as measured in terms of both salary and standard of living [47]) remained fairly stable throughout the 1990's, various demographic and societal changes had major structural repercussions, including changing job types, the arrival of more women in the workplace, the difficulties experienced by the young when trying to find a first job, the reaching of retirement age after a long, fruitful career, the increasing number of single-parents, etc. The impact of all these types of change on health is a particularly grey area in France.

Mortality between 25 and 65 years of age

There are two sources of information about death rates in France, namely the Insee and the Inserm.

The first source of information about mortality and social status (apart from studies that could be categorised as "historical" in approach [129]) is based on a huge sample assembled by the Insee following the 1954 Census [56]. Ever since then, data on deaths between 34 and 65 years of age correlated with social status have been regularly published. Results are calculated on the basis of cohorts of the population assembled on the basis of Census data, and then by "permanent demographic sampling" which makes it possible to derive statistics for one member of the population in one hundred from one Census to the next. The second information source for this age group is the Inserm Centre for the Epidemiology of Medical Causes of Death which stipulates the deceased's social status at the time of death as well as the cause of death.

Using the Insee data, a rigorous comparison can be carried out of mortality rates between different occupations, and the Inserm data gives information on the medical cause of death. A major drawback is that the occupation recorded is that declared which gives at best a superficial idea of a person's social status, especially in the case of women.

An executive can expect to live more than six years longer than a worker

Insee data for 1982 to 1996 [113] (table 1) show that the life expectancy at 35 years of age of male managerial personnel and professionals is 6.5 years longer than that of workers: whereas two in eight 35-year-old workers will die before reaching 65, only one in ten professionals will do so. Even within the worker class, differences can be discerned with qualified workers living 1.5 year longer than unqualified ones. Neither is the group of professionals and executives uniform in this respect: the life expectancy at 35 of managers working in the private sector is 43.5 years, shorter than the 46 years of public sector managers and professionals working in an intellectual or an artistic milieu. Socially based mortality differentials would seem to be less marked among women but are nevertheless significant between the extremes of unqualified workers (45.5 years) and public sector managers and professionals working in an intellectual or an artistic milieu (51 years).

Table 1 **Life expectancy and death probability by socio-occupational class in France (Insee cohort 1982-1996)**

Socio-occupational class in 1982	Life expectancy at 35 years of age (years)		Probability of dying between 35 and 65 (%)	
	Men	Women	Men	Women
Professionals/executives	44.5	49.5	13	6.5
Farmers	43	47.5	15.5	8
Intermediate professions	42	49	17	7
Craftsmen/tradesmen	41.5	48.5	18.5	7.5
Employees	40	47.5	23	8.5
Workers	38	46	26	10.5
Difference in life expectancy between workers and executives	6.5	3.5		
Relative probability of dying: worker-executive			2	1.6

Source: Mesrine, 1999.

Less inequality amongst women?

Table 1 only shows data for working women. For a global comparison of the female and male populations, social situation can be estimated in terms of the educational level attained. Taking all European countries together [99], greater inequality is observed among men than among women according to this criterion, with France following this general pattern. Comparisons carried out for three age brackets (35-50, 50-60, and 60-75) for the period 1980-1989 show that higher educational level is associated with longer life for younger male and female subjects, but that this pattern is not seen among the older men [91]. More recent data would make it possible to determine whether this difference is simply a generational effect.

Are socially-based mortality differentials increasing?

Socially-based disparities in mortality rate have been analysed over three time periods: 1975-1980, 1982-1987 and 1990-1995 [99]. The data concern three samples of French men, all in work at the beginning of the period and classified at that time according to their occupational group (table 2).

Table 2 — Changes in mortality in men of different socio-occupational classes between 1975 and 1995
(mortality risk compared with that of executives)

	1975-1980	1982-1987	1990-1995
Farmers	1.3	1.2	1.3
Craftsmen/tradesmen	1.4	1.3	1.3
Professionals/executives	**1**	**1**	**1**
Intermediate professions	1.2	1.2	1.3
Employees	2	1.9	2.2
Skilled workers	1.9	1.8	2
Unskilled workers	2.6	2.5	2.4

Source: Mesrine [113].

Although the death rate of employees compared with that of executives rose slightly between 1975 and 1995, the differential in mortality between executives and the other groups remained fairly constant. Nevertheless, such results may mask changes in socially-based differences in mortality if the relative proportions of the different groups significantly changed in the meantime. In fact, whereas executives and professionals accounted for just 10.7% of the population in 1975, this figure had risen to 16.7% by 1990, which modifies the situation of this group relative to all the others. Moreover, for valid comparison of different periods, it would also necessary to take into account the proportion of the population which was out of work at the beginning of the observation time, a variable which can change significantly from period to period, as can this group's mortality rate. Therefore, although the Insee results show that there is still a strong correlation between mortality and social status, it is difficult to monitor changes and trends on the basis of the data available.

The Inserm data do not help with this problem. When two periods are compared – 1979-1985 and 1987-1993 [91] – the differential mortality between male workers/employees and executives/professionals appears to have grown from 2.6 to 2.9, an increase which might be due to deterioration in employees' situations. However, the fact that the Inserm data suggest a more extreme disparity than do the Insee results bears witness to the fact that trying to quantify socially-based differences in mortality rate is a methodologically difficult endeavour, and that attempting to compare such results for different time frames is fraught with even more complications. For these reasons, any such results should always be interpreted with caution.

Social differences and medical causes of death

The Inserm data make it possible to attribute medical causes of death to the excess mortality in poorer social classes [91], so it is possible to calculate how many fewer active male employees and workers would have died between the ages of 25 and 54 (per 100,000) if the rate of mortality due to such and such a cause had been the same as that of male managers and professionals.

Of the total of 366 deaths per annum, there would be 240 (65.6%) fewer, specifically:
- 85 due to cancer, including 22 due to lung cancer and 29 to cancer of the airways or upper digestive tract,
- 34 due to cardiovascular disease,
- 67 violent deaths, including 25 suicides and 20 in traffic accidents,
- 22 due to alcoholism,
- 32 due to other causes.

As indicated by these estimates, the death rates of male workers/employees were greater than those of executives/professionals for all causes of death between 1987 and 1993. However, AIDS deserves special mention: from being more common in the managerial class in the period 1979-1985, by the period 1987-1996, AIDS-related mortality had become the same in both groups [57].

A similar analysis for women yields a more complicated picture because breast cancer accounts for a significant fraction of all deaths of women of working age, and breast cancer is more common in more privileged women [83].

France and other European countries

Across Europe, the mortality rate for manual workers is higher than that for other occupational classes, and a similar pattern is seen for most causes of death [99]. However, certain national differences are obvious (table 3): in France, there is particularly marked socially-based inequality in cancer mortality, especially cancer of the upper airways or digestive tract (the degree of inequality in deaths from lung cancer is similar to that seen in neighbouring countries); moreover, the excess death rate of French manual workers from digestive tract conditions (*e.g.* cirrhosis of the liver) is far higher than the excess mortality rate elsewhere in Europe. As a general rule, social differences in mortality due to cardiovascular disease tend to be lower in Southern Europe (including France). Geographical variations are also subject themselves to temporal variation, *e.g.* employees and craftsmen have only been more likely to die of heart disease since the end of the 1960's [101].

For two of the four medical causes of death dealt with by Kunst [99], the most pronounced socially-based disparity is seen in France. This is also true if all causes of death are considered together, with a ratio between the mortality rate in manual workers

Table 3 **Relative mortality rates in manual and non-manual workers of between 45 and 59 in different European countries**

	Lung cancer	Other cancers	Cardio-vascular	Digestive
France	1.65*	1.75*	1.14	2.20*
England and Wales	1.54*	1.07	1.50*	a
Ireland	1.95*	1.17*	1.23*	1.08
Finland	2.20*	1.14*	1.47*	1.37*
Sweden	1.46*	1.11*	1.36*	1.58*
Norway	1.62*	1.15*	1.35*	1.42*
Denmark	1.51*	1.09*	1.28*	1.65*
Switzerland	1.73*	1.29*	0.96	1.62*
Italy (Turin)	1.26	1.17*	1.08	1.85*
Spain	1.38*	1.31*	0.98	1.59*
Portugal	1.07	1.15*	0.76*	1.59*

* Ratio significantly different from 1.
a. Not available.
Source: Kunst [99].

and that in non-manual classes of 1.71 (compared with 1.33 in Denmark and 1.53 in Finland) [100].

So, inequality in health status (which tends to be most pronounced among men of working age) is a long-standing problem in France, and one whose dimensions are not improving (and may even be growing). Unfortunately, no useful, comparable indicators exist for children or people of over 65 years of age, and the data for women are much less comprehensive. However, it has been demonstrated in a comparative European study (in which social status was estimated in terms of educational level) [99] that overall, socially-based inequality as evidenced by differential mortality rates is worse in France than in either Finland, Norway, Denmark or Italy, and that this is true for both men and women.

Social inequality and morbidity

Life-threatening risk factors, handicaps, disability, deficiencies

There are not many sources of statistics on social inequality and morbidity. The last ten-yearly survey of Health and Medical Treatment was conducted by the Insee and the Credes in 1991-1992 on 12,000 ordinary households (not including any institutions). The Credes Insurance Coverage and Health survey (SPS, conducted every two years since 1998) gives information on those covered by insurance schemes for general, agricultural and self-employed workers and professionals [72, 73].

The 1996 SPS survey [73] estimates state of health based on two parameters, namely life-threatening risk factors and disability. These parameters were scored by physicians for the diseases

Table 4 **Life-threatening risk factors and disability in different socio-occupational classes in France (after normalisation for age and sex), 1996**

Social class*	Number surveyed	Life-threatening risk factors	Disability
Overall		1	1
Farmers	797	0.96	1.03
Craftsmen/tradesmen	1,130	0.95	0.94
Professionals/executives	2,694	0.93	0.86
Intermediate professions	3,308	0.97	0.97
Employees	2,122	1.03	1.06
Skilled workers	4,356	1.05	1.03
Unskilled workers	1,527	1.10	1.13

* Current or last position of the head of the household.
Source: Credes, 1998 [72].

stipulated by the investigators and on the basis of an overview of the responses to a questionnaire (table 4). By setting a reference value for the population as a whole at 1.0, social inequality was observed in terms of both life-threatening risk factors (0.93 for higher management *versus* 1.10 for unqualified workers) and disability (0.86 for management *versus* 1.13 for unqualified workers).

International comparisons can be made using responses to a question about perceived health status included in the item *"Do you consider your state of health as less than good?"*[1] in several different European studies. The figure of 2.24 for France signifies (approximately) that the proportion of workers replying "Yes" to this question is double that in the male population as a whole (table 5).

Table 5 **Differential between workers and the population as a whole in different European countries with respect to the question "Do you consider your state of health as less than good?"**
(men in the country of between 25 and 69 years of age)

Country	Differential
France	2.24
Denmark	2.19
United Kingdom	2.32
Netherlands	2.4
Germany	1.63
Switzerland	2.12
Sweden	2.79

Source: Cavelaars [19].

---

1. Based on logistical models comparing male workers (both skilled and unskilled) with the male population as a whole (after age-matching) [60].

Part two Health inequalities and disparities in France

In this respect, France is in the middle in terms of inequality rather than at the extreme, as was the case for mortality. Mortality and declared morbidity deal with very different issues and are calculated in very different ways, so comparison is difficult. However, comparison of disparities in both morbidity and mortality for certain specific, diagnosed conditions [68] gives a good correlation (thereby confirming that inequality exists), most clearly in the case of chronic bronchitis. However, non-life-threatening problems like influenza are more often declared by employees and executives even though their actual risk of dying of the infection is lower than that of workers and farmers. Moreover, it is known that how health problems are formulated depends on social status, *e.g.* where the borderline is placed between problems that have a medical dimension and those that do not [44]. For this reason, it is possible that certain problems – medical in nature but not identified as such and not therefore viewed as a reason to seek medical advice – are underestimated in surveys of health status, and these problems may be exactly those which are more common in the poor.

Figure 1 **Proportion of individuals in different social classes declaring deficiency (matched for age and sex)**
(indices compared with mean)

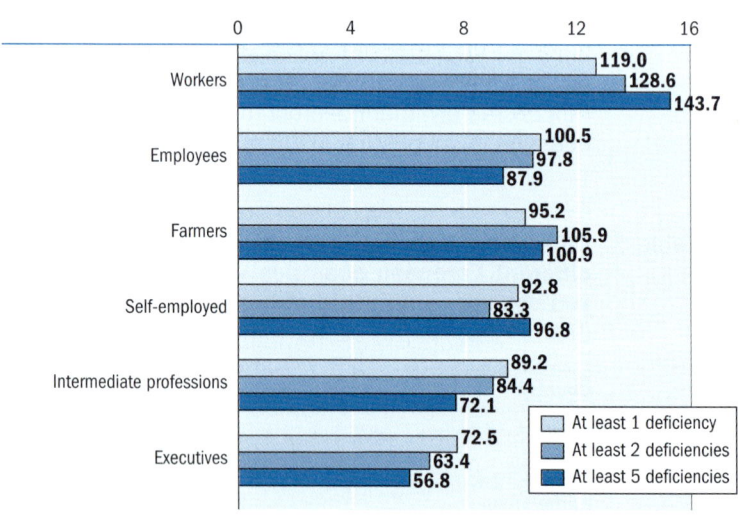

Source: HID Survey, 1999.

The Handicap, Disability and Dependency survey (HID) contributes information on this problem although people with significant impairment or recognised disability are over-represented in this study population. This survey has been set out to determine, for the first time, the number of disabled people in France, and describe their social condition, health status, the support they are given, and the kind of support that they need. The available data (figure 1) are from the 1998 survey which focused on institutionalised patients, and from the 1999 survey which focused on people still living at home [115].

This survey revealed that socially-based inequality is particularly pronounced in the case of disability. Of the total of 16,900 people of all ages living at home who were included in the survey, the proportion from the working class who declared at least one deficit was 1.6 time higher than that in the managerial class (after normalisation for sex and age). For those of under 20 years of age, this ratio was 1 to 2.

There was a major differential with respect to the ability to keep a handicapped child in the home: considering children with the same degree of handicap, the handicapped child of a worker is three times more likely to be institutionalised as the child of a manager or of someone in an intermediate profession. This latter pattern had already emerged in the survey focusing on institutions carried out the year before.

Inequality begins at birth

Inequality exists at birth – and even before birth, if one can say that. No successive, historical data exist linking infant mortality and social status because the latter information does not have to be given on death certificates. However, a series of recent studies show that inequality, having been demonstrated to exist prior to 1990, still persists, at least when evaluated in terms of the mother's educational level [92].

The 1995 national perinatal survey highlighted inequalities in the matters of premature birth and low birth weight (table 6), both of which are less likely if the mother is educated. Particularly at risk are farmers, tradespeople, craftsmen and the unemployed.

Certain factors are known to play a role in these perinatal indicators, including single motherhood, pregnancy in the very young and the very old, and inadequate medical monitoring (particularly for prematurity). Smoking also affects foetal growth. Even when all these factors are taken into account using multivariate analysis, socially-based differences are still in evidence. The other mechanisms involved probably include the way in which the community to which the mother belongs operates: such contextual factors not only have direct impact on health, but also dictate other key factors such as the likelihood of the woman working or not.

Taking dental health as an example

Socially-based inequality in the health of children and adolescents is generally poorly understood, apart from in the area of dental health. This is because a whole series of studies of schoolchil-

Table 6 **Premature birth and low birth weight broken down according to the parents' social status in France. 1995**

	Number	Prematurity[1] %	Low birth weight[2] %
Mother's educational level			
Primary[3]	709	5.4	9.9
Secondary, cycle 1	4,930	5.4	8.5
Secondary, cycle 2	2,474	4.0	8.3
Higher education	3,943	3.4	5.8
Unemployed[4]	196	9.2	11.3
Couple's socio-occupational class[5]			
Professionals/executives	2,042	3.4	4.4
Intermediate professions	2,552	3.6	6.4
Employees (office workers)	2,942	4.4	7.8
Farmers, tradesmen, craftsmen	745	5.4	10.0
Employees (shop workers), service personnel, workers	3,793	5.2	9.0
Unemployed (either member of the couple)[4]	492	5.7	12.1
Overall		4.5	7.6

1. Birth before 37 weeks of gestation.
2. Births in the lowest 10th percentile for the gestational age (based on a reference population).
3. Includes women with no schooling.
4. Unemployed people who declared a profession are classed under said profession.
5. Classified according to the highest-level occupation in the list (be it the mother's or the father's occupation) for couples; classified according to the mother's occupation for single mothers. PCS classification 1982.
Source: Enquête nationale périnatale 1995, naissances vivantes uniques.

dren have been conducted in this area over the years [65]. Between 1955 and 1970, the incidence of dental caries exploded in all children, irrespective of social class. Since then, dental hygiene has greatly improved across the board but to a greater extent in more privileged families so that now social inequality has become manifest in an aspect of health where previously it did not exist. Thus, although the global incidence of caries has decreased in France, the dimension of the social differences is the same in 1998 as it was in 1993 and 1990 (table 7). The children of farmers or of unemployed parents have twice as many teeth with caries as the children belonging to the managerial class.

Surveys of the dental health of adults reveal less social differences in the incidence of caries, be they treated or not. But in adults, social inequality in dental health is manifest in other figures. Table 8 is based on the French part of an international study in which the number of teeth with caries, missing teeth and filled teeth were recorded for two age brackets and then broken down on the basis of three socio-economic levels (high, middle, low).

Table 7 **Percentage of 12-year-old children without any caries at 12 years, by the parents' socio-occupational class**

	1990	1993	1998
Farmers	18	27	33
Tradesmen, craftsmen	24	39	38
Executives	34	43	47
Intermediate professions	23	31	43
Employees	24	38	43
Workers	21	31	32
Others	16	25	30
Overall	23	35	39

Source: Dental Health in France [85, 86].

Table 8 **Mean number of adults with teeth with caries or fillings and missing teeth, according to socio-occupational class: subjects of 35-44 years of age (1993) and 65-74 years of age (1995) living in the Rhône-Alpes region**

Age	Socio-occupational class	Number surveyed	Mean number of teeth		
			caries	missing	filled
35-44 years	High	146	0.9	2.0	10.8
	Moderate	342	1.2	2.4	11.1
	Low	512	1.3	3.6	9.9
65-74 years	High	76	0.9	10.2	8.4
	Moderate	154	1.1	14.2	6.7
	Low	373	1.2	19.4	4.0

Source: Hescot et al. [84], Bourgeois et al. [53].

The greatest inequality is seen in the number of missing teeth with a two-fold difference between the lowest socio-economic bracket and the highest. In the poorest subjects moreover, dental care had been more aggressive with 17% of those aged between 35 and 44 in the lowest socio-economic group carrying false teeth, as compared with just 6% in the other two groups. In contrast, the frequency of fixed prostheses (e.g. bridges) is comparable in all three groups. Among the older subjects, differences were even more marked: 22% of those in the lowest socio-economic group had had all their teeth removed, as against 0% in the highest group.

Socially-based inequality in dental health is at least partly due to inequitable access to care, largely due to the low rate of reimbursement by the insurance system. According to the 1997 Insurance Coverage and Health survey, fully 12% of the population forewent dental care entirely for financial reasons. Nevertheless,

Part two Health inequalities and disparities in France

studies conducted in the United States and Canada as well as France have shown that removing financial obstacles does not completely solve the problem of reluctance to seek dental treatment [65].

An unknown relationship: social differences and accidents

How social status correlates with the occurrence of accidents is unknown. No data are available on accidents among children, neither on traffic accidents nor home accidents, although it is well established that the likelihood of the latter is intimately linked with housing conditions [133]. National statistics on accidents in the workplace are compiled on the basis of type of activity rather than the victim's social characteristics, so it is difficult to assess to what extent the risk of accident in this context is linked to class [124].

For road accidents, no study taking the number of kilometres driven into account has been conducted in France in the last ten years to investigate social status as a risk factor. However, some useful light is shed on this question by the figures presented in table 9 which are based on police reports on over 200,000 accidents in which injury occurred in 1997, and in which social status was detailed [124]. These figures are compiled by the Inrets (National Institute for Research on Transport and Safety) and data on the seriousness of the accident only concern injury to the driver.

Table 9 **Seriousness of injuries to the driver in road accidents according to socio-occupational class. 1997**
(percentage)

	Killed	Injured	Lightly Injured	Lightly uninjured
No reply	1.6	6.3	39.4	52.7
Professional drivers	*1.5*	*6.7*	*22.2*	*69.5*
Farmers	4.0	11.4	22.4	62.1
Craftsmen, tradesmen, self-employed	2.8	8.3	29.1	59.8
Executives, professionals, senior managers	1.6	5.9	30.0	62.5
Mid-level managers, employees	1.5	6.9	40.4	51.3
Workers	2.7	12.3	38.5	46.5
Retired	4.7	12.0	31.6	51.7
Unemployed	3.0	10.4	39.7	47.0
Other	2.6	14.9	47.9	34.5
Overall	**2.5**	**10.6**	**38.9**	**48.0**

Source: Cermes, IFRH, data from the Inrets department of Accident research and evaluation, 1997.

On average, for every 100 drivers involved in an accident which had to be dealt with in a report by the police or gendarmerie, 48 were unharmed, 39 suffered mild injury, slightly over 10 were seriously injured, and 2.5 were killed. These figures are then broken down according to the driver's occupation: professional drivers were most likely to escape injury, followed by the group consisting senior managers, professionals and executives. If the categories are classified according to the likelihood of being seriously injured or killed, those at highest risk fall into the "Others" group (17.5%) followed by retired people (16.7%), farmers (15.4%), workers (15%) and the unemployed (13.4%), with managers, professionals and executives at relatively low risk (7.5%). These figures have not been analysed in depth to probe reasons for the differences, and more work is indicated in this area.

Geographical inequalities in health

France is one of the most varied landscapes in Europe, with respect to human, social and cultural features as well as physical ones. This heterogeneity is reflected in disparities in health status, about which a geographically based analysis can reveal much. Thus, high-risk populations can be assimilated to high-risk geographical units, and the epidemiological profiles of different populations can be represented cartographically. For this report, four health indicators have been mapped and analysed:
- life expectancy at various ages together with standardised mortality ratios which illustrate inequality in respect of death in the most direct manner;
- rate of premature death (before the age of 65): most premature deaths can be considered as avoidable (being due to high risk behaviour or failure to exploit the health care system), and as such represent a priority area for immediate action;
- mortality profile by age and cause of death which illustrates the particularities of various different geographical units in regard to these key parameters;
- body mass index, which acts as a general lifestyle indicator as well as being strongly predictive of future health problems.

Differential life expectancy: growing disparities

Life expectancy at birth

Figure 2 shows cartographic representations of life expectancy at birth in different employment zones for the periods 1973-1977 and 1988-1992. Between these two periods, the difference between the highest and lowest life expectancy figures in different places increased dramatically for both men (from 6.6 to 10.1 years) and women (from 3.6 to 6.9 years). The pattern more or less follows the administrative regions within which the towns and their surrounding countryside share similar characteristics (although life expectancy in town is globally higher than that in the country). In 1990, a T-shaped zone of relatively low life expectancy is seen extending from the Channel coast in the north down through the Rhine, the Ardennes and the Auvergne. This is surrounded by a U-shaped zone of relatively low mortality stretching down from the lower Seine valley, around the Pyrenees, back up along the Mediterranean coast and finally up through Burgundy. Two main concentrations of excess mortality (notably the area extending from the coast of Nord-Pas-de-Calais to Alsace, and the part of Brittany west of the Saint-Nazaire-Saint-Brieuc line) are obvious, as are two concentrations of relatively long life expectancy (in and around the Pays de la Loire region [apart from around

Geographical inequalities in health

Figure 2 **Life expectancy at birth for both sexes during the periods 1973-1977 and 1988-1992 in France (scale: employment zone)**

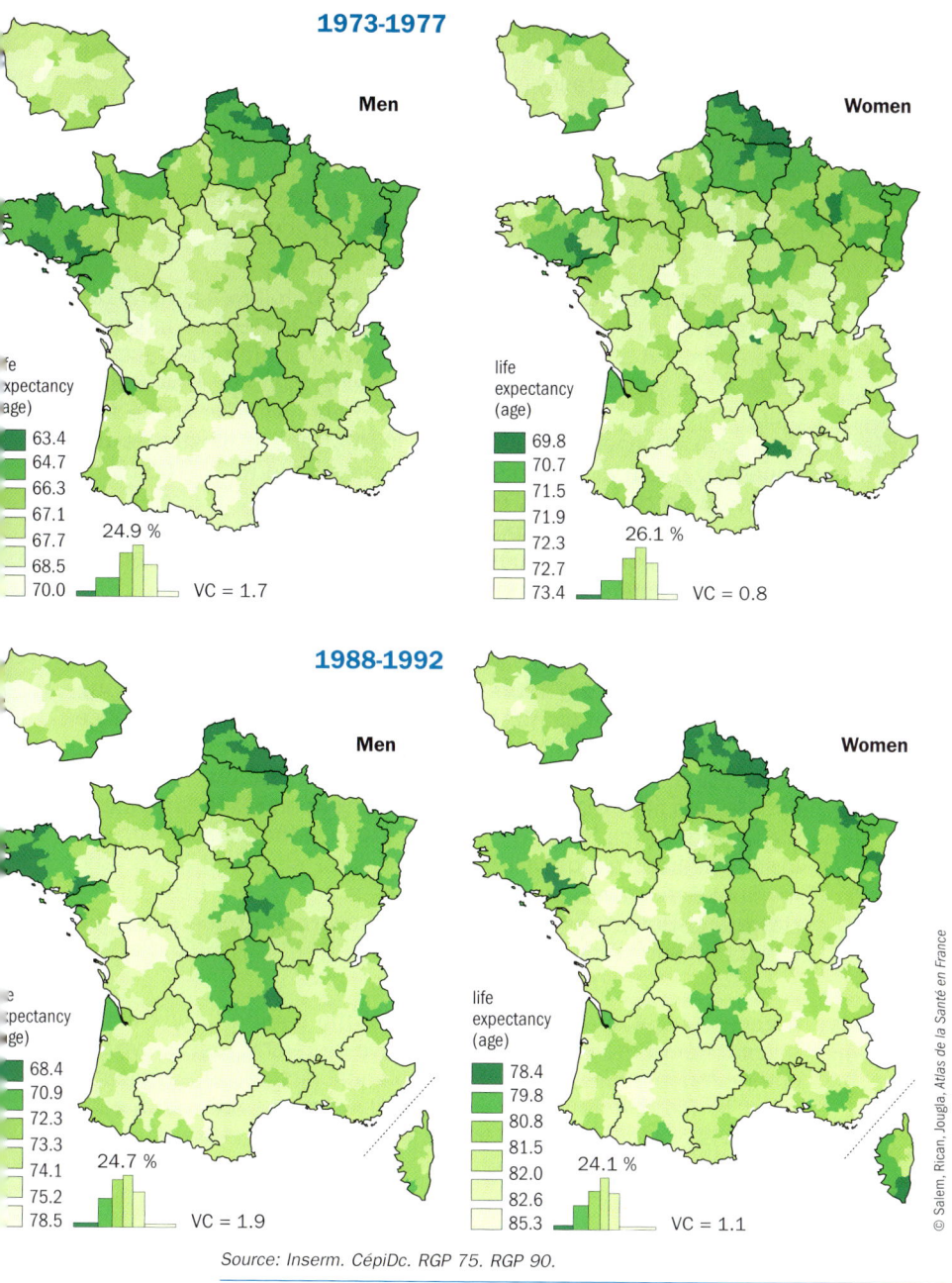

Source: Inserm. CépiDc. RGP 75. RGP 90.

the city of Nantes], west of the Centre region and the deep South-West).

In Eastern France, it can be seen that excess mortality is on the increase along a meridian running down from the Ardennes to the Auvergne, and that east of this line (towards the Italian and Swiss borders), life expectancy is relatively high. Finally, the Île-de-France region around Paris is apparently split into two with life expectancy in the northern edges relatively low like that in the neighbouring areas of Champagne and Picardy, whereas elsewhere it is relatively high. A similar division of the Île-de-France is observed whatever particular health indicator is being considered.

A similar pattern of disparity for life expectancy at 65 years of age

Geographical discrepancies in life expectancy follow a general (as opposed to age-specific or gender-specific) pattern of mortality differentials. A similar pattern is seen whether life expectancy at birth, at 35 years of age or at 65 is being mapped. However, a map of life expectancy at 65 (figure 3) bears witness to the fact that such changes are subject to inertia, and it illustrates the impact of death at advanced age on overall mortality. The maps drawn up on the basis of employment zones show a similar pattern to that of life expectancy at birth, and there is still a considerable discrepancy between the highest and the lowest values, both for women (4.9 years) and men (6.3 years).

Life expectancy is relatively high in four particular areas, namely the South West (centred around Auch and Castres), the Centre-West (centred around Tours), the Centre-East (centred on Dijon), and the South East (centred on Alpes de Provence). Île-de-France is again partitioned in the same pattern as for life expectancy at birth. Paris, Lyon, Marseille, Bordeaux and Nantes fall in the middle, and life expectancy at 65 in Toulouse and Nice is relatively high. Other towns follow the regions to which they belong with the lowest figures (almost all below 15 years) observed in big and medium-sized towns located north of a line drawn between Le Havre and Belfort together with those towns scattered along the coasts of Normandy and Brittany.

Disparities between town and country (and the relevance of the parent region)

A geographical analysis at the level of the canton (a unit in the second tier of the French administrative hierarchy, just above the commune) produces a higher resolution picture. The indicator used in figure 4 is the standardised mortality ratio and each canton is graded according to the French average (100) after normalisation for age. This approach highlights features that are not apparent at a larger scale.

Mortality rates are particularly homogenous in the administrative regions of Nord-Pas-de-Calais, Picardy, Lorraine and Alsace which are all densely populated and heavily urban. Little disparity is seen between rural and urban zones in these regions. This picture

Figure 3 **Life expectancy at 65 years of age for both sexes during the period 1988-1992 in France (scales: employment zone and towns with more than 20,000 inhabitants)**

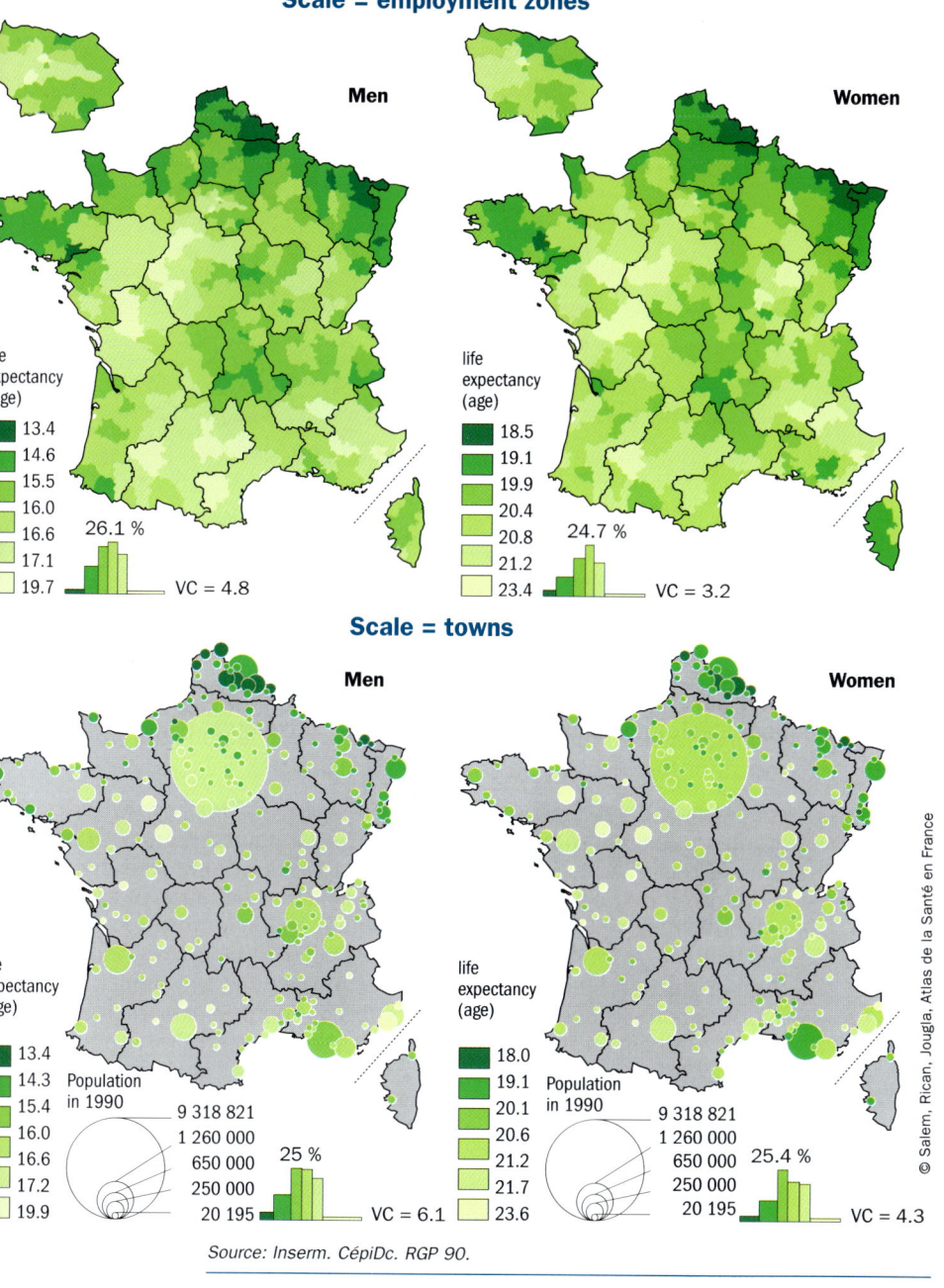

Source: Inserm. CépiDc. RGP 90.

Figure 4 **Standardised mortality ratios for the period 1988-1992 (scale: canton; integrated figures)**

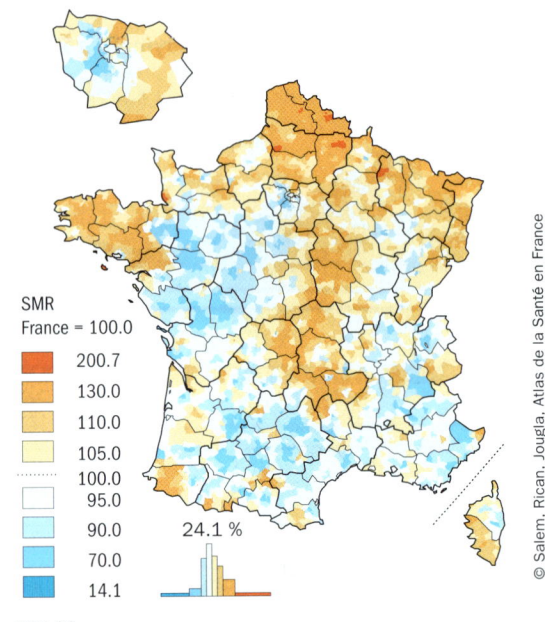

Source: Inserm. CépiDc. RGP 90.

reflects regional particularities, on the one hand cultural (eating, smoking and drinking habits) and on the other social and environmental (these are centres of mining and metal works in which the working classes predominate and which have undergone the worst effects of the industry and manufacturing crisis).

In contrast, clear discontinuities are evident in Brittany, in the Limousin region and in the Pyrénées-Atlantiques region. The Rennes basin in particular has a distinctly lower death rate than is observed in the rest of Brittany, and a similar situation is seen around Limoges. The Pyrénées-Atlantiques region is frankly cut in two, with high mortality in the west echoing that in the neighbouring Basque country, and far lower mortality in the east (the Béarn region). These discontinuities follow contours which cross different administrative regions, *e.g.* as far as mortality is concerned, Brittany extends down as far as Nantes, and mortality rates in the Creuse and Corrèze regions are closer to those in the Auvergne region than to that in Haute-Vienne (which is officially part of the same region). These geographical patterns are probably due to social and cultural divisions, some of which are characterised to some extent. Although it is impossible to rank all such factors, an example could be analysed for the purposes of illustration, namely why the death rate in the Basque part of the

Pyrénées-Atlantiques region is frankly higher than that in the Béarn region just to the east: Basques feel a strong cultural identity, which is a strong determinant of eating and drinking habits, and profound industrial and rural roots. Similarly, there has been significant implantation of service industries in the towns of Rennes and Limoges meaning an influx of executives and office workers (whose life expectancy is higher), thereby introducing discontinuity with respect to the surrounding predominantly agricultural lands. Rennes in particular has benefited from major socio-economic changes fostered in Brittany.

Apart from in the northern band of excess mortality (where there is little apparent difference between rural and urban zones), death rates are systematically lower in towns, and they are often particularly low in bureaucratic centres (*e.g.* regional capitals). This pattern is particularly marked in a central diagonal running down from Reims to Bordeaux.

In contrast, as one moves away from the centre of regions towards the periphery, the death rate tends to rise, a pattern which is particularly evident in the Pays de la Loire and the Midi-Pyrénées regions. This is due to the way regions are organised at the spatial level which follows on from the objectives set when these administrative entities were set up in 1789. Delegates to the Revolutionary Constituent Assembly wanted structures in which every single citizen lived within a day's journey of the power centre (*i.e.* the capital of the region ("département")), a policy which engendered massive polarisation of the regions around the regional capitals (the Préfectures). This polarisation was exacerbated when jobs began concentrate in towns, leaving the cantons located around the periphery of the region profoundly rural and isolated. This excess mortality-promoting pattern is especially important in mountainous areas such as the Pyrenees, the Alps and the Vosges.

In summary, many of the geographical disparities in mortality in France cross regional borders so that analysing this question on a region-by-region basis (as is a common practice) is inappropriate. Disparities between urban and rural areas deserve special attention because these differences do not just arise as a result of different living conditions in town and country, but also – mainly? – as a result of social differences between country and townspeople.

Differences in the age at which people die

Excess mortality during working age is far higher in France than in neighbouring countries: between 1988 and 1992, 80,000 people were dying at between the ages of 15 and 59 every year, corresponding to 15% of all registered deaths in mainland France. Most of these deaths were due to behavioural factors, including

Part two — Health inequalities and disparities in France

Disparities between different regions and within regions

suicide, accident, smoking and excessive drinking. The economic and social consequences of this excess death rate alone make this a serious public health problem.

Studying male mortality rates (broken down into five-year age brackets and at the level of employment zones) reveals the existence of seven different types of zone, each quite distinct from the others. Mapping these zones reveals a significant geographical pattern (figure 5).

Type I is characterised by low mortality at all ages: this is seen in the South West of France, urban employment zones in the South (Bordeaux, Toulouse, Lyon, Grenoble and Dijon), and a broad western band stretching from Caen to Nantes and taking in Rennes.

Type II is characterised by excess mortality between the ages of 15 and 24, and low mortality in all other brackets: this covers mainly rural employment zones around the Type I areas mentioned

Figure 5 **Employment zone profiles based on mortality rates during the period 1988-1992 (by five-year age brackets from 15 to 59 years of age)**

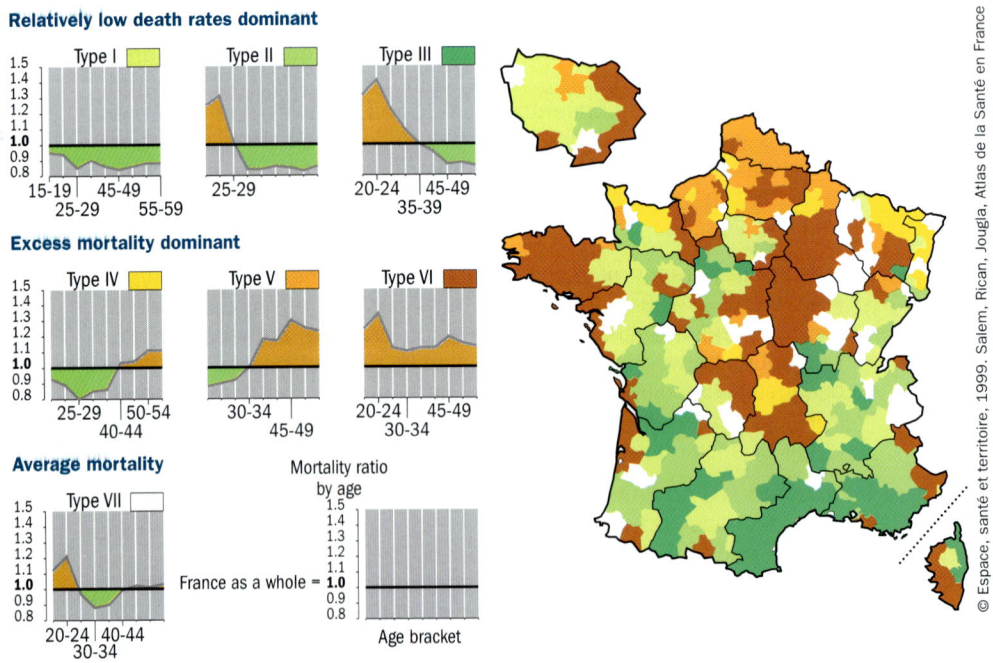

Source: Inserm. CépiDc. RGP 90.

above: rural areas in the Poitou-Charentes, Aquitaine, Midi-Pyrénées and Rhône-Alpes regions.

Type III is characterised by excess mortality between 15 and 35, and low mortality between 40 and 59: this mainly corresponds to employment zones on the Mediterranean coast.

Type IV is characterised by inversion of the preceding pattern, *i.e.* by low mortality before 45 and high mortality thereafter: this pattern is mostly seen in the industrial basin in the east of France.

In Type V, the features are the same as Type IV but more marked with the borderline between relatively low and relatively high mortality located at 35 years of age (instead of 45): this describes the urban, industrial north (the Nord-Pas-de-Calais, Picardy and Haute-Normandie regions), Paris and the regions to the north of the capital.

Type VI is exceptional with excess mortality in all age brackets: covered are rural zones in Brittany together with a central diagonal running from the Champagne-Ardenne region to the Auvergne region, and certain zones on the Atlantic coast.

Finally, Type VII more or less represents the French average, and does not follow any particular geography.

From a demographic point of view, it is the 15-29 age bracket which gives the best statistical resolution when it comes to analysing geographical disparities in premature death. Typing of the employment zones is based on this parameter, independently of the absolute level of premature death. In this age group, suicide and road accidents account for a large majority of deaths. From a geographical point of view, the key differentiating factor is the level of urbanisation in the employment zones. The heavily urbanised north of France is characterised by relatively low mortality between 15 and 29, in contrast to Brittany, the central diagonal and the rural South-West in all of which there is excess mortality in this age bracket. Conversely, in these same regions, the mortality rate among those younger in age living in an urban environment (*e.g.* Rennes, Bordeaux, Toulouse, Lyon and Grenoble) is relatively low. Above and beyond regional particularities with respect to premature death, the degree of urbanisation therefore plays a major role in determining mortality profiles, a situation which is largely accounted for the fact that there are far more deaths on roads in rural areas.

Nevertheless, the special characteristics of the eastern part of France and the Mediterranean coast deserve mention. The first is a mainly urban and industrial area and the relatively low mortality between 15 and 40 seen in Alsace and Lorraine perhaps represents inversion of the general trend in premature death. A retrospective study of figures taken from towns with more than 20,000 inhabitants and employment zones collected between

1973 and 1977 showed that the earliest evidence of this change appeared in the towns in the 1970's, before it subsequently spread out over the entire region.

In the area along the Mediterranean coast, which is dominated by service industries, mortality between 15 and 35 is relatively high: this is due to road accidents and AIDS. The excess mortality rates recorded at all ages in the employment zones corresponding to Nice and Marseille are more difficult to explain, but they can probably be assimilated to the similarly high mortality rates observed along the Atlantic coast. An overall analysis of mortality indicators in coastal zones points to generally poor health status, a situation which has to be seen in the context of the heavy industrialisation common around sea-ports.

Disparities between large and small towns

Mortality profiles for different age brackets have also been investigated for towns with over 20,000 inhabitants (figure 6). As a general rule, the geographical pattern remains unchanged: excess mortality at all ages along a central band running from the Champagne to the Massif Central regions, in Brittany and in the Atlantic ports; relatively low mortality before 29 and excess mortality after 35 in the Nord region; low mortality up until 35 and excess mortality after 40 in the east; and excess mortality up until 35 and low mortality after 40 along the Mediterranean coast. It appears that the local mortality rate between 15 and 59 years of age depends more on the region being considered than on the size of the town.

The novel information from this map is that, in many regions, mortality rates in secondary towns are not always the same as in the main towns in the region. Thus, whereas mortality in general in this age range is relatively low in the cities and towns of Rennes, Caen, Orléans, Limoges, Toulouse, Lyon, Grenoble, Dijon and Besançon, it is higher than the average in most of the neighbouring small towns up until the age of 30 (or even 40 in many). Again, road accidents are one factor, coupled with differences in social make-up, notably the larger proportion of workers and employees in small towns as against a larger proportion of managers in larger towns.

Therefore, analysis of mortality rates at different ages and at different scale yields information on differences in health status between towns, rural areas and coastal zones.

Differences in terms of cause of death

Public health policy involves defining – in a certain place and for a certain population – health priorities, and then identifying ways of improving the situation. Figure 7 represents the results of multifactorial analysis of male and female mortality at the scale of employment zones and towns with more than 20,000 inhabitants.

Figure 6 **Town profiles based on mortality rates during the period 1988-1992 (by five-year age brackets from 15 to 59 years of age)**

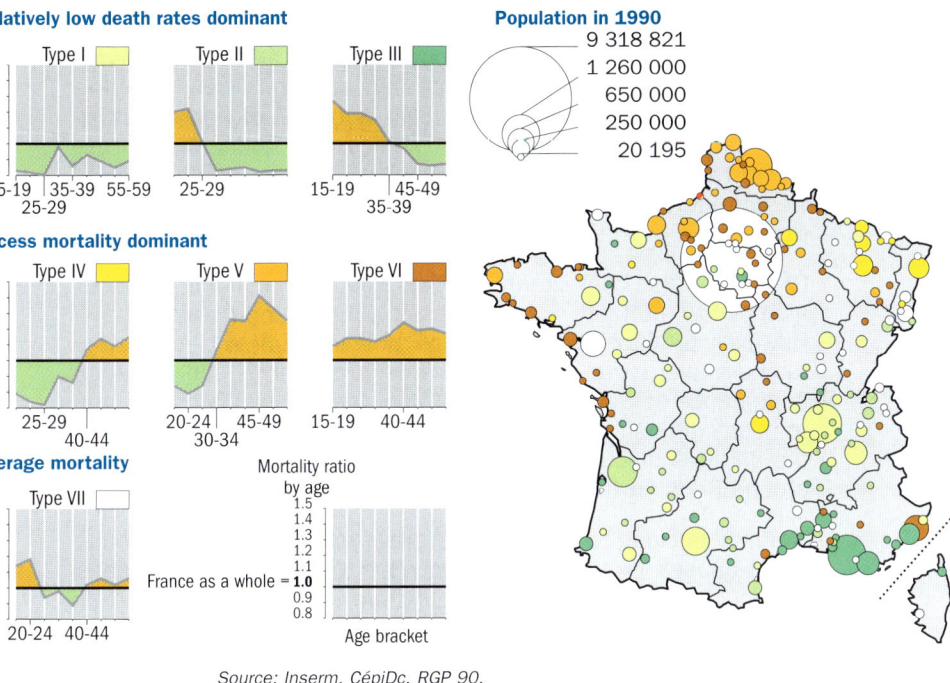

Source: Inserm. CépiDc. RGP 90.

Seven different mortality profiles which follow a clear geographical pattern

For male mortality, seven different types of profile were identified at the employment zone scale. For all causes of death, three of these profiles were characterised by relatively low mortality and four by relatively high mortality.

Cartographic representation of these statistically differentiated groups shows certain very pronounced geographical patterns, which are somewhat reminiscent of the patterns seen in the context of life expectancy. Again, mortality is low in the south and high throughout the northernmost parts of France as well as in the Lorraine and the Auvergne regions (although within these areas, the picture is by no means homogenous).

In group I, mortality is particularly low for causes of death related to smoking or possibly pollution, *i.e.* cancer of the airways, chronic bronchitis, etc. In contrast, the number of deaths due to suicide, road accidents and stomach tumours is slightly elevated. This kind of profile is characteristic of rural, non-industrialised areas such as those located in the Centre region, the Pays de la Loire region, Southern Normandy, the Rennes basin, the Poitou and the Limousin regions. Nevertheless, a similar pattern is observed in the regions of Franche-Comté and Rhône-Alpes.

Group II is characterised by relatively low mortality for causes of death associated with alcohol consumption (alcoholic cirrhosis and psychosis, cancer of the upper airways, and diseases of the digestive tract). This mortality profile is typical of non-industrialised areas in the South-West of France (the Aquitaine and the Midi-Pyrénées regions), the Mediterranean coast and the south-western part of the Paris basin, all areas with a high general life expectancy.

Group III is also characterised by low alcohol-related mortality, but also by low mortality due to road accidents and prostate cancer. However, fatal infectious diseases (notably AIDS) and respiratory tumours are more common in this group. The simultaneous appearance of low mortality due to suicide and high mortality due to poorly defined causes raises a question about the reliability of the data (as discussed above). This mortality profile is observed around Paris, in the town of Nice and on the island of Corsica.

Group IV is close to the French average except that mortality due to all causes is slightly elevated. This group describes a band running diagonally down the country from Champagne in the north-east in a south-westerly direction to the Auvergne. This is also the pattern in the mountainous areas of the Vosges and the Alps which are already under-populated and are experiencing further, steady depopulation.

Group V is characterised by excess mortality for all causes of death, especially those associated with heavy drinking (alcoholic cirrhosis and psychosis, cancer of the upper airways and digestive tract, and stomach cancer). The suicide rate in this group is also relatively high. This profile is found in agricultural areas in Brittany and along the Normandy coast into Picardy.

Relative mortality is even higher in Group VI which is marked by excess mortality due to circulatory disease, heavy drinking and respiratory disease (associated with smoking). The number of deaths due to road accidents and AIDS is relatively low. This pattern is typical of the old industrial heart-lands of the Nord region, the Lorraine region and the industrial East.

Group VII is rather special with the worst mortality indicators for almost all causes of death apart from road accidents. The incidence of respiratory diseases and diseases associated with heavy drinking is particularly high. This pattern is confined to employment zones in the traditional mining country of the Nord-Pas-de-Calais region.

Geographical inequalities in health

Figure 7 **Employment zone profiles based on comparative mortality rates and cause of death for both sexes (1998-1992)**

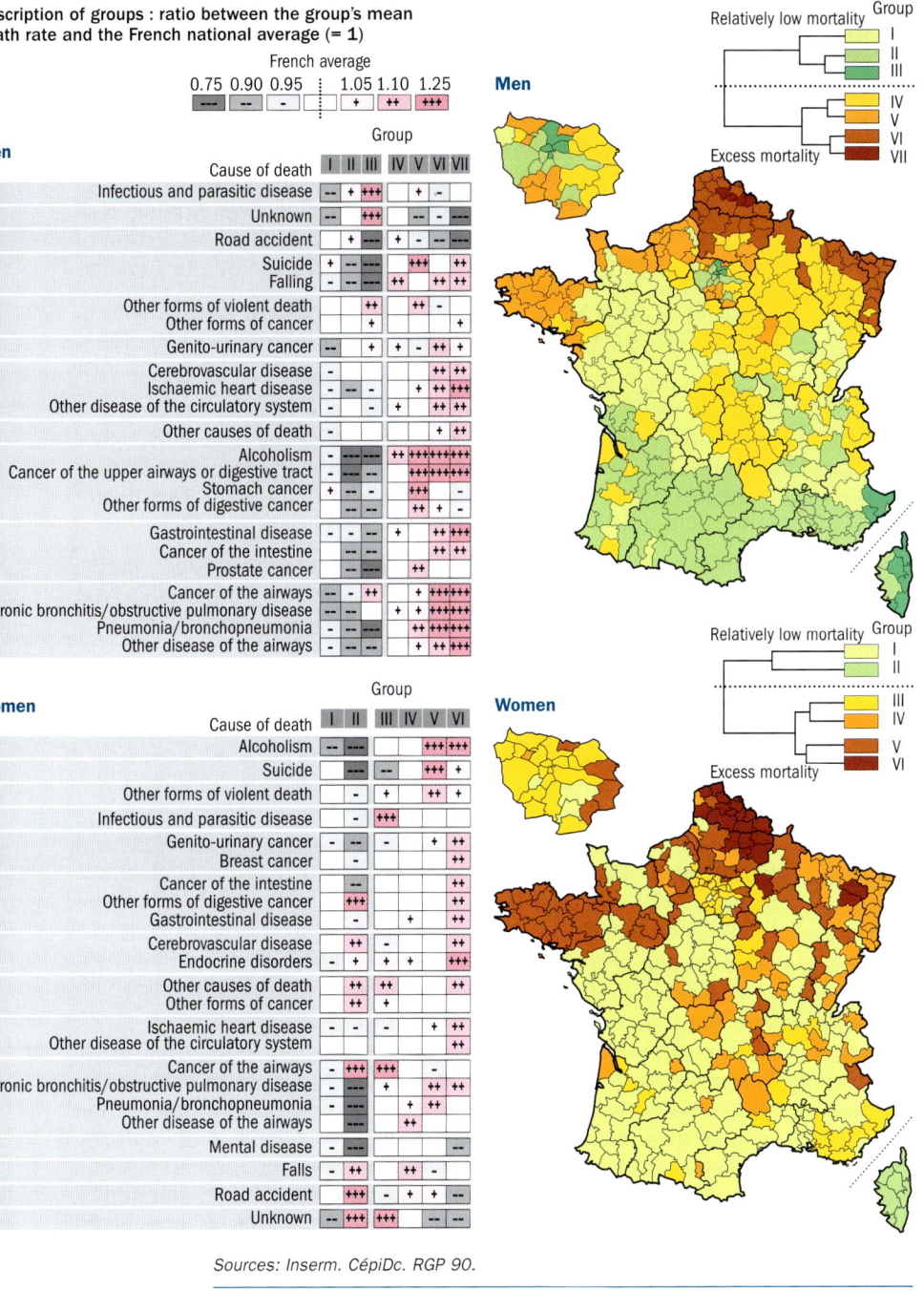

Sources: Inserm. CépiDc. RGP 90.

Part two   Health inequalities and disparities in France

Female mortality gives a far less clear-cut geographical pattern

As well as being far lower generally than male mortality, female mortality does not show the same north-south distinction, and in fact no very clear-cut patterns are obvious at all. The trend is as if lower overall mortality were resulting in homogenisation of the picture throughout France. However, six different patterns can be distinguished.

Group I is characterised by relatively low mortality for all causes of death: this applies to most parts of the country.

In Group II, death from digestive and respiratory cancer, cerebrovascular disease and road accidents are slightly over-represented. However, interpretation is made difficult by the high proportion of deaths from unknown causes. This pattern is unique to Corsica.

Group III is characterised by marked excess mortality due to airways cancer: this profile typifies the urban areas of the Paris basin and the Mediterranean coastal zone and reflects the fact that many more city women smoke.

In Group IV, mortality due to all causes of death is slightly higher than the average. Mainly in the east of the country, the across-the-board excess death rate amongst the females of this region is far from being as pronounced as that of their menfolk.

Generalised excess mortality is similarly seen in Group V, particularly with respect to alcohol-related causes. As for men, this type of mortality profile predominates in Brittany and Normandy.

The female Group VI corresponds to the male Group VII, characterised by marked excess mortality for all causes of death: this pattern is seen in employment areas in the north which were formerly centres of mining and industry.

Region is a major factor

Both of these analyses reveal a strong north-south dichotomy in health status in France. Health is better in the Centre-West and South-West, and globally worse right through a crescent drawn over the north of France. However, the factors which determine health status are not the same everywhere: the relative importance of smoking, drinking, occupational factors and general life style determinants probably varies enormously from region to region.

It has been pointed out that certain profiles are specifically associated with an urban setting, especially Paris and the Mediterranean coast. Analysis at the scale of towns with more than 20,000 inhabitants makes it possible to relate local mortality profiles with both town size and regional context. The first obvious pattern is again that of disparity between groups characterised by excess mortality for all causes of death and groups of generalised low mortality. In a general way, the profiles remain the same with excess mortality in the northern crescent, thereby suggesting that mortality indicators are more closely related to the local regional pattern than to town size. However, certain particular features deserve attention.

Mortality is generally relatively low in the bigger towns (*e.g.* the regional capitals of Nantes, Toulouse, Lyon, Grenoble and Dijon, Paris, and towns on the Mediterranean coast), apart from for infectious and parasitic causes of death (mainly due to AIDS).

Towns in Brittany and the East (Nancy, Metz, Strasbourg, Colmar and Mulhouse) do not have the same mortality characteristics as their surrounding areas: although male mortality is slightly higher in these towns, it is nevertheless fairly close to the French average (whereas it is significantly above the average in the areas around all these towns). And female mortality in these towns is even below the average. The high excess mortality due to alcoholism and associated causes observed in Brittany at the employment zone scale, or the high mortality rate due to respiratory disease in Eastern employment areas is not reflected in towns in these areas. This finding illustrates the differences between town and country in these regions with respect to life styles and behaviour patterns.

On the other hand, the patterns in the ports of Normandy and the Nord region (from Cherbourg to Dunkerque), and the towns in the former mining centres in the latter are quite consistent with the patterns observed at the employment zone scale.

The importance of regional affiliation with respect to mortality profile reproduces therefore, to a lesser extent, particularities linked to the level of urbanisation of population centres. Health status is generally better in larger towns than in either small urban units or peripheral zones.

Mapping mortality types shows that health status follows marked geographical patterns. Known disparities between north and south emerge, but this type of analysis also makes it possible to determine different, geographically specific components. Excess mortality in the North-West is not the same as excess mortality in the North-East; the reasons why mortality is relatively low in the South-West are not the same as the reasons it is so in the South-East. Geographical typing reveals particular combinations of different environmental, behavioural and socio-occupational risk factors. The causes of death which are, in every case, the most discriminating with respect to geographical disparity are those associated with smoking and drinking, and to a lesser extent AIDS. This is ample evidence that pertinent public health measures need to be implemented in all these areas. Integrating these mortality profiles with other indicators (*e.g.* related to morbidity or care consumption) might be useful when it comes to devising policies to remedy geographical inequality and promote optimum public health.

AN INSTANCE OF GEOGRAPHICALLY-BASED INEQUALITY IN MORBIDITY: OBESITY IN THE YOUNG

Body Mass Index (BMI) represents one of the most reliable succinct measurements of a person's overall state of health. It contains information about past eating habits, present social and health status (the risk of medical problems and also employability difficulties), and is predictive of future problems (cardiovascular disease, bone and joint problems, diabetes, etc.). Obesity is largely associated with poverty and is a growing problem in France.

A problem of epidemic proportions between 1987 and 1996

Data recorded in young men presenting for National Service constitute the most complete data base on this question in France. Between 1987 and 1996, a total of more than 4 million individuals were examined in this context.

BMI* figures (table 10) show that the prevalence of obesity rose steadily throughout the period, whatever the threshold chosen to define obesity. The percentage of young men with a BMI of over 25 (a particularly relevant threshold in young people) increased from 11.5% in 1987 to 16.5% in 1996. A similar trend is seen if the threshold is set at 27 (from 4.7% in 1987 to 8% in 1995). Extreme obesity (BMI ≥ 30) doubled between 1987 and 1996. Preliminary data for 1998 indicate that the percentage of young males with a BMI of over 25 had further risen to 16.8%.

Table 10

Body weight profiles among conscripts presenting between 1987 and 1996
(percentage)

	Thin	Normal	Overweight		Obese
	BMI < 18.5	18.5 < BMI < 25	BMI ≥ 25	BMI ≥ 27	BMI ≥ 30
1987	5.8	82.7	11.5	4.7	1.5
1988	6.3	82.0	11.7	5.0	1.7
1989	6.0	81.5	12.5	5.4	1.9
1990	5.9	80.6	13.5	6.0	2.1
1991	6.4	80.3	13.3	5.9	2.0
1992	5.8	79.7	14.5	6.5	2.2
1993	5.3	78.9	15.8	7.2	2.5
1994	5.5	79.0	15.5	7.1	2.5
1995	5.6	78.8	15.6	7.3	2.7
1996	5.5	78.0	16.5	8.0	3.1

Source: Cetima, 1987-1996.

High prevalence in the countryside, large numbers in town

Two major patterns emerge from obesity figures (BMI ≥ 25) broken down by commune type (table 11). Firstly, prevalence is inversely proportional to commune size in a remarkably tight correlation, a

---

* Nutritionists classify nutritional status on the basis of body mass index: this is defined as an index of below 18.5; over 25 is overweight and between 27 and 30 is classified as pre-obese; over 30 is obese.

relationship that has always been true. Secondly, the prevalence of obesity in all types of commune has been growing regularly and at a precipitous rate, rising by 40 to 45% more or less everywhere between 1987 and 1996 [131].

Obesity has become a mass phenomenon in France. Although in relative terms obesity may be more common in the countryside, it is of course in town that the highest numbers of obese people are found and, in particular, in the biggest towns. Obesity is therefore a major public health problem in both rural and urban settings.

Marked regional disparities

Comparing regional maps for 1987 and 1996 (figure 8) shows identical rate amplitudes, in a 1:2 ratio, but a major increase at the low end of the scale (from 8.7% in 1987 to 11.2% in 1996) and, to an even greater extent, at the high end of the scale (from 17.4% in 1987 to 24.2% in 1996). It is rare that any kind of regional analysis reveals such major disparities. France is divided in three according to the 1987 map:
– a unit composed of Brittany, the Loire Valley and the Basse-Normandie regions, characterised by very low prevalence;
– a rectangle of moderate prevalence with corners at the Nord-Pas-de-Calais, Alsace, Midi-Pyrénées and Aquitaine regions;
– a Mediterranean rim of low prevalence composed of the Languedoc-Roussillon and Provence-Alpes-Côte-d'Azur regions.
Two regions do not fit into this pattern: Corsica where obesity is particularly common, and the Île-de-France region where it is particularly low.

By 1996, high prevalence had massively spread out from the South-West to cover almost the whole country apart from Brittany and its immediate neighbours. The dramatic degeneration around the Mediterranean rim is particularly alarming – quite at odds with triumphalist vaunting of the benefits of the Mediterranean diet.

Table 11 **Prevalence of excess body weight (BMI ≥ 25) in conscripts presenting between 1987 and 1996, according to the size of their commune of origin**
(percentage)

commune size	1987	1988	1989	1990	1991	1992	1993	1994	1995	1996
under 2,000 inhabitants	13.1	13.2	13.9	14.8	14.5	16.1	17.7	17.2	17.4	18.1
from 2,000 to 5,000 inhabitants	11.7	11.9	12.7	14.1	13.6	14.7	16.2	15.9	15.5	16.2
from 5,000 to 10,000 inhabitants	11.4	11.7	12.6	13.5	13.4	14.5	15.9	15.2	15.7	16.5
from 10,000 to 20,000 inhabitants	11.1	11.1	11.8	12.7	12.9	13.9	15.0	15.1	15.4	15.9
from 20,000 to 50,000 inhabitants	10.9	11.2	11.8	12.8	12.7	13.9	15.2	15.1	14.9	16.2
from 50,000 to 100,000 inhabitants	10.3	10.3	11.6	12.6	12.6	14.2	15.0	14.4	14.5	15.7
over 100,000 inhabitants	10.0	10.3	11.0	12.2	12.0	13.0	13.8	13.8	13.9	15.0

Source: Cetima, 1987-1996, Insee 1990.

Part two Health inequalities and disparities in France

Figure 8 **Prevalence of obesity (BMI ≥ 25) in men of between 17 and 25 years of age in 1987 and 1996 (scales: region and towns of over 20,000 inhabitants)**

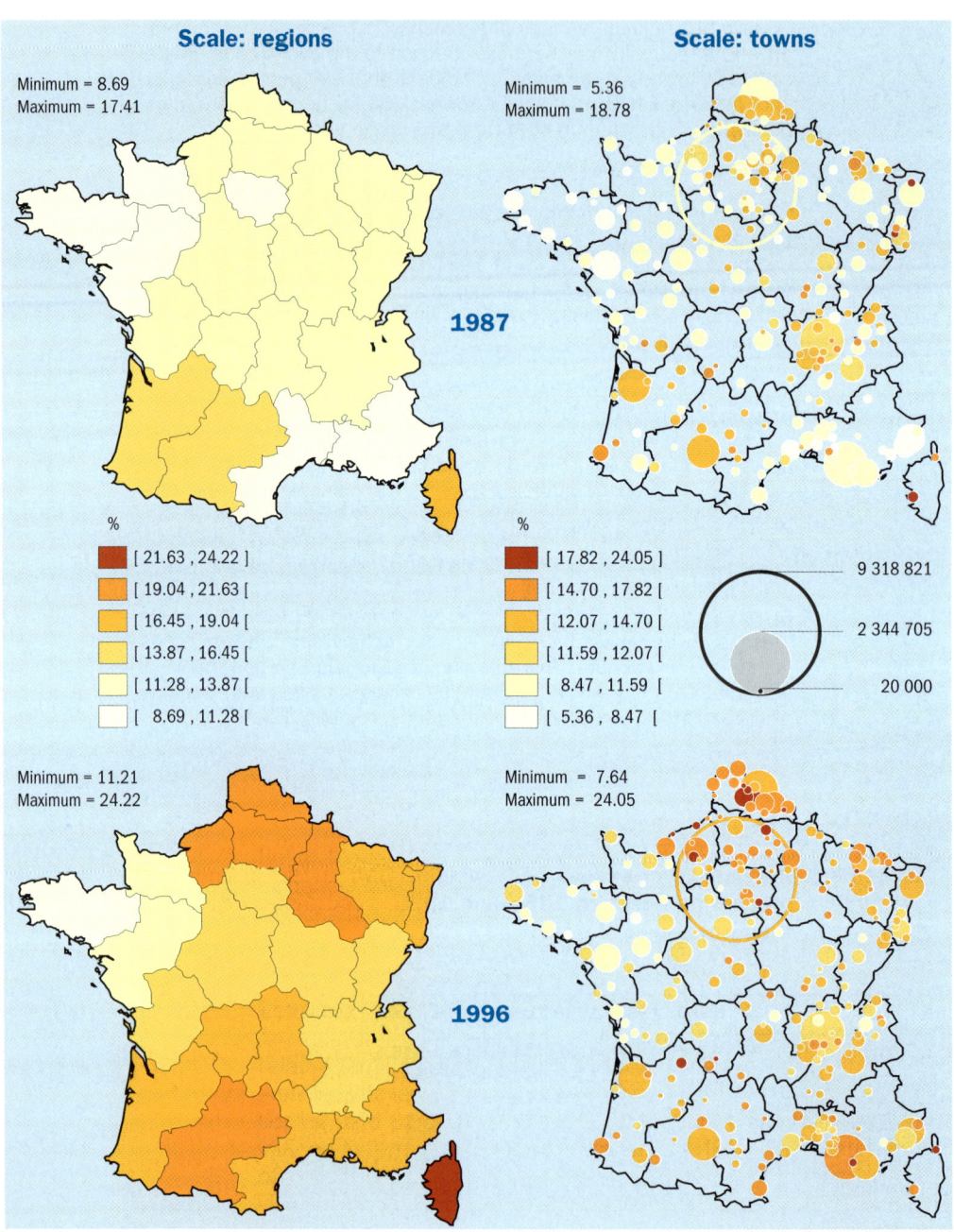

Source: Cetima. Insee.

Higher-resolution analysis of obesity at the level of urban units containing more than 20,000 inhabitants has been conducted. These maps show that obesity is more dependent on region than on town size, *i.e.* a town in the Provence-Alpes-Côte d'Azur region (or the Nord region, Brittany, etc.) is likely to have a similar prevalence of obesity as another different-sized town in the same region, rather than resembling a similar-sized town in a different region. This finding is compatible with the idea that behaviour patterns are regionally conditioned, a topic which remains little investigated and which seems to contradict the widespread idea that eating and drinking habits are becoming more uniform throughout France.

The 1996 map clearly shows the generalisation of high percentages of obesity in urban centres (apart from in Brittany and neighbouring regions). Prevalence can be seen to be increasing in those towns where obesity was already common in 1987 (in the Haute-Normandie, Nord-Pas-de-Calais, Champagne, Aquitaine, etc., regions) but, even more worrying is the fact that obesity in the Mediterranean regions – where it was rare in 1987 – had, by 1996, reached levels comparable to those seen in the Nord. It is difficult to avoid the temptation to compare this pattern with that of areas of worst poverty on the corresponding economic map: the relationship between economic hardship and obesity could be tested by integrating information on nutritional status, educational level, professional training, etc.

Analysis of the geography of obesity in France reveals an alarming trend among young men, the most striking aspect of which is the dramatic increase in the prevalence of obesity more or less throughout the country. The suddenness of this growth precludes an exclusively genetic mechanism in that it would be difficult to understand why any all-important genetic factor had not been expressed previously. Explanations must also be sought in the increase in poverty: as shown in the United States, obesity is a disease of the poor.

Socio-geographical inequality in health

Little work has been done on the question of inequality in health in the context of both geography and social status at the same time, *i.e.* the health of people of similar social status living in different geographical units has not been compared [89, 124].

Analysis of regional disparities in mortality among workers and employees does not change the general geography of mortality. Death rates are higher in this class in the northern crescent, and lower in this class in the Midi-Pyrénées and Languedoc-Roussillon regions. This group therefore presents a geographical pattern which is independent of the proportion of the local population as a whole which they represent. This finding is less clear-cut for executives and professionals among whom the level of general mortality varies far less, although those living in the Provence-Alpes-Côte d'Azur region, in Corsica and around Paris are more likely to die prematurely (which must be considered in the light of AIDS which caused many deaths in this group in the 25-44 age bracket, at least up until 1995). If the analysis is confined to causes of death associated with smoking and drinking, the northern crescent of excess mortality emerges, thereby emphasising the weight of regional factors in this type of behaviour whatever specific social class is under consideration (figure 9).

Social disparities in mortality are common to all regions: the ratio of the mortality rate of workers/employees to that of managers/professionals is over 1.0 throughout the country. However, this figure also follows a certain geography which seems to follow the pattern of disparities in general mortality between different regions. The highest values are seen in Brittany and the Nord-Pas-de-Calais region then the Alsace, Pays de la Loire, Picardy and Haute-Normandie regions, and the lowest values are observed in the South. In other words, the regions where general mortality rates are highest are also the regions where social disparity is most marked, and in the regions where mortality is relatively low, there is not as great a differential between the upper and the lower classes (figure 10).

Therefore, the regional context (environmental, socio-economic, cultural, etc.) constitutes a major factor in socio-geographical disparities in health status. Ecological analysis indicates that it is socio-occupational considerations which are the main determinant underlying geographical disparities in mortality, but it also shows that disparities persist between different geographical units even after compensation has been made for this type of variable. Therefore, in order to investigate interactions between socio-occupational class and social, environmental and health contexts, it is necessary to make the analyses on the basis of smaller, more relevant units.

Socio-geographical inequality in health

Figure 9 **Comparative mortality rates among people of between 25 and 54 years of age between 1987 and 1993 (all causes of death); broken down according to social class at the regional level**

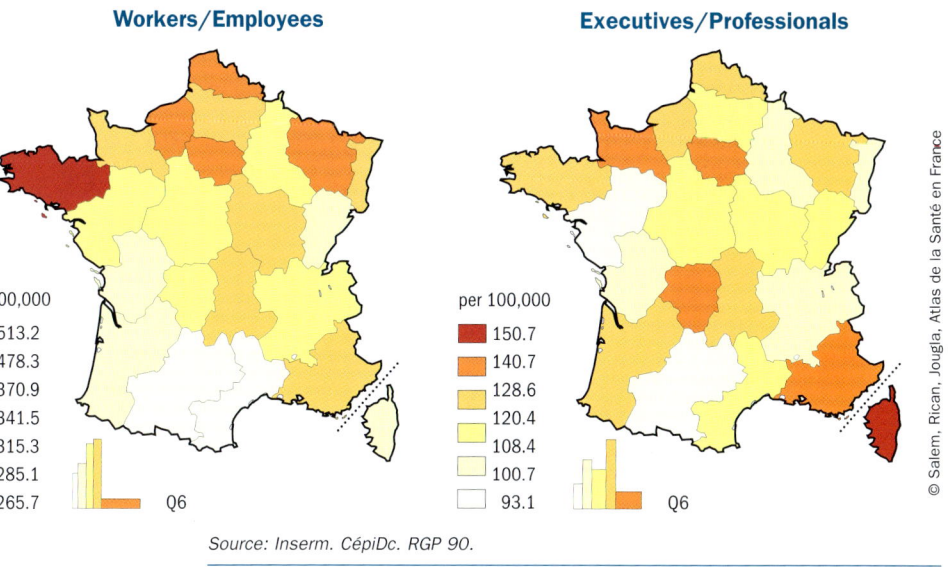

Source: Inserm. CépiDc. RGP 90.

Figure 10 **Ratios between comparative mortality rates for the "worker/employee" class and the "executive/professional" class**

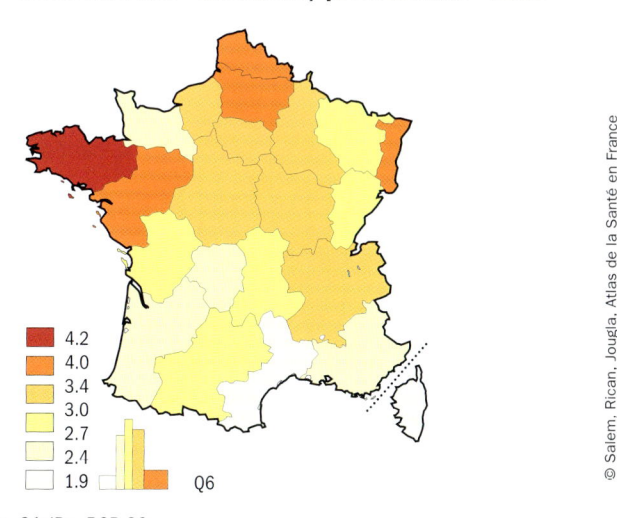

Source: Inserm. CépiDc. RGP 90.

AN INSTANCE OF SOCIO-GEOGRAPHICAL INEQUALITY: OCCUPATIONAL HAZARDS AND CANCER

It is estimated that about one-third of the socially-based mortality differential due to cancer in industrialised countries is due to occupational exposure to carcinogenic substances, and that this figure rises to about one half in the case of lung and bladder cancer [95]. And this is in a context in which cancer, as was discussed above, is the single most important medical cause of death with respect to excess mortality in male workers and employees. The fact that cancer is so commonly induced by exposure to toxic substances in the workplace means that the list of occupational diseases needs revising because only a small proportion of occupational cancers are actually treated as such: only about 500 cases in 1999 (taking all forms of cancer into account) whereas the true figure would be of the order of several thousands.

Both the importance of occupational exposure and the extent to which it is under-estimated are particularly evident in the case of lung cancer. A 1996 study of new cases of lung cancer referred to one Île-de-France hospital showed that 24% of the 123 patients who had been interviewed by an occupational health specialist were eligible for compensation for occupational disease, *i.e.* 15% of all the new cases in the department concerned in that year [103]. Although the statistics show that the number of cases of occupational disease being recognised by the social security system [55] has been steadily rising (from 7 in 1981 to 26 in 1991 and 205 in 1998), the number of cases of occupationally-induced lung cancer remains massively underestimated.

At this point in time, no French data are available to make it possible to estimate the fraction of the main diseases on the list of occupational diseases which could be caused by occupational exposure. Estimates are therefore usually based on published data from other countries. One exception is asbestos and mesothelioma: the results of the National Mesothelioma Surveillance Programme show that at least 80% to 90% of all cases of mesothelioma in France are due to occupational exposure [123].

Only 413 cases of cancer attributed to asbestos (208 cases of mesothelioma and 205 of lung cancer) were recognised as occupational in origin by the national insurance system in 1998 (with reference to tables 30 and 30bis), whereas a "low" estimate of real asbestos-related mortality in France in 1996 is of 1,950 deaths (750 from mesothelioma and 1,200 from lung cancer) [75]. Therefore, only about one-fifth of all cases of occupational, asbestos-induced cancer are recognised as such.

The likelihood that a disease induced by occupational exposure to asbestos will be recognised as an occupational disease varies enormously from place to place, *e.g.* in 1995, in the Rouen Regional Health Insurance area, 22.9 out of 100,000 employees were recognised as having fallen ill due to occupational exposure to asbestos and awarded compensation, whereas the corresponding figure in Lille was 7.9 despite the two areas being comparable in terms of risk in this respect, *e.g.* both are among those with the highest mortality rate due to pleural cancer (a good indicator for occupational exposure to asbestos) and the related death rates in each are similar. A recent study showed that the probability that a case of mesothelioma will be recognised as occupational in origin varied by a factor of as much as 13 between different regional health insurers [81].

Understanding and correcting socially-based inequality in health

A review of the literature shows that our understanding of socio-geographical disparities in health status remains very fragmented compared with that in other European countries. In particular, the social classes which have traditionally been used and the available statistical information are both inadequate in the light of the complexity of causes, as was discussed earlier in the context of geographical and socio-occupational disparities.

Understanding socially-based inequality in health is a key issue in France if the efficacy of current policies is to be gauged, and if new, better strategies are to be devised to attenuate inequality and control the effects of doing so on general health status. Such understanding will depend on research into these questions, but it will also – and perhaps primarily – depend on understanding the representations of health and its determinants in the minds of the various people concerned, *i.e.* researchers, professional health care providers, policy makers, health insurers, patients and the general public as a whole. In this perspective, an effective multifactorial model to represent all the many different health determinants is far from complete. However, we have enough information about inequality in health to begin to advance certain explanations and propose recommendations.

As discussed in the review above, since the first development of various different fields in public health, the objective has been to identify links existing between how society is organised and how disease and death are distributed within the population on the one hand, and between individual life styles and health status on the other [69]. After a century of enormous progress in both social conditions and health status-including the establishment of the health insurance system, extraordinary therapeutic advances and, more recently, hope for the future based on the field of genomics-analysis shows that significant social inequality in health persists. This France has in common with its European neighbours, *e.g.* historical analysis of mortality figures compiled in Great Britain since the 1920's (figure 11) shows:

– mortality in general – taking all causes of death and all social classes together – declined throughout the 20th Century, at a particularly fast rate at the beginning of the period (due to major advances in living conditions and standards of hygiene). It continued to fall at a lower rate in the second half of the century as a result of biomedical progress, *i.e.* improved diagnosis and treatment;

Figure 11   **Standardised mortality rates per 100,000 inhabitants in England and Wales for the richest percentile of the population and the poorest percentile between 1921 and 1983**

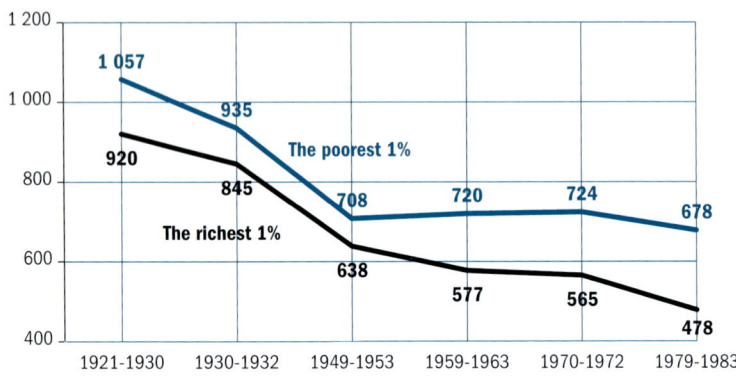

Source: taken from Najman [117].

– the differential in mortality between the richest and the poorest has been steadily growing since the 1960's, a trend which has accelerated recently so that, in relative terms, the differential is more extreme today than it was in the 1920's;
– the differential reached a minimum at a particular point in history, namely during the post-war period of reconstruction, since when they have further deteriorated despite the construction of the Welfare State and even before the economic recession of the 1970's.

Review the social classes used and identify other determinants

Whether the spotlight is on death, disease, health-related habits and behaviour patterns or individual or general care consumption, the available social indicators which are currently emphasised describe socio-economic position (in the "Weberian" sense of the term [105]) in at best an approximate fashion, and they describe living conditions even less adequately [62].

The classes usually used

Socio-economic status is classified on the basis of:
• Occupational class, *e.g.* the classic socio-occupational classes (CSP, *catégorie socioprofessionnelle*) used in France. This system has two major limitations. Firstly, it does not easily lend itself to comparison with other countries; and secondly, it tends to ignore two groups among whom health needs are particularly acute, namely those who are not in work (the unemployed and retired people) and women in general. Finally, this system fails to take

into account recent increasing disparities within the various classes, concerning salaries, forms of work (notably part-time working) and working conditions [114].
• Income, which can be normalised to a variety of denominators (per capita, per family or per household) or expressed in monetary units per consuming unit (number of adults plus number of children in the household). At the individual level, these data are difficult to obtain since total revenue includes not only stable income sources but also irregular sources of revenue, conditional revenue sources (*e.g.* social security payments), undeclared income (*e.g.* cash-in-hand work), etc.
• Educational level: analysis of this variable must necessarily take into account a person's age, their generation, historical events which occurred during their childhood (conscription, war, migration, etc.), especially when it comes to comparisons with other countries or over long periods of time, or for surveys of entire populations containing groups of all ages.
• Integrated index: all three of the above-mentioned indicators can be summarised in the form of a single, integrated index or score, *e.g.* the Duncan Socio-economic Index [74] or the Nam-Powers Socio-economic Score.
• Administrative classification systems, *i.e.* classes based on formally established legal and/or social security instruments, *e.g.* minors (those of under 18 years of age), the elderly (with a lower age limit corresponding to that of minimum ageing), retired people, those eligible for social security assistance, those benefiting from the provisions of Universal Health Insurance Coverage, the disabled (*i.e.* those who are receiving Disability Payments), etc.

Fragmentary appreciation of the situation

Even at the level of these traditional classification systems, our understanding of socially-based inequality in health in France is at best fragmented and at worst non-existent. For children, few data on health status are collected after the first few months or years of life, although the Handicap, Disability and Dependency survey has gone some way towards illuminating the situation of disabled children. Similarly, there is little data on the elderly.

In other fields, extensive amounts of data have been collected but they do not necessarily give much information about inequality because the narrow classes used were chosen for specific relevance to a certain end and often do not correspond to social class differences. This is true, for example of AIDS for which the existing results are formulated in terms of mode of transmission. The same problem affects studies of other contagious diseases like tuberculosis in which the analytical approach adopted is a "biomedical" (or etiologic) one rather than a socially based one. The presentation of road accidents and accidents at work similarly follows a logic specific to the field in question, *e.g.* for accidents in the workplace, compilation of figures on incidence per type of activity is designed to help work out the contribution different types of companies must make towards the financial burden entailed by such accidents.

Therefore, in a general way, health-related information systems are not organised to yield regular information about inequality in health in a reactive way so that data can be rapidly made available, published and compared (*e.g.* over time in order to identify trends). As a result, it is very difficult to follow changes in such inequalities, and in consequence, it is likewise difficult to judge the impact of either changing working conditions or reforms to the social or health care system. The same gaps are apparent in national exhaustive monitoring systems and in more specific monitoring and research instruments which focus on a single disease, a single mechanism of action or a single geographical sector.

The limitations of these approaches

The limitations of the approaches is that they remain basically descriptive. Although they make it possible to point up the constancy of inequalities over time and social class, they give little information, at the personal level, on the reasons why people fall into poor health and, at the collective level, on "new" determinants and social risks, *i.e.* new forms of vulnerability and inadequate social and health-related security.

From a political point of view, these class-based descriptions (sometimes, as was discussed above, calculated on the basis of categories established for the purposes of social assistance), although they make it possible to evaluate the impact of existing assistance policy and draw attention to its deficiencies, are ineffective when it comes to renewing these instruments and means of public action. In the field of health – and particularly with respect to primary prevention and access to instruments and policies of secondary prevention – higher-resolution appreciation of personal and collective social determinants and behaviour patterns is necessary to renew the approaches and implement measures which address exactly these specific situations and sets of circumstances associated with vulnerability.

Finally, at this time, accumulated knowledge in France and public health research concern the *effects* of observed inequalities (and possibly the evaluation of instruments and processes designed to control such effects) rather than the *causes* thereof. The result is, to quote a recent article in the *International Journal of Epidemiology*, *"as is demonstrated in the limited but growing literature on social inequalities in health, ignoring the social determinants of socially-based disparities in health leads to incomplete accounting for observed changes in the morbidity and mortality of populations and, in consequence, hindrance of any efforts made in the matter of prevention"* [98].

The need to take other determinants into account

The need to extend the conventional approach to inequality is perfectly illustrated by certain epidemiological results obtained by multivariate analysis of a whole series of "classic" socio-economic variables. One of many North American studies addressing racial inequalities in health shows that, even after adjustment has been made for race, income, educational level, marital status and disability, the chance that a Hispanic subject will declare (perceive) his or her state of health to be poor is still over 1 [136] (figure 12). Other variables – as yet uninvestigated – probably account for this "excess" risk. What are they?

In the last twenty years, epidemiological surveys – mostly conducted in America and Britain – have addressed social determinants using sociological and psychosocial approaches (figure 13), e.g. numerous articles have indicated that low level of social integration (as measured by a social network index) correlates well with high-risk behaviour (smoking, alcoholism, eating disorders, sedentary life style, etc.). Other articles focus on the strong association of an individual's social network with both the incidence of stroke and its specific mortality [134].

Although these hypotheses are old and were actually originally French ideas (e.g. Durkheim's research into suicide and the writings of Cassel who was the first to suggest that there might exist an epidemiological link between social support networks and morbidity), they have not yet been statistically tested in France (as they have in America and Northern Europe).

Figure 12 **Declaration of poor state of health: odds ratio estimated by multivariate analysis**

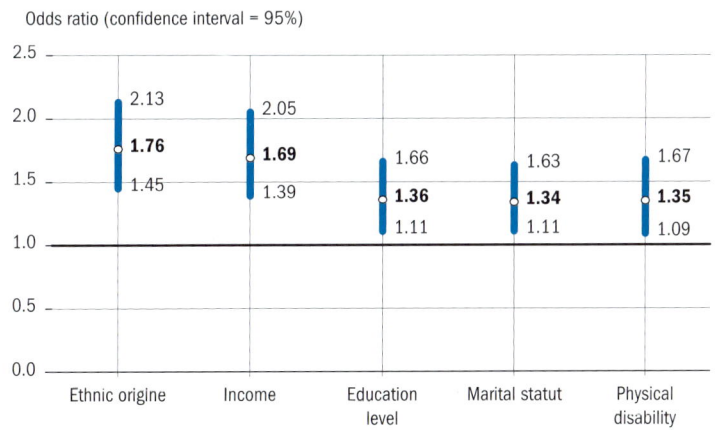

Source: US Agency for Health Care Policy and Research, 1999.

Figure 13 **Theoretical outline of health-related social and psychosocial factors**

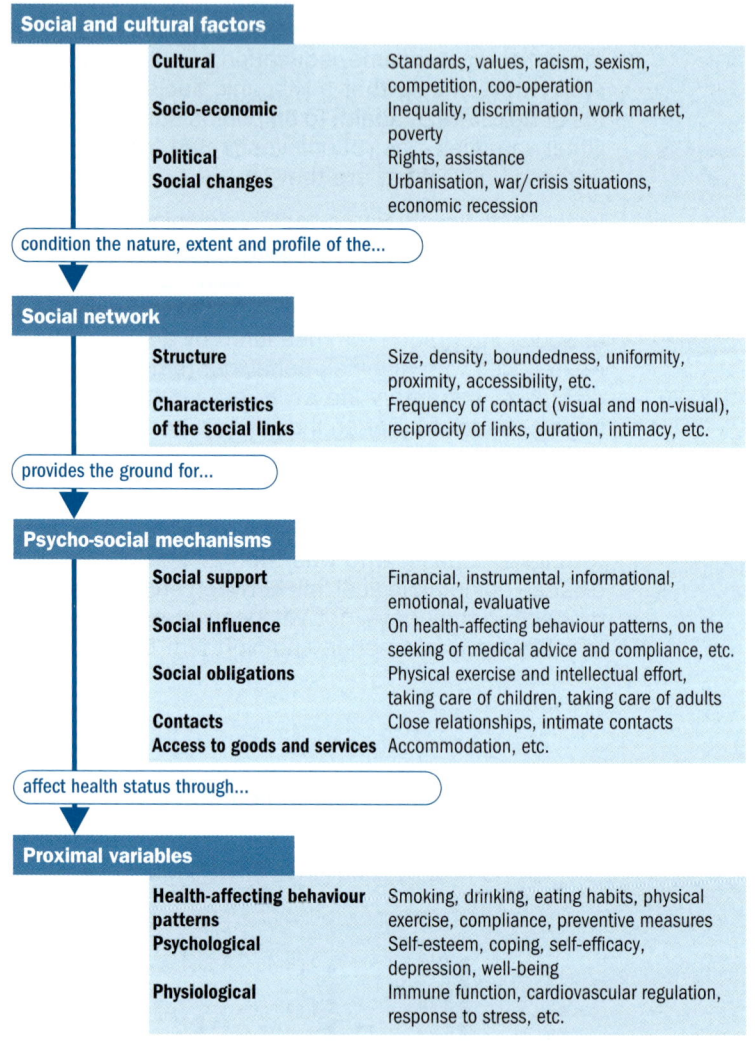

Source: taken from Berkman et Glass [50].

Epidemiological research into the impact of living conditions is also profiting from the integration of new approaches, in particular concerning working conditions and, more specifically, new forms of work-related precariousness [46]. Numerous studies on stress in the workplace and its consequences on health have been conducted in the context of a model based on "job decision latitude-psychological demand" such as that proposed by Karasek [94]. This proposes that the combination of little latitude together with strong demand is the most prejudicial to health. Another model based on "effort-compensation" (*e.g.* that developed by Siegrist [128]) takes into account effort – both extrinsic (to meet a demand formulated by co-workers) and intrinsic (to meet a demand fixed by the person him or herself) – and compensation, which may be in the form of either money, status or self esteem.

Outside of the workplace, recent epidemiological studies have attempted to take stock of what Kaplan and Lynch referred to as "neo-material conditions", *i.e.* those associated with current life in post-industrial society: eating habits, leisure activities, vacation habits, the possession of material goods, etc. [105]. In a number of recent papers, relationships – not of course necessarily causal – have been detected between these factors and personal health. Their value is to refresh the perspective and create new tools to investigate socio-economic inequalities and also situations of social precariousness and exclusion. The approach is no longer one of measuring the impact on health of belonging to some specific social class, or of being in a state of poverty or complete exclusion from society; the issue is rather "relative" or "intermediate" exclusion affecting a large fraction of the population (and an even larger fraction at some time or another), specifically the inability – even temporary – to access material goods and services which are not fundamentally necessary in the strict view but which bring pleasure and a feeling of well being, and which, in symbolic terms, constitute a sign of belonging to the leisure-centred consumer society.

An unknown factor in France: the health status of immigrants

Finally, we will address a topic on which scientific data are practically non-existent in France, that of the health of immigrants in general [77] and, in particular, the influence on access to preventive and curative health care of different emigration histories, cultural backgrounds, past and current living conditions, etc. This almost complete vacuum is explained in terms of the difficulties inherent in obtaining such scientific data and the political taboo and prejudices (both ill and well-intentioned) associated with all questions of immigration. The first explanation does not hold water given the abundant work done in other countries on this subject which could be used by French scientists for inspiration. For example, international results suggest that it is not national origin *per se* (nationality being a sensitive piece of information in the sense defined by the National Information Technology and Privacy Commission *[Commission nationale informatiques et libertés]*) which is the key factor, but rather emigration history or even past history of stigmatising experiences. On the last point, a recent literature review covered twenty-odd studies, all of which pointed to statistical links between the frequency of episodes of perceived racist treatment or discrimination and poor health (depression, psychological problems, cardiovascular disease, etc.) or failure to seek medical advice [97]. Politically, our point of view is that such research needs now to be encouraged, for a number of reasons. With respect to public health policy, it is inadmissible (and potentially dangerous for the health of the population at large) that we know nothing about the health status – specific or non-specific – of immigrants. From a more general political point of view, taboos and prejudices feed ignorance, so this priority must be clearly signalled, profiting from the fact that global economic improvement in our country raises, both more acutely and also more passionately, the question of public solidarity issues in the context of the most vulnerable individuals and populations.

Consider health determinants at the level of both the individual and the community

Among the various indicators used for area-based analyses, the most common are median income per inhabitant, the proportion of the population living below the poverty line, median educational level, the unemployment rate, the proportion of households receiving assistance from the social security system, the proportion of manual workers, etc. Any of these may be considered in isolation, or combined in the form of an index [130]. Used massively whenever personal information is unavailable to investigate links between socio-economic situation and state of health, these measurements are nevertheless often criticised, in this case, for the methodological bias introduced in the demonstration.

Multi-level analysis...

However recent studies have shown that it is useful to combine – using multi-level statistical analysis methods [135] – such community variables (*i.e.* to describe a context to which the individual is exposed) with personal variables [93]. One of the first studies to use this type of approach was carried out in 1987 in the County of Alameda in the United States and it showed that those living in a poor neighbourhood were more likely to die prematurely at adult age, even after adjustment for a whole series of personal socio-economic variables [82].

However, even in such multi-level analysis, the distinction between a contextual explanation (which is what one is looking for) and a "skewed composition" (introduced by how the data were collected) remains difficult to pin down [70]. Some European studies have shown that, in contrast, there is little link between local socio-economic differences and the frequency of abusive smoking and drinking or psychiatric morbidity, once the subjects' personal characteristics had been taken into account or if community characteristics were integrated otherwise [66, 71, 125].

... for comparing different countries or different regions

Many experts attest to the value of the multi-level approach when it comes to trying to compare different countries [106], and it is true that the physical and health environment, the quality and availability of services (not just health-related services) and socio-cultural characteristics probably have a "collective" influence on the links detected between personal socio-economic characteristics and health status (as well as modes of care consumption). Collective in the sense that these characteristics do not simply correspond to the sum of the personal characteristics [110]. This type of work also contributes to the attempt to regionalise health policy currently underway in many other European countries as well as France. It provides detailed information (at the relevant local socio-economic scale) to decision-makers responsible for defining health needs and allocating resources for regionally-based care provision.

Integrate inequality in health into the analysis of precariousness and exclusion

Among researchers, decision-makers, health professionals and the public in general, there is an implicit prejudice underlying reflections, positions and active measures: that of distinguishing between the question of inequality in health from that which deals with the health status of those in the direst straits (precariousness or social exclusion) and their access to treatment and care.

Exclusion, precariousness and inequality

In France, certain experts have perfectly described the success – at the level of both media and politics – of the idea of social exclusion which term became synonymous with "area for public action" in the 1980's [49] while the question of inequality (especially in the field of health) still represents a public taboo, confronting not only cherished ideas in our welfare state but also the objectives of redistribution of our social coverage system at a time when the priority is to reduce government expenditure and taxation [111].

Strong personal, collective and professional representations respond to these distinctions: it is always someone else who is excluded – a research subject, a patient, a beneficiary – never me. From this point of view, the concepts of precariousness, marginalisation and vulnerability [45, 58, 59, 121] (which are often used synonymously although each describes something else: cumulative and often transient processes) have probably not succeeded in changing these representations.

These experiences of precariousness or vulnerability (financial, economic, professional, familial, emotional, etc.) concern a large part, probably the major part, of the population whereas the most serious outcome (poverty or full-blown social exclusion) only affects a small number of people right at the bottom of the social ladder, this ladder representing a continuum – with poorly defined rungs – between social integration and social exclusion. Therefore, studying those who are excluded and evaluating the instruments which are supposed to take care of them – and also those responsible for people in a situation of precariousness – seems to us worthwhile, not only for what it will reveal about these people but also for what it will reveal about social risks (conventional or "novel") in the field of health, the extreme diversity of paths towards precariousness and the (un)suitability of our health care and social coverage systems with respect to the needs of people in general [61].

An integrated approach based on "social determinants of health status" in the broadest sense

If, on the one hand, studies of the health status of people in a precarious situation raise the question of *"why people in the most precarious position prioritise other values at the expense of their health"* [51] and if, on the other hand, the question raised by observation of the persistence of inequalities in health is indeed one of knowing what, in people's lives – from the point of view of the conditions of their social, familial and professional lives, and their social environment and how they interact or do not interact with this environment, their past history, etc. – determine (to what extent and in which direction) their health status, it appears that these two approaches must necessarily be integrated into that, more global, of research into the social determinants of health status.

In terms of political action, such integration seems equally necessary. Above and beyond the urgency with respect to health and society represented by situations of acute exclusion (the homeless [78], illegal immigrants, desocialised drug addicts [52, 87], etc.) and, even if specific measures ("low threshold" access instruments, outreach programs, medical shelter programmes, etc.) are necessary to take care of these populations, these programmes cannot and should not dispense with the need for an overall policy which, at the same time, attempts to reduce socially-based inequality in health and, in the end, reduces the risk of social exclusion. As pointed out by the British experts M. Shaw and G. Davey Smith, *"in the long term, the best way to grasp the compromised health of excluded people is to pursue policies which lead to the greatest possible equality [...]. All the studies show that the most economically egalitarian societies – those in which social cohesion is at a maximum – are the healthiest"* [127]. Thus, in the above-mentioned continuum between vulnerability, precariousness and exclusion, long term global policies are required, policies which take into account the disparate (if such is the case) needs of all under consideration.

Broaden the theoretical model of health and its determinants

A better understanding of social inequalities in health is necessary in our country if we are to be able to evaluate the impact of current policies and develop new ones to mitigate inequality and/or control the effects on health. Such understanding necessarily comes from research into these questions, but also – and perhaps primarily – from considerations of the representations of health and its determinants among all the various players concerned, *i.e.* researchers, professional care providers, political decision-makers, health insurers, patients and the general public.

Beyond seeking medical advice and treatment

It is striking how extraordinarily limited the scope of the theoretical models of health is for many professionals, decision-makers and scientists in France. In the mid-1990's, Evans and Stoddart criticised the poverty of a conceptual approach based on simple feedback – if rather simplistic – between health and the health care system (figure 14) and proposed an alternative model which has the double advantage of repositioning the question of access to care (and therefore to biomedical technological progress) in the context of questions – important in another way – about social determinants of health, and putting in perspective the concept of health and its determinants with respect to the more general question of personal well-being. They also emphasised that *"from the point of view of personal well-being and social performance (including economic productivity), the key factor is the individual's perception of his or her own state of health and functional capacity"* [76].

This, apart from the classic epidemiological approaches which are limited in that they are essentially descriptive, as discussed above, alternative approaches – novel in France – aimed at conceiving health from the point of view of attitudes and behaviour patterns seem promising to us for research into the particular causes and/or determinants to be taken into account in a perspective of public health and public action.

The role of psychosocial and behavioural characteristics

This objective requires research based on gathering original personal information from the general population or from people belonging to specific social groups, taking into account, as well as characteristics (personal or of the community) relevant to living conditions or conditions of social integration, what are referred to as *"intermediate variables"* [61], *i.e.* personal psychosocial or behavioural characteristics such as representations of health, the attention paid to personal health, the ranking of health among other personal priorities, self-esteem, adaptability, interiorisation of medical norms and prior or familial experiences of disease and care consumption, etc.

Such research into health-related behaviour patterns is well established in Britain and America, in particular research into Health

Figure 14 **From a simple model based on feedback between state of health and the health care system, to models which incorporate social determinants of health**

The simple feedback model

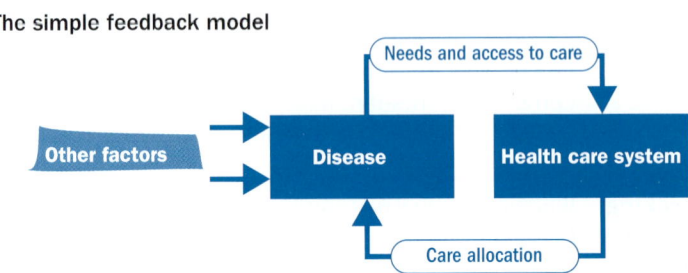

The social-determinant-based model

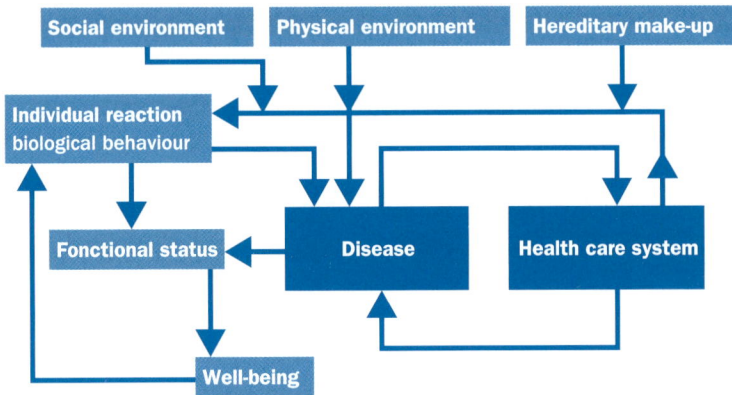

Source: taken from Evans et Stoddart [76].

Belief Models which, since the 1950's, has been accumulating evidence to show a close relationship between beliefs and seeking medical advice or following medical instructions, the use of prevention programmes, the modification of prejudicial behavioural traits (addiction, sexual behaviour patterns, etc.).

Reference can also be made to other research in Britain and America, still in the field of health, into the influence of health-related familial behaviour patterns – or "family production" [132] – on the interactions between representations in terms of control, coping, and perceptions of self-efficacy, between fears and motivations in terms of health protection, etc. [80]. The accumulation of such results – mostly from North America – shows in a convincing fashion, on the one hand the extent to which these determinants are distributed in society (if determined) and, on the other hand, to what point behavioural and psychosocial factors are linked to state of health and the willingness to seek medical advice. Conducted in social frameworks quite different from France, their conclusions and limitations cannot be simply transposed and these factors deserve systematic investigation in this country.

The value of the longitudinal approach

Longitudinal approaches are also worth developing, in particular those aimed at, by means of following (ideally in a prospective fashion) cohorts over a long period of time in order to investigate the long-term effects on health of the accumulation of periods (possibly retrospectively) during which individuals have been having problems. Although some retrospective French studies have suggested that serious events in childhood may have an adverse impact on adult health [112] and many others have described, in a transverse way, the state of health of populations in difficulty, little is known about outcomes in people who have had transient experiences of poverty or social exclusion.

Understanding and prevention

When it comes to public health, the essential objective of conducting research into the social determinants of health status remains prevention. It is often forgotten that, apart from in the case of contagious disease and immunisation, despite the successes of clinical epidemiology and prophylactic treatment, medical risk factors – detectable test abnormalities of exposure to toxic substances – have only ever been able to account for a fraction – and a relatively small fraction at that – of the overall incidence of disease and causes of death (in particular chronic disease).

The "grey area" of personal inequality in health

To re-examine an example reported by Marmot in 1998 [110] concerning the relative risk of death from cardiovascular disease with respect to risk factors according to rank in the British Civil Service, it emerges, after stock has been taken of known (and today very well-characterised) cardiovascular risk factors, that an extremely large fraction of the risk remains unaccounted for, and that this fraction increases with decreasing rank.

On the basis of this seminal finding, it appears that part of this "grey area", these unknown risk factors, is probably genetic in origin, and that the other part is socially determined. It is nevertheless important to remember that the characterisation of genetic risk factors in the case of chronic diseases which are dependent on multiple genes (and to an even greater extent their applications in public health and preventive medicine strategies and programmes) constitute a long-term endeavour and that (even if interindividual variability with respect to susceptibility to disease and chance of cure is shown to be genetically determined in the future) only a fraction – probably very small – of social inequality in health will be accounted for by such genetic variability. It remains then that a significant fraction – probably most in some diseases – of cases could be avoided if the effects of social determinants of disease were known and could be controlled.

Scientific ...and political challenges

From the point of view of research, many studies in the field of the social epidemiology and sociology of health are yet to be conducted if we are to put ourselves in a position of being able to describe and understand the various determinants of health, provide decision-makers with the information they need to develop public health policies specifically aimed at reducing observed areas of inequality, and evaluate such policies, programmes and instruments. In practice, although certain research issues remain unresolved at this time (*e.g.* research into underlying biological mechanisms, as yet poorly characterised apart from the relationship between physiological responses to stress on the one hand and coronary heart disease or immune responses on the other [54], but also, as has already been discussed, research into interactions between social and genetic determinants of disease, or again the construction of novel hypotheses and their demonstration using the methods of social science), the political challenge, in the end, is how to improve our understanding so we can better act and prevent disease.

Although overcoming inequality in health goes well beyond the scope of health policy (of course, employment policy, urban policy, the National Education system, redistributive fiscal policy, etc. all have an impact on inequality in health which is probably greater than that of strictly defined health policy), it seems to us that generalisation of the political approach leads to a risk of fatalism and inertia. In contrast, certain health-related measures, even if they are insufficient in themselves to eradicate inequality, may contribute to the problem and deserve to be made priorities, as some of our European neighbours have done.

For example, controlling the impact on health of situations of social vulnerability involves improving the efficiency with which such situations are detected by the existing care and assistance instruments; by improving the accessibility and effective exposure to prevention programmes; by expanding screening programmes to include, above and beyond contagious and chronic diseases, mental problems, health problems in adolescents, violence (both within and outside of the family); by a general reformulation of care provision to create a rational set of integrated services (of health promotion and social support for preventive and curative care) and matched to the demands and needs of people, rather than a fragmented system which requires on the part of its users the initiative to identify, adapt and learn. From this point of view, health strategies and policies to reduce inequality are a priority because they are intimately interconnected with another priority, that of ensuring equitable, high-quality health care in the broadest sense. Although throughout the industrialised countries of Europe there is a unanimous feeling that equitable access to high-quality primary curative health care and the most modern specialist care is not enough, reducing inequality in health will involve prevention and compensating for the effects of social determinants of health status.

Take-home lessons now

Globally therefore, inequality in health constitutes one of the aspects (and consequences) of general social inequality, with particular reference to income, housing conditions, educational level, employment and working conditions.

The effects of these parameters on health involves many different and diverse mechanisms, but these are to a large extent identifiable even if their social differentiation is not fully demonstrated.

Thus, for dental health, certain eating habits and certain preventive measures are key factors in children whereas for adults, the seeking of (or failure to seek) help has a major impact on observed inequality. Eating habits and differential participation in sporting activities likewise plays a role in childhood obesity.

Certain forms of behaviour are associated with various causes of death in adults. An ever-increasing body of evidence is accumulating of the negative effects of what can be referred to as "social stress" and stress in the workplace, whether it be on the outcome of pregnancy or (for stress in the workplace) cardiovascular and musculoskeletal problems.

Care – which has for a long time been mistakenly put to the fore among all the various determinants of health status – is nevertheless a major factor, but as important are the factors which determine whether medical advice is sought in the first place (and the accessibility of such care, either in geographical terms or, in particular, in financial terms) and the quality of the care provided (which is itself geographically diversified if not socially determined[2]).

In certain areas, care does not in any way account for the observed inequality (the risk of accident, for example). In other examples, *e.g.* heart disease and cancer, questions about the role of care must be preceded by determination of the factors associated with

---

2. It has been shown in American and English as well as French studies that social discrimination in medical practice can result in differential care provision (including preventive care) according to patients' sociological backgrounds.

the incidence of the lethal problem (whether the problem is fatal or not once the diagnosis is established). Thus, for coronary heart disease, social inequality in terms of incidence refers back to primary prevention when social differences in lethality are less obviously interpreted, with questions about the seriousness of the initial disease, the use and dispensing of care, and the psychosocial context [101].

Nevertheless, as was seen for mortality (in particular, premature death in men), it is clear that a significant fraction of the observed social inequality cannot be attributed to inequitable curative care but to certain forms of behaviour (themselves associated with living conditions) and working conditions. This does not mean that more ambitious prevention instruments – in particular primary prevention – which have been accorded more resources and are better matched to needs (specifically targeting those social groups which are at the highest risk, but also broadly integrated into medical and social care structures) might not make a key contribution to reducing observed inequality in health status.

MENTAL HEALTH, SOCIAL INEQUALITY AND LIVING CONDITIONS

If mental health is seen as a component of a person's social life, the question of the relationship between mental health and living conditions – taking both in the broadest possible sense – is right at the heart of the question of inequality in health. In analogy to other forms of health, mental health can be seen not only as one of the consequences of past difficulties but also as one of the "causes" of current social and financial problems.

Much has been written about social inequality in mental health but the field remains poorly characterised, partly because it is so difficult to investigate. As Lovell pointed out, it has been shown in something like one hundred epidemiological surveys (in both America and Europe) conducted since the 1940's that mental disease (psychosis, antisocial behaviour, substance abuse, depression, etc.) tends to be more common in deprived communities [104]. In the intervening years, the way in which mental disease is defined – and therefore studied – has changed significantly. Up until the 1980's, mental problems were seen in the context of a continuum between health and disease. A person's psychosocial environment can affect his/her position in this continuum and thereby trigger disease. Since then, in particular with the publication of the Version IV of the Diagnostic and Statistical Manual of Mental Disorders (DSM IV) by the American Psychiatric Association, the tendency has been to treat mental problems as discreet entities in which the individual is either affected or not by a set of specific, serious symptoms which define a certain mental pathology.

The scarcity of data on the general population

In the last twelve years, three major epidemiological studies have been conducted in France on representative cross-sections of the general population, all based on a standardised psychiatric diagnostic approach. Of these, only two provide data on socio-economic status. In the first (conducted in the Île-de-France region), serious depression was found to be more common in people receiving the RMI (twice as common among the men, and 1.4 time as common among the women) [96]. The other data comes from the Credes Health and Social Coverage survey. Work status was the socio-economic factor most closely related to the incidence of depression: compared with an incidence of 8% in working men, 32% of those not currently in work (including 24% of all unemployed men) were suffering from depression; in women, depression affected 44% of those not working, and just 19% of those in work. The prevalence of depression is particularly closely related to socio-occupational status among women, affecting 23% of working class women, 16% of craftswomen and managers, and 15% of farmers. In men, educational level gives the most convincing correlation: 17% of men at the lowest educational level were found to be suffering from depression, a level which is 2.5 times higher than that seen among university graduates.

Mental health, and living and working conditions

Various explanations are proposed to account for these links. The first is that they result (at least in part) from artefacts of the measuring process: certain behaviour patterns or experiences might be mistakenly taken for evidence of mental problems, *e.g.* because certain cultural groups are over-represented among the poor or because of extreme cases (*e.g.* sleep quality is unsurprisingly poor among the homeless, or because of the suspicion and fears of illegal immigrants).

The second involves genetic determinism, *e.g.* it has been extensively shown that schizophrenia has a considerable genetic component (although environmental factors may well be key in triggering the disease).

The third involves social causality, *e.g.* it has been shown in cohort studies of groups of people confronted with difficulties that unemployment is associated with an increased incidence of depression and alcoholism. Other studies have revealed other factors linked to depression, *e.g.* major upheavals (divorce, separation, etc.) and extreme stress (rape, war, serious accidents, environmental catastrophes, etc.). Finally, research conducted in the workplace has revealed links between work-related stress (particularly the combination of strong psychological demand coupled with little job decision latitude) and psychological distress or depression. Gazel's cohort study of employees of the French Electricity utility (EDF/GDF) showed that the incidence of depression in both the men and the women depended on the extent of the social support they received and the level of stress associated with their work, and this independently of other risk factors [120].

As Lovell observed, *"social class needs to be defined better with respect to this analytical criterion. It would be interesting to see whether employment classes redrawn according to this criterion rather than on the basis of social prestige, income and educational level would give a different gradient for the prevalence of mental disorders [...]. As well as developing classification systems which correspond to the reality of social divisions in the modern work place, it is also important to examine new characteristics: the demand for productivity, the need to handle uncertainty, and flexibility of independence coupled with isolation"* [104].

From the "syndrome of exclusion" to "ordinary depressive problems"

Much qualitative sociological and psycho-sociological work has been carried out on the relationship between mental health and living conditions.

At the extreme end of poverty, certain authors talk about the "syndrome of exclusion" which results from a "process of rejection", *i.e.* *"processes of abasement and mistrust – whether introspective or social in origin – as a consequence of which persons cease to recognise themselves and cease to be recognised as independent subjects, and, as such, worthy of respect"* [109]. This syndrome with its triplet of features of shame, despair and emotional/cognitive inhibition corresponds to a particular mental condition which is different from any described in conventional psychiatry, and which is often complicated by alcoholism and/or drug addiction [108]. Its prevalence in at-risk populations remains to be established on an epidemiological basis, and how to manage the problem – at both the psychiatric and the social level – also remains an as yet unanswered question.

Other studies have specifically addressed psychosocial suffering and conditions which do not correspond to any recognised mental disease (ill-being, relational problems, depressive symptoms, etc.). One such study based on in-depth interviews tackled the kinds of difficulty associated with degraded working conditions (precarious situation, risk of redundancy, moral pressure, etc.), principal among which difficulties are the feeling of uselessness, culpability and exhaustion. It found a link between extreme working conditions and feelings of tiredness, loss of energy and shame or humiliation. The author concluded that understanding mechanisms of "self-destruction" (those which lead the most vulnerable to wear themselves out thereby paving the way for frank depression) *"is not designed to encourage the tendency to treat (either psychiatrically or with drugs) the small upsets of everyday life but might, in contrast, contribute to consolidating the social resources which help build social identities and interpersonal relationships"* [88]. This type of work-aimed at prevention and treatment-deserves emulation.

Finally, in the field of mental health – to a greater extent than in that of somatic health – knowledge which is currently sparse and fragmented needs to be integrated even though the "social question" on these subjects appears clearly primordial. In the same way and for many different reasons – which are as much to do with specific professional cultures and methodological difficulties as they are to the resources invested and, generally, to the place reserved for mental health in French health policy – original experimental initiatives are emerging (*e.g.* centres for exchange and advice, centres for the unemployed, integrated social and psychiatric units, etc.), both in the scientific literature and in public health strategy, although thus far, there has been little evaluation of the results and not many reproducible models have been established.

HEALTH AND INEQUALITY/ HEALTH AND POVERTY: THE NEED FOR A UNIFIED APPROACH

Research into inequality in health and the impact of precariousness is based on one of two different approaches.

The existence of social inequality in health has long been recognised and quantitatively monitored in France, specifically by means of mortality indicators since the 1970's. But this approach itself was the secondary product of research into mortality: it was not undertaken in response to a social demand; the only social demand – essentially addressed to the Insee and Credoc and then the Credes – concerned unequal care consumption. And for thirty years, the awareness of socially-based differential mortality patterns had little impact other than on the rhetoric of decision-makers and representatives of the poorest in society. Neither did it stimulate further research. The question of "how and why do such disparities appear?" was long attributed – without any firm evidence – to "poor living conditions". French researchers certainly contributed information on the disparities, but more through research into risk factors and determinants of such and such a disease, rather than directly addressing the victims of inequality. This meant that no specific instruments were established to identify and rank the main types of inequality, nor to try to construct frameworks of thought on the conditions and social and physiological factors which promote inequality. On the other hand, much research has been conducted abroad especially following the Black report in Great Britain. France is behind in this new field of intense national research, the objectives of which are not primarily social but rather seek to deepen our theoritical approach to the central question "Why are some people healthy and others not?*"

In contrast, operational perspectives are very present in work concerning the relationship between precariousness and health. In the second half of the 1990's, the man in the street could see for himself every day how degraded was the state of health of the homeless, social workers could cite health problems as one of the most important difficulties of a broader circle of people and families in a situation of "precariousness", and hospital doctors could only react with perplexity and pragmatism to the change in some groups of their patients, whose situation and attitudes they failed to completely understand. The social demand for knowledge comes from many sources, including medical and social institutions, politicians, patient support groups and other non-profit-making organisations, etc. The investigative approach is not characterised by the same questions as the issue of inequality. The first operational objective is "What can be done?" with "How can precariousness and health be co-ordinated" second, and the theoretical question far behind. The approach of the researchers themselves, be they sociologists or epidemiologists, is characterised by this context: by concentrating on a particular population and its own concrete problems, they are led to identify more accurately, to examine what, for the population, health means and to study its relationship with the health care system.

Research carried out in these two contexts contributes a consistent and complementary overview of phenomena which are obviously not unrelated.

Precariousness and vulnerability

Populations in a difficult financial situation, for whom tomorrow is uncertain, are mostly at the bottom of the social ladder by whatever standard is used for assessment (educational level, income, relational capital, etc.). What emerges most strongly from international and French research into inequality, taking the entire social scale into account, is that there exists an overall gradient, all disease included. Not only is mortality higher at the bottom of the scale, but almost all diseases are more common. Independent of any question about relationship with the health care system, it is therefore reasonable to concentrate on those populations in situations of precariousness and vulnerability, i.e. those people who are at highest risk of disease.

In France at least, smoking and drinking figure among the reasons for social disparity in health: workers smoke and drink more than managers. The situation of precariousness (risk of redundancy, unstable employment, lack of resources, homelessness, etc.) generates enough anxiety in and of itself to exacerbate these types of behaviour. In Great Britain and Canada, analyses [110] adjusted to take stock of this phenomenon have led to a particularly interesting conclusion which directly concerns populations living in precariousness: working in a subordinate job with no room for manœuvre or initiative is a risk factor for poor health, a phenomenon for which the underlying mechanisms are beginning to emerge, particularly in the field of cardiovascular disease.

In terms of state of health, situations of precariousness can therefore be continuously analysed across all social classes and, in a fairly consistent way, we can expect to see links between poor social situation and poor health. This would make it legitimate to require those responsible for formulating public health policy to pay more attention to those who every body agrees are the most vulnerable.

Health problems and the vicious circle of precariousness

The fact of the existence of a vulnerable population living in precarious conditions is reinforced by two other facts, qualitatively confirmed by extensive sociological research (notably into disability) conducted in the milieu concerned but difficult to quantify. Three observations can be made.

1. Effect of selection, notably in the world of work, affects sick people or those in delicate health. This effect is probably all the more important now the economic situation affords employers choice of those that can be expected to be the most productive from an abundant pool of manual labour. Looking for a job can involve health information which is incompatible with stable, integrated working life (part time work, the inability to cope with physical effort or prolonged mental strain). If it can be considered as a "product" of precariousness, delicate health can therefore be at its root. It is easy to see how a vicious circle can become established between health problems, financial difficulties and professional insertion. Thus, in many cases, managing a health problem can enable the person to break the vicious circle and find more stable employment.

2. In such self-propagating phenomena, mental health plays a central role. All social workers and non-profit-making organisations involved in the fight against precariousness have long talked about the frequency among those in difficult living conditions of depression, other psychological problems, and the taking of psychotropic drugs, usually associated with "feeling bad" rather than frank mental disease. The picture is consistent (although imprecise) between these on-the-ground observations, confirmed by epidemiological and sociological research, and hypotheses advanced to understand instances of socially-based inequality in health, in which mental health may be an important component of the causal factors.

3. These observations explain why the term "destabilising" is to be preferred to the word "precariousness": the ongoing, adverse process with its accompanying uncertainty as to the future is as likely to endanger health as an installed state of poverty or exclusion. Talking about processes leads, among other things, to including in the observation, not only a more confined circle of excluded people, but a broader group of financially and socially threatened populations at risk because of their economic situation, their immediate environment in poor neighbourhoods, and cultural factors. Measures to help them break out of the above-mentioned vicious circle can therefore be addressed to all these populations.

---

* R. Evans and Th. Marmor *"Why are some people healthy and others not?"* [76].

THE RELATIONSHIP BETWEEN POVERTY, HEALTH AND HEALTH CARE

Finally, studying questions of health in those living or on their way to a situation of precariousness yields data which support the importance of health problems. These data concern the attitudes of the people and groups concerned, and the difficult characteristics of their relationship with the health care system. Two observations illustrate the specific attitudes of those living in precariousness vis-à-vis the health care system.

Whereas it is implicitly understood in today's developed societies that "good health is the most precious commodity" (sub-text: how to preserve good health in both the short and the medium term comes before any other priority), questions of health may be pushed back to the second rank if there is doubt about survival or in an atmosphere of general uncertainty (*e.g.* due to a lack of resources or accommodation, or difficulty in close relationships). The poor and those living in precarious conditions are not the only ones to have an ambiguous attitude to health in the long-term (whence various well-documented problems such as the fact that not all populations have the same attitude to prevention). And this phenomenon may even go as far as the failure to take into account immediate health alerts, rare in better integrated milieus.

The corollary to relegating health to a secondary priority is the frequency of high-risk behaviour. Apart from the best characterised instances (smoking and drinking), other forms of high-risk behaviour (dangerous driving, violence, addiction, etc.) are often associated with poverty. Qualitative analysis reveals the complex etiology of such behaviour patterns. These attitudes can contribute to erecting a bar-

rier between patients in a situation of precariousness and professional health care providers:
– Consistent with the above-mentioned attitudes is the delaying of seeking medical advice. Most of the relevant data were acquired prior to the installation of Universal Medical Coverage, at which time financial obstacles certainly represented the most significant component of such reluctance, including poor compliance with the prescription, often notified by the care providers. The financial problem is now largely overcome but, in proportions which it is obviously not at the moment possible to measure, other obstacles probably remain, consisting of a combination of questions of money, culture, attention to health, confidence in care providers, and understanding of drugs and therapeutic procedures.
– This set of behaviour patterns, which are fundamentally at odds with medical culture and the philosophy of the profession, are difficult to understand for the professionals. Studies of people attending specialist centres established to cater to the uninsured clearly reveal a double need, corresponding to different histories of precariousness: for some, a need to be treated like an ordinary patient in an ordinary, non-humiliating setting; and for others, a need for care providers who "understand" patients with unusual histories or behaviour patterns. Only the patients themselves are in a position to decide which suits them – which probably justifies leaving the choice of which type of structure to consult to them. This therefore means establishing – despite the existence of measures to guarantee universal health coverage – special units to treat those living in precariousness who become sick.

Public policy to mitigate inequality in health

As we have seen, disparities and inequalities in health status have multiple causes, the most important of which have nothing to do with the health care system. Policy in almost any field designed to mitigate social inequality and regional differences is likely to have some effect – direct or indirect – on health status. In general, the effects of these policies on health are not evaluated because this is not their primary purpose.

Although combating inequalities and disparities in health necessitates global policies, nevertheless, players in the health care system have a role to play in broadcasting their point of view in democratic debates on policy in other areas (employment, housing, transportation, leisure activities, environment, culture, etc.) and, most of all, by initiating measures designed to push the health care system towards increased fairness because, as we have seen, it is itself a source of inequality and disparity.

In confrontation with socially based disparities in health, mention could be made of four public policy areas in addition to charitable initiatives: the establishment of social security coverage for the long-term unemployed (RMI, *Revenu minimum d'insertion*) in 1988, the 1998 Law against exclusion, the establishment of Universal Medical Insurance Coverage in 1999, and the December 2000 Ruling of the Ministerial Municipalities Committee to support the creation of municipal health units. Patient support groups are showing an ever-increasing willingness to take the health problems of underprivileged people into account and, although they are already playing a significant role in this area, this role can only grow in the future.

According to some experts, these policies are designed to combat exclusion, not inequality. However, it can be defended that policies against exclusion, *i.e.* those that specifically target the needs of people at risk of exclusion, namely populations in a precarious situation, are essential tools in the fight against inequality. This for two reasons:
- if they improve the situation of the most under-privileged, they may reduce inequality;
- by targeting excluded people or people in a precarious situation, these policies may also have an impact on broader populations, if only as a result of consideration of the ways in which the health and social systems are operating poorly.

The 1998 HCPH Report on the link between precariousness and health has it that those who are currently affected by the phenomena of precariousness – who have been recently and who are at risk of being so in the near future – represent a significant fraction of the population (between 12 and 15 million people, according to different estimates, *i.e.* 20 to 25% of the population as a whole). Working directly with this population is essential if inequality in health is to be overcome. However, this should not preclude broader consideration on the causes underlying such inequality and the ways of correcting it.

Let us briefly review the four above-mentioned policies designed to combat exclusion.

Creation of the *Revenu minimum d'insertion*

Receipt of the *Revenu minimum d'insertion* affects the long-term unemployed people at whom it is targeted in three different ways. By ensuring a stable income, the RMI helps people organise their lives better and meet their most urgent needs. Therefore, they eat better and can find accommodation more easily. All policies aimed at providing for minimum needs (adult disability benefit, single parent benefit, minimum old age pension, etc.) have the same objective. The RMI represents a safety net, a differential income which adds on to other resources to provide the recipient with a minimum. In addition, health care costs for RMI beneficiary are reimbursed at 100%. Finally, payment of the RMI depends on a reinsertion contract which covers the person's health care needs: the signing of the reinsertion contract makes it possible to seek, together with the beneficiary, responses to his or her specific problems, notably with respect to health problems. Moreover, it is the occasion for the various collaborators to identify the needs of the most under-privileged and allocate the major resources required for re-insertion (610 million euros) to construct suitable responses for local needs. It is therefore possible to formulate measures aimed at social and occupational re-insertion which cover the health needs of those concerned: a consultation with a psychologist or a dietician during courses, occupational reinsertion initiatives integrated with the monitoring of subjects who are tackling their alcoholism, facilitated access to free mental health consultations, help with parentality, etc.

The Law against exclusion (July 29 1998)

The Law against exclusion (July 29 1998) also has a dual advantage with respect to health problems. It is a global political initiative to tackle the causes of exclusion across the board. By providing for instruments in the fields of employment and housing policy, it has an impact on the health of the people concerned. In the field of health policy, the Law includes six sections, not all of which are equal in importance (regional programmes to enhance access to prevention and care (Praps, *Programmes régionaux d'accès à la prévention et aux soins*), the establishment of Health Care Access Offices (Pass), alcohol-related issues, lead poisoning, a report on the school medical service, and a comparison of the performance of different administrative divisions in the fight against tuberculosis) and are announced in Article 67: *"improving access to prevention and care for the least privileged in society constitutes a primary objective of health policy. Public health programmes implemented by the State, more local administrative structures and health insurance institutions take into account the specific difficulties of the least privileged"*[3].

The Law launches regional programmes to enhance access to prevention and care[4], the design and implementation of which are the responsibility of the Prefect of the corresponding Region. These programmes were conceived in a three-step process: analysis of the problems encountered by people in a situation of precariousness with respect to accessing prevention and care, and the resources available for remedying these problems; definition of priority areas for action in the period 2000 to 2002; and scheduling of measures to be implemented at the local, departmental and regional levels. Evaluation of the first generation of 26 such programmes [131] shows that:
– they have created a regional dynamic by virtue of the direct participation of players on the ground who are concerned by these problems; they make it possible to improve co-ordination of the various existing forms of intervention and promote "bridges" between social, medico-social and medical structures, between care provision, prevention and re-insertion, and between hospitals and care provision outside of hospitals;
– they have provided the means to test a genuine example of political regulation of regional health programmes by creating the Regional Health Policy Committee.

More than 10,000 people have been involved in the setting up of these regional programmes which have resulted in 1,100 different initiatives. The programmes and initiatives are due to be evaluated in 2002 when the second generation of such programmes are going to be prepared (the programmes to run from 2003 to 2005).

In the Spring of 2000, the Health and Social Affairs Inspection Bureau (Igas, *Inspection générale des affaires sociales*) published a report on how implementation of the Law against exclusion is going ahead, in which it judged that the regional programmes are *"a useful instrument, the scope of which needs to be specified"*. The opinion was that *"State services have set up a system to identify all the needs at the Departmental level, but the mobilisation of partners-as provided for in the regional programmes-is unequal"*. The report recommended enhancing communication and co-ordination, developing better links with regional health

---
3. Article L. 1411-4 of the Public Health Code.
4. Article L. 1411-5 of the Public Health Code.

plans, and recognition of the central role of such programmes in health-related prevention and education policies.

In the hospital field, the Law against exclusion consolidated the hospitals' social functions and provided for the creation of Health Care Access Offices (Pass, *Permanences d'accès aux soins de santé*[5]) which are intended to ensure that hospital structures take better stock of the social problems of the people referred to them, from admission through care provision to post-discharge follow-up. This means modifying both how hospitals work and how they relate to the general social and health network in the outside world. Three hundred hospitals were given an extra 38,112 euros of funding to this end. An evaluation of these offices carried out by the management teams of the hospitals, and specifically a progress report compiled under the supervision of Dr. Jacques Lebas, state that establishment of these offices has been progressing relatively slowly, *e.g.* by the end of 2000, numerous hospitals had not yet drawn up an agreement with external collaborators, despite the fact that such agreements are essential to the success of the instrument. The Igas report on implementation of the exclusion law recognised that in quantitative terms, results had been fairly good but that overall readability was inadequate and that openness to the outside could be improved, notably by the systematic appointment of *"steering committees open to patient support groups and non-hospital-based health care professionals"*.

During the debate in Parliament on the exclusion bill, delegates wanted to introduce an Article to bring the Safe Food and Alcohol Centres (CHAA, *Centres d'hygiène alimentaire et d'alcoologie*) into the Law (of June 30 1975) pertaining to social and medico-social institutions (Article 72)[6]. This renamed these Outpatient Alcohol Severance Centres (CCAA, *Centres de cure ambulatoire en alcoologie*) which were thenceforth to be finance by the health insurance system. Since that time, the number of such centres and their operating costs have significantly grown.

The exclusion law also gave prefects new powers to combat paediatric lead poisoning (Article 123). The Prefect can oblige a private landlord to carry out any construction work necessary to protect the health of children who might be threatened with lead contained in old or damaged paint work. Implementation of the provisions of the law has been slow, in particular in those areas where the public authorities have had trouble finding alternative accommodation for the families concerned during the work.

Finally, the law provided for the compilation of a report on *"the role of the school medicine service in policy related to prevention*

---

5. Articles L. 6112-1 7° and L. 6112-4 of the Public Health Code.
6. Article L. 3311-2 of the Public Health Code.

and how to consolidate the system to improve the monitoring of schoolchildren, especially in those places where medical advice is not sought as often as it should be" (Article 70), and *"a report on the feasibility and modalities of transferring the responsibility for the fight against tuberculosis from the regions to the State"* (Article 77). Both of these reports were compiled but little concrete action resulted. The Igas report on implementation of the exclusion law mentions a few experimental measures[7] and expresses the desirability of integrating the school medicine service into the care access network.

Universal Health Insurance Coverage (the Law of July 27 1999)

The Law of July 27 1999 provides for Universal Health Insurance Coverage (CMU, *Couverture médicale universelle*) and profoundly changed many of the pre-existing instruments of medical assistance as well as giving millions of people access to free health care without too much paperwork. CMU provides medical coverage to those who were not hitherto covered at all, and provides complementary health insurance (*i.e.* 100% reimbursement) to those on low income. More than 5 million people benefit from CMU, of whom, nearly 3 million had previously benefited from medical assistance. In 2000, 1.5 billion euros (including 1.07 billion from State funds) were allocated to CMU. Over 750 mutual companies and insurance companies have been accredited. According to the Spring 2000 Igas report, *"CMU was launched successfully: information was broadly disseminated to its target audience, both at the national level (thanks to the early establishment of collaborations with non-profit-making organisations) and at the local level."*

More attention to health in municipal policy

Over the last two years, there has been a move towards taking more stock of health-related issues in municipal policy. This is manifest in two ways:
– most municipal contracts covering the period 2000-2006 include a health provision, unlike prior contracts,
– the Ministerial Municipalities Committee has encouraged local policy makers to establish "municipal health units" in order to help professional health care providers and residents in particular neighbourhoods to work together on access problems (access to both prevention and to care) and formulate solutions. This corresponds to an initiative similar to the Regional Programmes for Access to Prevention and Care (Praps) but at the local level.

These are positive changes but nevertheless warrant a re-examination of the role of local authorities in health, and how health-related measures are to be designed and implemented at the municipal level.

---

7. The working protocol for the project to monitor medical and social parameters among pre-school children and elementary schoolchildren in Pas-de-Calais, and the initiative to enlarge the scope of the school medicine service to improve access to care in Seine-Saint-Denis and Oise.

Support groups Support groups often play an essential role in focusing attention on social problems:
– they propose solutions – often experimental – to problems that they observe,
– they solicit the administrative authorities so that more global solutions can be identified,
– they often contribute to the implementation of public policies so that they reach specific populations which are ignored or inequitably considered by the institutions.

When considering how inequality in health can best be combated, support groups could be playing a more important role. It is they who have the best idea and the most global perspective of the problems of those living in precarious conditions, so they could make a concrete contribution when it comes to designing and implementing appropriate policies. To do this successfully, they need adequate resources to be able to analyse their operations, evaluate any innovative measures that they conduct, and compare their experiences, at the international as well as the national level.

HEALTH IN FRENCH OVERSEAS DEPARTMENTS

Life expectancy at birth has significantly increased over the last twenty years so that now, in the French West Indies, it is close to the national average. In Guiana, it has increased particularly over the last seven years although, in 1997, it was still lower than in the French West Indies. In Réunion, after rising up massively until 1990, it has since slowed down; in 1997, male mortality was significantly higher than on the mainland, and the overall difference in life expectancy between the two was nearly four years, a figure which seems to be on the increase (table 12).

These satisfactory results are associated with a steady drop in infant mortality (death before one year of age) since the 1970's (figure 15). However, this parameter has stabilised or even slightly deteriorated since the 1990's with a resultant effect on overall life expectancy, so the recent improvement in the latter statistic is due to improvements at more advanced ages of life.

Table 12 **Life expectancy in mainland France and its overseas departments. 1990 and 1997**

	Year	Men	Women
Guadeloupe	1990	70.2	78.3
	1997	73.3	80.4
Martinique	1990	72.9	79.8
	1997	74.9	81.3
Guiana	1990	65.5	73.9
	1997	72.4	78.7
Réunion	1990	69.0	78.3
	1997	70.1	78.5
Mainland	1990	72.8	81.0
	1997	74.2	82.1

Figure 15 **Infant mortality in mainland France and its overseas departments**
(rates per 1,000 live births)

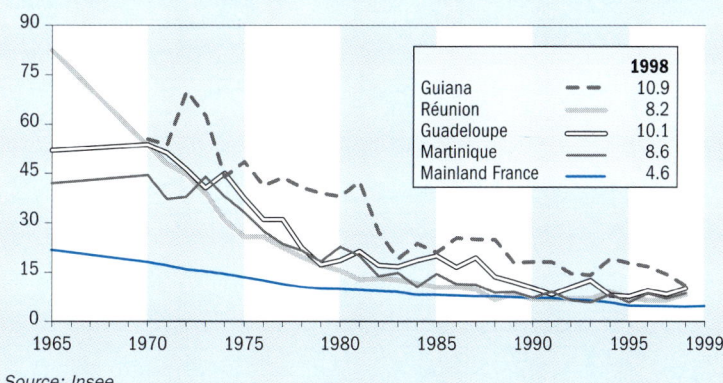

	1998
Guiana	10.9
Réunion	8.2
Guadeloupe	10.1
Martinique	8.6
Mainland France	4.6

Source: Insee.

Perinatal mortality

Since 1996/1997, spikes of perinatal mortality[1] have been observed in the various departments (apart from Guiana where the original level was relatively high) (figure 16).

The relative weight of perinatal disease in infant mortality dropped between 1987 and 1990 then rose again. Between 1993 and 1995 in the French West Indies, it then rose again back up to the level of the 1980's, accounting for 53% of all infant deaths. In Guiana, it almost tripled to 60%.

The same phenomenon is seen in Réunion, although not to the same extent (perinatal disease accounting for 52% of infant mortality).

To investigate this phenomenon, larger populations were investigated in the 1998 Inserm perinatal survey in the French departments of America (table 13).

Table 13 **Premature birth and low birth weight in mainland France and its overseas departments (1998 National Perinatal Survey)**

	Mainland	Guadeloupe	Martinique	Guiana	Réunion
Premature birth (< 37 weeks)	6.8	11.4	10.3	14.0	10.2
Birth weight below 2,500 g	7.2	11.4	11.1	13.7	10.7

The figures for Réunion are based on a national sample of 226 mothers and are comparable to those of the 1995 survey. A larger population is currently being analysed.
Source: Insee.

Figure 16 **Perinatal mortality in mainland France and its overseas departments**
(rates per 1,000 births)

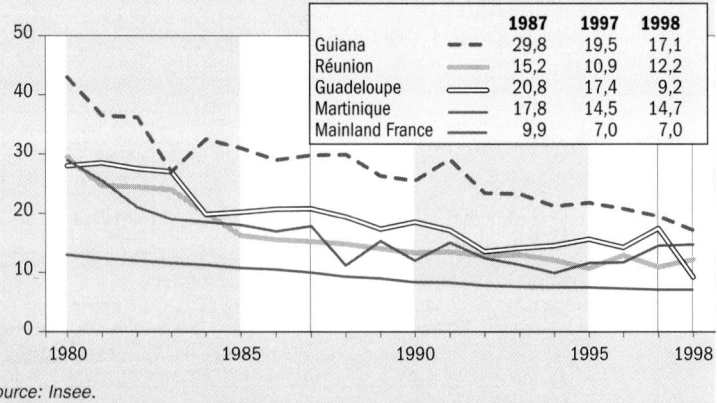

	1987	1997	1998
Guiana	29,8	19,5	17,1
Réunion	15,2	10,9	12,2
Guadeloupe	20,8	17,4	9,2
Martinique	17,8	14,5	14,7
Mainland France	9,9	7,0	7,0

Source: Insee.

---

1. Number of still births and deaths within 7 days compared with total number of births.

This showed that, in the French departments, mothers tended to be younger, smoked less, and were living alone during pregnancy (28% in Guiana and 40% in Martinique, compared with just 7% on the mainland). Two special factors in Guiana are the fact that prevention and care are inaccessible for part of the population, and the large numbers of foreign women who come to the country to give birth. Pregnant women are more admitted into hospital more often, but this does not compensate for the lack of prenatal consultation.

Mortality

In 1997, 5,400 deaths were recorded in the French West Indies – Guiana region, the mean for 1991-1992 having been 5,060. In Réunion, the rise in the number of deaths (from 3,200 in 1993 to 3,620 in 1997) is partly due to the ageing of the population.

Death before 75 years of age

External causes – physical injury and poisoning – are the main cause of death in men of under 75 in all the departments (table 14). These account for more than one-third of all Possible Years of Life Lost (PYLL) among men in the French West Indies, half in Guiana, and nearly one-third in Réunion. Among women, these causes of death are in first place in Guiana but third in the other overseas departments. Road accidents dominate this category of causes of death, accounting for more than one-third of fatal injuries in Guadeloupe, and one-quarter in the others.

Table 14 **Possible years of life lost (PYLL)* (1993-1997)**

	Guadeloupe		Martinique		Guiana		Réunion	
	Rank	%[1]	Rank	%[1]	Rank	%[1]	Rank	%[1]
Men								
Injury and poisoning	1	41	1	34	1	51	1	31
Cancer	3	13	2	17	4	7	3	16
Disease of the circulatory system	2	13	3	16	3	9	2	17
Infectious and parasitic disease	4	10	4	9	2	16	8	4
Total number of PYLL	5,080		63,116		25,871		149,095	
Women								
Cancer	1	22	1	29	3	12	2	20
Disease of the circulatory system	2	21	2	25	4	11	1	27
Injury and poisoning	3	19	3	15	1	27	3	16
Infectious and parasitic disease	4	10	4	6	2	27	10	3
Total number of PYLL	49,994		44,983		16,896		106,197	

* The PYLL indicator is mainly used in public health to give a measure of deaths before the age of 75 which does not have the same weight as deaths after 75. This indicator excludes infant mortality
1. Percentage of PYLL due to a given cause compared with all PYLL (all causes)

Source: Inserm, Antilles-Guiana Statistical Unit figures.

Part two Health inequalities and disparities in France

Table 15 **Rates broken down between men and women and causes of death* (1993-1997)**

	Guadeloupe		Martinique		Guiana		Réunion	
	M	W	M	W	M	W	M	W
Infectious and parasitic disease	40.4	26.6	35.5	21.5	76.5	78.1	26.9	19.9
including AIDS and HIV infections	21.5	8.2	15.7	4.7	44.7	41.8	4.7	1.5
Cancer	237.4	156.6	231.0	165.2	244.9	146.5	270.2	160.6
Endocrine disorders and immune system problems	35.0	57.4	36.6	44.7	32.7	53.3	40.3	65.2
Mental disease	38.2	18.1	32.7	16.4	30.3	21.7	61.3	24.5
Nervous system disease	31.0	18.2	27.8	21.9	26.2	14.0	31.1	20.1
Disease of the circulatory system	293.6	361.8	265.5	323.4	296.2	390.5	391.5	442.4
including cerebrovascular disease	117.4	142.4	106.1	119.4	114.9	150.0	139.0	162.1
Respiratory disease	60.8	44.0	56.6	56.0	56.2	35.4	128.5	91.7
Gastrointestinal disease	51.7	41.4	38.9	36.2	39.8	29.7	69.7	57.1
Genito-urinary disease	18.4	15.8	18.7	12.1	10.9	12.7	21.4	22.4
Problems originating in the perinatal period	6.2	5.5	5.4	3.8	12.7	13.2	5.6	3.1
Ill-defined symptoms and morbid states	47.7	72.3	37.9	51.6	51.2	72.6	54.9	71.8
External causes of injury	125.0	45.8	84.3	36.4	139.6	53.6	117.8	52.7
including road accidents	40.3	7.6	19.8	5.4	36.2	10.6	25.2	5.7
and suicides	16.2	5.3	16.0	4.7	17.3	9.9	32.6	7.9
Other diseases	12.6	19.6	13.9	13.5	20.1	30.4	10.5	15.6
Total (all causes)	**998.0**	**889.0**	**884.8**	**807.6**	**1,037.0**	**950.1**	**1,230.0**	**1,047.0**

* These rates have been calculated using the age profile of the mainland population in 1994 for reference. This bypasses the effects of different age profiles in the various geographical units studied.

Infectious and parasitic diseases are the second cause of death for both men and women in Guiana. The proportion has risen since 1987-1990, particularly among women. In the French West Indies, infectious disease is only the fourth cause of PYLL, although the proportion has doubled since 1987-1990. These rises are mainly due to an increasing incidence of AIDS. In Réunion, infectious disease is the eighth cause of premature male death, and the tenth with respect to women.

Although cardiovascular disease accounts for a significant fraction of premature death, this needs to be put in context in that such deaths tend to be at more advanced age. Nevertheless it is the second cause of PYLL in Guadeloupe and for women in Martinique, the third for men in Martinique and Guiana; in Réunion, it is the first cause of PYLL for women and the second for men. In all departments, high blood pressure is the main risk factor for cardiovascular disease. In women cancer is the first cause of PYLL in the French West Indies, the second in Réunion and the third in Guiana. In men, cancer is in fourth place and only accounts for 7% of all PYLL. In Martinique, it occupies second place (17% of all PYLL), and third place in both Guadeloupe (13%) and Réunion (16%).

Réunion is differentiated from the other French overseas departments by a relatively low mortality due to infectious and parasitic disease, and cancer here accounts for only half the national average of PYLL. However, circulatory system disease is relatively more important. The fourth cause of PYLL is:

– mental problems in men (8.3%), mostly associated with heavy drinking;

– digestive disease in women (8.3%), three-quarters of these cases being alcoholic cirrhosis.

Although its consequences appear to differ in men and women, alcoholism is a genuine social scourge in this departments and the Regional Health Conference has declared this problem a priority area for action and launched a corresponding specific Regional Health Programme.

- Diseases involving the circulatory system are clearly in the lead with men and women in Réunion most affected, followed by those in Guiana. Compared with 1987-1990, levels have dropped among the men in the French departments of America. In Réunion, excess mortality is 1.5 time higher than on the mainland for both men and women.

- Compared to 1987-1900, the cancer death rate in the French West Indies has somewhat dropped in men and risen in women; in Guiana, it has increased in women and not changed in men. In Réunion, compared with the 1988-1992 period, it seems to have increased among women and dropped in men.

- Among women in Guiana, the number of AIDS-related deaths has exploded since 1987-1990 (multiplied by a factor of 5) to go well above the level among men. In the French West Indies, the rates increased among both sexes, but to a lesser extent in women. In Guiana, a large number of children of under 5 years of age die of AIDS, and this is also true in Guadeloupe although the situation has improved here since the implementation of certain, effective measures in 1996 (HIV testing of pregnant women, prenatal therapy, etc.). Over the last four years, Martinique seems to have almost brought the problem of infantile HIV infection under control.

- Although there has been a decrease since 1987-1990, a higher proportion of men still die on the roads in Guadeloupe than in the other departments. As in the previous period, the rate is still highest in the 75-84 age bracket. In the other departments, it is the 15-34 age bracket which accounts for the most road deaths. In Martinique, annual figures sometimes fluctuate enormously but mean rates were identical in the two periods 1993-1997 and 1987-1990.

- In Réunion, after a drop in 1992-1996, the number of road deaths has been climbing again since 1997 due to increased car ownership and overcrowded roads. However, although fatal accidents are common, the total number of accidents in which injury occurs is falling, a result of government measures to improve road safety.

- Since 1987-1990, the mean annual death rate due to perinatal conditions has double or even tripled in Guiana, with girls more affected than boys. Under one year of age, the rate went up from 4.9% to 9.9% in boys, and from 3.7% to 12.2% in girls.

• In the French West Indies, although the death rate of girls has steadily dropped, that of boys has substantially dropped in Guadeloupe and increased in Martinique. In Réunion, rates in both are on the rise over those in 1988-1992: by a factor of +74% in boys under one year of age (to 4.4%) and of +28% in girls (to 2.5%).
• For deaths due to complications of pregnancy, delivery or postdelivery, it is better to use the maternal death rate, *i.e.* the number of deaths per 100,000 births.

Maternal death rate

Period	Guadeloupe	Martinique	Guiana	Réunion
1987-1990	51.4	54.4	64.6	27.0
1993-1997	46.9	24.4	79.3	26.0

Although it only represents a small number of deaths, this indicator gives the worst differential with respect to the overall national average.

Compared with the-unsatisfactory-situation in 1987-1990, there was no change in Guadeloupe in the 1993-1997 period and significant improvement in Martinique. But the trend in Guiana is really worrying: the problem may be one of inadequate access to care or one of poor performance of the system.

In Réunion, this rate improved at an earlier stage, from 200 in the 1960's, 170 in the 1970's, and 45 at the beginning of the 1980's. It seems now to have stabilised at a similar level to that seen in Martinique.

Taken from [48].

Summary and recommendations

Geographical and social inequality in health is greater in France than in most other European countries and, far from decreasing, both problems persist and there has been deterioration in the picture according to some of the indicators over the last two decades.

Excellent performance in the curative care system has long obscured this reality, not only in the minds of the general public but also in those of professional health care providers, decision-makers and researchers. The net result has been that inequality has not been given the priority attention that it deserves in terms of health policy, and more specifically, public health policy.

Notably, the rate of premature death (before 65) among French men is far higher than in neighbouring countries and this is partly due to behaviour patterns which can be addressed (suicide, accidents, smoking, heavy drinking, etc.). At 35 years of age, the life expectancy of a member of the managerial or professional class is 6.5 years longer than that of a member of the working class, and this trend is manifest through all the intermediate classes, be they categorised in terms of occupational status or income. Socially-based inequality in the incidence of cancer is also more deeply entrenched than in many countries, especially with respect to cancer of the upper airways and digestive tract.

After 65 years of age, differences associated with mortality largely disappear, although there is little information available on inequality with respect to morbidity in general and quality of life (*i.e.* life expectancy with unimpaired health). Some research done in these areas (*e.g.* the studies commissioned by the Credes, and the Handicap, Disability and Dependency survey) has revealed marked socially-based inequality with respect to life-threatening risk factors, disability and deficiencies.

Such inequality is installed at birth, despite perinatal health being an area into which massive resources are invested through both public health policy and social measures: the incidence of premature birth and low birth weight correlates closely with the mother's educational level or the socio-economic class of the household.

In geographical terms, the great economic and social diversity of France is associated with parallel geographically-based inequality in the matter of health. Differences are apparent already at the regional level but analysis at the employment zone level reveals even greater discrepancies.

Although the situation is generally better in town than in the country, neither population density nor degree of urbanisation can fully explain the great variability seen in health status within any given region. Social factors explain some instances of continuity between contiguous regions and, inversely, changes in pattern within the same region. Analysis at an even smaller scale can help point up specific environmental and social factors underlying inequality.

Reducing inequality will involve action in a number of different areas.

Recognition of the problem

Inequality raises questions about the egalitarian principles of our health care system, including about how equitably curative and prophylactic care are provided.

Therefore, inequality needs to be recognised by all the various players: researchers, professional health care providers, health policy makers, health insurance schemes and the funding agencies.

Whenever health priorities are being identified (especially by the National and Regional Health Conferences), inequality – a central public health issue – must be systematically and comprehensively examined and taken into account.

Monitoring

Monitoring instruments need to be consolidated.

In particular, the system should be reorganised so that data generated by different institutions (*e.g.* the Insee, Inserm, Ined, InVS and the health insurance scheme) can be integrated and shared. Of course, this must be done in such a way as to protect confidentiality, but such integration of data from diverse sources would make it easier to detect and characterise specific instances of inequality.

Existing public health surveillance instruments (*e.g.* the notifiable disease, morbidity registers, occupational health and death certificate systems) should systematically be used to collect data on individuals' social status.

In addition, specific surveillance systems should be established to follow trends in inequality over time and in space.

Understanding

Above and beyond simply describing areas of inequality, it is important to understand the underlying factors, and identify ways of remedying the situation. This means:

Summary and recommendations

- research into the social determinants of health in the broadest sense: health implies not only the absence of disease but a general perception of well-being, and also requires that the health care system respond to generally felt needs and expectations; in parallel, to describe the social component, it is important to include not only people's personal psychosocial and behavioural characteristics but also the social and economic characteristics of their community and immediate environment;

- detailed evaluation of the extent to which medical and social services are responding to real people's needs and expectations, and this for everyone, whatever their position in the social continuum going from frank exclusion (recognised as such) to apparent social integration (which might be masking unidentified but negative social or health factors).

Implementation

If inequality is to be reduced, novel, well conceived measures will have to be implemented which are specifically aimed at remedying the problem.

The concept of "priority zones" in health policy could be developed in an analogous way to the zones delineated for educational policy or urban planning. Specific resources could be allocated to such zones to run health education programmes, to promote the integration of medical and social services, and to consolidate care provision and prevention. This would contribute to reducing both social and geographical inequality where social segregation is associated with geographical separation.

This objective also means consolidating existing public health services, the resources and performance of which leave much to be desired. Boundaries, responsibilities and practices need to be re-defined, in particular those of the school and prison medical services, the occupational health system and the Mother and Child Protection programme (PMI, *Protection maternelle et infantile*).

Providing sustained support

Sustained support is key in the form of ongoing evaluation and monitoring of the measures implemented in the context of the Law against Exclusion. Thus, Universal Health Insurance Coverage – the first review of which has just been completed – must be genuinely accessible to all eligible; Health Care Access Offices (Pass) need to be established in all public hospitals; and every effort must be made to ensure successful functioning of the Regional Programmes for Access to Prevention and Care (Praps) in all regions (which will involve establishing a specific monitoring instrument).

If socially-based inequality in health in the broadest sense is to be eradicated, measures cannot be confined to just the poorest or most profoundly excluded in society. From this perspective, the train of thought which starts with those situations of acute exclusion which bring the fairness of the overall health care and social coverage systems into question, needs to be taken through to its logical conclusions. This will involve addressing the extension of Universal Health Insurance Coverage to illegal immigrants, the threshold effects of the law, definition for all covered of a set of rights and health services reimbursed by the community, and harmonisation of health insurance schemes; all these represent areas which cannot be considered separately from inequality in health.

In conclusion, with the same underlying rationale as the three preceding points, the working group offers one final recommendation to policy makers: always take health into account in all areas of public policy (not just health policy but also fiscal, industrial, agricultural, municipal, educational, urban planning policies, etc.). And this consideration should be extended to predicting the impact or evaluating the effects of any such measures on socially-based and geographically-based inequality in health.

PART THREE

Resource allocation in the health system

Part three
Resource allocation in the health system

Composition of the Working Group

President Simone Sandier, High Committee on Public Health

Rapporteur Isabelle Durand-Zaleski, High Committee on Public Health

Members Jean-Marc Aubert, Social Security Directorate,
Ministry of Employment and Solidarity
Alain Coulomb, High Committee on Public Health
Stéphanie Deschaume, General Health Directorate,
Ministry of Employment and Solidarity
Gérard Duru, Lyon 1 University, CNRS
Francis Giraud, High Committee on Public Health
Claude Gissot, Directorate of Research, Studies, Evaluation
and Statistics, Ministry of Employment and Solidarity
David Herlicoviez, Directorate for Hospitalisation
and Care Logistics, Ministry of Employment and Solidarity
Jean Langlois, National Council of the Order of Physicians
Alain Letourmy, Centre for Research into Medicine, Disease and
Social Science
Dominique Polton, Centre for Research and Documentation on
the Economics of Health
Juan Vinas, Social Security Directorate, Ministry of Employment
and Solidarity

Co-ordination Claudine Le Grand, General Secretariat of the High Committee
on Public Health

The Working Group wishes to thank for their contributions Bruno Chénais, Directorate for Hospitalisation and Care Logistics,
Ministry of Employment and Solidarity
Christine Freyermuth, Directorate for Hospitalisation
and Care Logistics, Ministry of Employment and Solidarity
François Lemaire, Henri-Mondor Hospital, Créteil

Introduction

The resource allocation problem presented itself to the planners at a very early stage with the need to set a figure for the number of medical students to be trained and the introduction of the health map in the 1970's. Many other measures relating to the supply of or demand for health commodities or services are also evidence of this.

Addressing how resources can be most efficiently allocated involves making certain conceptual and methodological choices concerning how to monitor and analyse current allocation within the system with a view to finding ways to improve it.

In principle, the best way of allocating resources will be that which affords the best state of health at the lowest cost, although of course, one has to define both what one means by better state of health in the context of populations and the types of cost under consideration (public, individual, care costs, costs in terms of human life, absolute value, percentage, etc.).

When allocating resources which are necessarily limited, a satisfactory approach would involve evaluating care needs, determining priorities, and taking as a basis the relationship between care needs and the services necessary to meet them. It is important to be aware of the complexity of the approach and exercise prudence when executing it and drawing conclusions. On the one hand, the concept of need is usually a theoretical and dynamic one; and on the other hand, the means for meeting given needs vary in time and space (being regularly changed as a result of medical progress or economic factors). Short-cuts between general targets and means are to be avoided because they are often misleading. Thus, the annual National Health Insurance Expenditure Target (Ondam, *Objectif national des dépenses d'assurance maladie*) set by Parliament should reflect the relationship between the sums provided by the health insurance system and public health priorities; in reality, this relationship remains mysterious.

When allocating resources, both present and future need to be considered because, while certain forms of investment have an immediate pay-back, others may not bear fruit for several years. In this respect, the inertia associated with the long duration of medical studies or major material commitments (like building hospitals) needs to be taken into account in order to avoid wastage associated with technical obsoleteness and changed needs. For example, new treatment modalities are tending to shift care from the hospital setting towards independent practitioners, thereby to some extent rendering acute care facilities redundant.

Another major problem with resource allocation is ensuring that it is consistent enough to allow implementation. Consistency is key in many different respects, *e.g.* between the initial situation and the target, between physical means and available funding, and between different care sectors.

Conditions for "efficient" resource allocation include clear, consensual targets, adequate and suitably distributed means, and agreement on the level at which decisions are to be taken and by which institution (*e.g.* national, regional or sub-regional) within a microstructure. It could be wished that the enormous progress made in the matter of information at both national and regional levels through the regular compilation of statistics, and through data collected in the course of regular and one-off surveys in France and other countries, might be used to inform resource allocation more effectively than in the past.

Post facto observations can be made of how resources are allocated in the system but the value of such observations is limited, *e.g.* it is known that health care professionals are distributed unequally through the various regions but this gives information about neither the efficacy of the distribution nor alternative allocation modalities which might improve it. *Post facto* observations are often incomplete and do not make it possible, for example, to determine the distribution of the system's human resources between biomedical care and prevention. Is it satisfactory? How can it be changed?

In the quest for efficiency – since a population's state of health does not exclusively depend on health care and preventive modalities – decisions about resource allocation to improve health need to be extended to other areas such as economic and social policy.

Thus, we will first present a overview of the system's current resources and then analyse possible ways of changing their allocation in the medium and long term, finally presenting recommendations with a view to reorganisation of the medical apparatus in order to improve the population's health.

Health system resources: the current situation

In the following, an attempt is made to review recent changes in how resources are being attributed in the health system. The selected period of 1990 to 2001 covers the years since the publication in 1998 of the previous HCPH "Health in France" Report, and will help give a longer term perspective.

This review covers the total financial sums invested, health care system productivity factors, and the regulatory framework in which the various different types of resource are currently allocated.

General remarks

What "health system resources" means is all the factors which contribute and interact to improve the population's health, with respect to either the diagnosis and treatment of health problems, or in the matter of preventing such problems.

This vast assortment includes different types of personnel, expensive pieces of equipment, various forms of intermediate consumption which come under the health sector in the strictest sense (*e.g.* the salaries of medical staff, health care establishment costs and pharmaceuticals) or which relates to other sectors in which part – but only part – of the activity contributes to better health, *e.g.* water quality, airborne pollution, food, housing conditions, improving the road network, etc. The first group is more easily identified than the second, and is therefore more fully characterised in statistical terms.

Health system resources can be expressed in physical quantities in terms of production units which are generally not commensurable (*e.g.* the number of doctors and the number of hospital beds). To transform them into a set of commensurable parameters, they have to be expressed in monetary units with reference to a valid system of prices or costs. On this basis, global resource indicators can be established and analysed from various perspectives (by region, by disease, etc.).

Resources can be broken down into capital resources and operating costs which are complementary but do not involve either the same allocation procedures or the same kind of medico-economic evaluation. Capital resources represent material investments (*e.g.* hospital beds and equipment) and other investments which, although not material, are nevertheless as important, *e.g.* the moneys spent on staff training structures, and funding for technical and scientific research to develop new diagnostic and therapeutic modalities (and thereby to enhance productivity).

In the field of resources – as in that of needs – decisions taken at various times in the past are still having major repercussions. Their effects touch not only on capital resources but they also limit the possibilities for operating costs. In the same way, any decisions taken today might have an effect on the marginal variation (flow) of the system's current resources (stocks) although in general, consequences only become apparent in the longer term, sometimes not for many years.

Regional inequalities in health care provision could be taken by way of example: these result from past decisions as to where to invest and where not to invest, and current policy can only compensate for their effects gradually.

Health accounts: an instrument of macro-economic analysis

When talking about the financial resources deployed for the health care system, what is usually being referred to is the national health account, a satellite of the national accounting system. Without going into details about the underlying methodology, it is important to bear in mind the relationships between the accounting system's assessments and the health system's resources as described above.

Each year, the national health account presents an assessment of current expenditure which does not include the capital resources of the health care sector. Certain forms of investment in health – especially those financed at the local level – are not covered in this aggregate process.

The main aggregate, current expenditure on health, gives a measure of the overall amount of funding devoted to the health sector by all the various agencies.

The health sector includes commercial and non-commercial medical activities, associated activities (*e.g.* occupational medicine, military medicine, prison medicine, etc.), teaching, medical research, community-based prevention measures, and health administration in both the private and the public sector. This definition has the merit of delineating a clear field but excludes measures designed to improve working conditions or environmental problems when the objectives of the measures in question are not explicitly and primarily health-related. Thus, the definition is too restrictive to cover the entirety of the health system's resources.

Moreover, some aspects of national health expenditure are more accurately known than others. In particular, expenditure on prevention is under-estimated in the accounts because this type of measure will only appear if it can be isolated in statistical terms (*e.g.* immunisation campaigns, specific public health policies, etc.). Thus, a large part of the efforts of professional health care providers in this respect such as advice on preventive measures given in the course of a consultation – the primary reason for which is treatment of a disease – remain unidentified and are ascribed to care, not prevention.

The health accounts make it possible to answer questions put in the context of the relationship between resource allocation, the restrictions acting on those providing the funds, and their efficiency. "Who pays and how much do they pay?" "Who gets it and how much do they get?"

In the accounts, expenditure (receipts) is broken down according to source of funding (obligatory protection, complementary protection, public sector, households) and agent of production (establishment, personnel, pharmaceuticals, other medical commodities, transportation, etc.).

Using health accounts for resource allocation with public health in mind is complicated by the fact that expenditure is not broken down in such a way as to allow analysis of expenditure on a disease-specific basis. This is particularly important when it comes to tracking expenditure on chronic diseases which is going to represent a major public health issue in the coming decades. Serious methodological problems are associated with complex factors such as temporal links between different diseases or combinations of diseases which often occur intercurrently in the same patient. Nevertheless, preliminary work is underway with a view to establishing disease-specific accounts (*i.e.* the annual sum of expenditure devoted to the prevention and cure of one specific disease). If the approach yields fruit, an attempt could be made to compare the efficiency of resource allocation on a disease-by-disease basis, *i.e.* evaluate the expenditure on different diseases in terms of the resultant degree of improvement in health.

A few figures based on the idea of health accounts will illustrate the level and changes of financial resources in the health system.

In 2000, the national expenditure on health in France was estimated at 140.6 billion euros, corresponding to 10% of the Gross National Product (GNP). Care costs and medical commodities account for the major part of this aggregate figure but it also includes collective prevention measures, the operating costs of research, and health administration. Care costs and medical commodities alone account for 86.8% of the total, 122.2 billion euros which represents an average of 2,016 euros per capita. According to the 1998 OECD figures, this puts France in 11th position with respect to per capita health-related expenditure and 4th with respect to the fraction of the GNP devoted to this area.

It is important not to jump to any conclusions about whether France is spending too much or too little on the basis of such figures. In practice, although comparisons with other countries can be useful when it comes to analysing parallel changes in different countries, it is impossible to set standards in this respect given the uncertainties of the evaluation process (which are pointed out by the experts themselves) and the need to avoid restricting the analysis to the single factor of the general economy.

Still according to figures for 2000, 72.8% of the national expenditure on health came from the Social Security system, 9.7% from households, 4.3% from the State and local institutions, and 12% from various complementary insurance organisations (7.8% from mutual insurance societies, 2.4% from private insurance companies and 1.8% from life assurance institutions). If the breakdown is confined to care costs and medical commodities, larger parts of the expenditure fall to the Social Security system (75.5%) and households (11.1%), with the public sector only contributing a small fraction (1%). The contributions of mutual insurance societies, private insurance companies and life assurance institutions were respectively 7,5%, 2,8% and 2,1%. Although the proportion of costs paid by the French patient is relatively high compared with other countries in Europe beyond any doubt, comparison in this respect between different countries is difficult because of disparity in the complementary insurance systems.

On the basis of type of service, expenditure on care and medical commodities breaks down as follows:

– 46.5% for patients staying in health care establishments, including 45.0% for hospital care in the public or private sector, and 1.5% for long-term care establishments;

– 26.1% for outpatient services (including 12.5% for physicians, 5.3% for dental care, 5.3% for auxiliary medical services, 2.3% for medical tests and 0.7% for treatments in specialised establishments (*e.g.* alcohol withdrawal, spa therapy, etc.);

– 20.5% for drugs and 5.4% for other medical commodities, *e.g.* ophthalmologic, diverse prostheses, dressings and consumables.

In France, as in many countries, health costs have been rising faster than the national wealth for many years (although this was not true in 1997 or 1999). The rate of increase in health care expenditure in relative terms (*i.e.* index-linked) has slowed down over the last twenty-five years although this trend has somewhat reversed over the last four years of sustained economic growth (figure 1).

Figure 1 **Expenditure on medical materials and services (1970-2000)**
(mean annual rate of increase in relative value per period; inflation-index-linked figures)

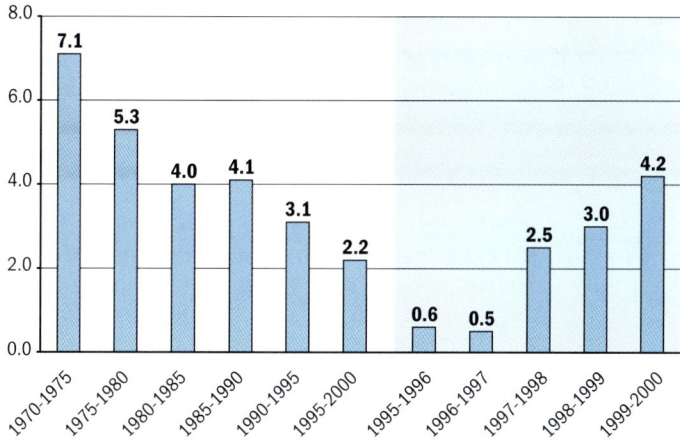

Source: National Health Accounts

The profile of expenditure on different types of care has changed over time and the structure of overall expenditure has evolved in parallel. Up until the beginning of the 1980's, hospital care was the growth area whereas since, it has steadily declined. This trend which can be seen in many countries is not just a result of French policy to cut hospital budgets but also due to patient demand, the development of new techniques whereby patients can be treated in an outpatient context, and the expansion in recent years of the medical network which has enhanced the viability of outpatient care.

The trend for medical commodities is opposite to that of hospitalisation: in 2000, they accounted for one-quarter of all expenditure on care and medical commodities from just 19.4% in 1980 (having been 28% in 1970). These changes reflect both the increasing role of pharmaceutical treatment at the expense of hospital care, and technological innovations which have resulted in the development of many new drugs which are effective but expensive. The proportion accounted for by outpatient medical services has remained fairly constant.

Changes in the share of the burden borne by different funding bodies reflects the changes in the rules of care coverage, the two most striking phenomena having been the transfer of responsibility for coverage from the State to the health insurance system, and the extension of complementary insurance which has lightened the load on households and partly compensated for the decrease in the rates of health insurance reimbursement for certain forms of care.

Production factors

Professional health care providers of various types play an essential role, not only a technical role in care production, prescription and counselling but also in terms of their economic weight. There are estimated to be about 1.6 million professional health care providers, and their salaries account for 70% of health costs.

In any given year, a breakdown on the basis of profession and specialism gives an idea of the volume of human resources available (table 1). This volume is mainly linked to resources allocated years before in the form of funding for different forms of training. To complete a description of the capacity of the supply to meet the demand of a population, it is useful to correlate the numbers with technical environmental indicators (the availability of equipment in the vicinity, encouragements to good practices), indications of activity and remuneration, data on geographical access factors (spatial distribution).

Table 1 **Changes in the density of different professional health care providers**
(per 1,000 inhabitants)

	1985	1990	1995	1996	1997	1998	2000
Physicians	2.66	3.06	3.24	3.25	3.26	3.28	3.32
Including							
General Practitioners	1.51	1.62	1.64	1.64	1.63	1.63	1.62
Specialists	1.55	1.44	1.60	1.61	1.63	1.65	1.70
Dentists							0.69
Nurses							6.54
Midwives							0.24
Pharmacists							1.00
Medical students							0.86
Student nurses							0.86

Source: Ministry of Employment, Drees.

Physicians On January 1 2000, there were 331 doctors per 100,000 inhabitants in France, a total of 197,224 more or less equally split between General Practitioners and specialists. However, the real number of generalists and specialists is not the same because a fraction of doctors classified as generalists are really specialists (about 22,000 of the total of 95,000 classified as generalists), *e.g.* in problems of the vessels, allergy, diabetes or acupuncture.

The most common specialists are (in decreasing order) psychiatrists, anaesthesiologists, radiologists, paediatricians, ophthalmologists and cardiologists.

In comparison to other countries (1997), the density of the medical network in France is lower than the European average (373), below that in Italy, Greece, Austria, Germany and Belgium, but above that in Sweden, Finland and the United Kingdom.

Mean national density does not say anything about the major disparities at the geographical level which result in inequitable access to health care for different people in different parts of the country.

Taking all disciplines and modes of practice together, the density varies as much as two-fold from department to department (figure 2), from below 200 doctors per 100,000 inhabitants to 400 per 100,000. Particularly well furnished are the Mediterranean rim and those departments where there is a medical school,

Figure 2 **Density of physicians and specialists in 1999**
(per 100,000 inhabitants)

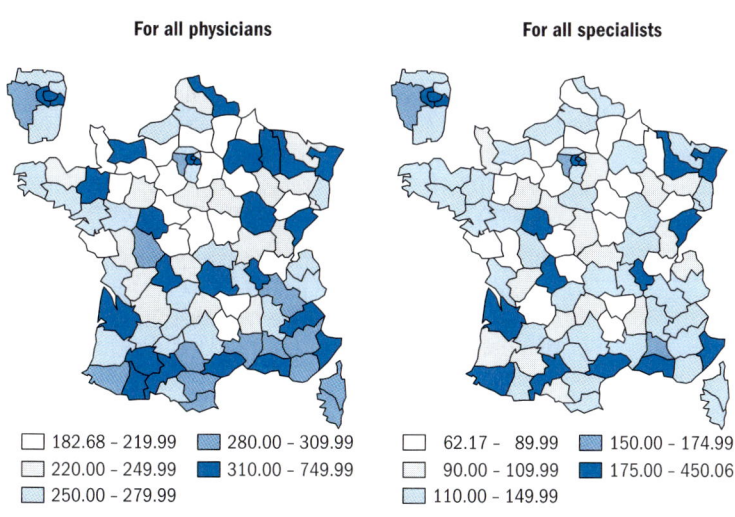

i.e. Haute-Garonne (Toulouse), Bas-Rhin (Strasbourg), Rhône (Lyons), etc. In contrast, the density of doctors is low in the Centre region and north of the Loire. Inequality is still more marked between urban and rural communities, and between the centre of towns and suburbs.

Disparities between departments are even more marked when it comes to specialists for whom, proximity to a teaching institution is particularly important (figure 2). Even ignoring the special case of Paris, the difference between departments is as great as three-fold (compared with two-fold for General Practitioners and specialists). The maximum density is around 220 specialists per 100,000 inhabitants in Haute-Garonne or Alpes-Maritimes, and the minimum is under 70 specialists per 100,000 in Lozère or Haute-Loire. Nevertheless, a recent poll showed that the French are in general satisfied with the distance of the nearest medical services, although 36% of those living in the countryside said that there were no specialists near enough to their homes. In fact, 84% of French people live in a commune where there is at least one generalist in practice, and the mean distance to the nearest office is seven kilometres (taking an average of eight minutes to get there).

Between 1968 and 1998, the number of practising physicians tripled as a result of the deferred effect of an increase in the number of medical students admitted in 1971. Since then, the number admitted has steadily declined (from 8,661 in 1971, to 6,400 in 1980, 4,000 in 1990 and 3,700 in 1999) and the rate of increase in the number of practising doctors has slowed down to the point that numbers are now almost constant.

Changes in the medical community have been accompanied by a small but significant decrease in differential density between the departments for General Practitioners, although this is not true for specialists.

From a demographic point of view, more women are practising today (in 1999, 35% of all physicians were women as opposed to just one-quarter in 1980) and the profession has aged, with fully one-quarter of doctors being over 50 years of age whereas this age group represented less than a third of doctors 30 years ago.

Some of the density predictions based on the current situation and hypothetical projections of future medical student numbers are frankly alarming, a point which will be expanded upon later on in the section of this chapter devoted to conclusions and recommendations.

Other professional health care providers

Apart from medicine, the other medical professions are dental surgery, midwifery and pharmacy.

Dental and orthodontal care is provided by 40,500 dental surgeons, most in independent practice with just over one-third of independent dentists being members of a group practice. Just over 1,500 of these specialise in orthodontal treatment. Between 1985 and 2000, the number of dentists rose by a factor of 17%, *i.e.* at a rate half as fast as that of physicians.

There are 14,400 midwives providing pre-natal and post-natal counselling in external consultations, for the most part based in a health care establishment. However, there are about 1,900 independent midwives who provide pre-natal and post-natal monitoring, and perineal treatment either in an office or in the home.

In 2000, there were 58,400 pharmacists of whom 72% owned or were working as an assistant in a high street pharmacy dispensing drugs and accessories (*e.g.* dressings) to non-hospitalised patients.

Medical tests are usually conducted on outpatients at one of 4,000 medical test laboratories which are supervised by physicians and/or specialised pharmacists.

The demographics and activities of the paramedical professions have been studied much less than those of physicians.

The largest group is that of the 383,000 nurses. Of these, 56% are employed in public hospitals, 13% in private establishments, and 31% practice independently. This profession is marked by a wide range of different types of situation, *i.e.* the nurse's position relative to that of the physician and other health care auxiliaries. The nursing profession together with other related occupations (*e.g.* nursing auxiliaries, home assistants, etc.) are highly regulated in all European countries but in different ways. This leads us to think that it is not simply technical exigencies which condition the circumstances of a profession but also historical particularities, *e.g.* the overlap between what is seen as health-related and what is seen as more the remit of the social services, the relative place of the State and local institutions or players, the importance of private initiative and public policy, and the resultant regulations, especially financial modalities.

Various paramedical professionals are involved in forms of rehabilitation, including physical therapists (52,000), orthophonists (13,500), orthoptists (2 100), podiatrists (8,800), psychomotor specialists, occupational therapists and dieticians.

Hospitals On January 1 2000, there was a total of 486,000 hospital beds in France. Just over half of these were for medicine, surgery and obstetrics, 90,400 were for follow-up care and physical therapy, 83,400 for long-term care, and 67,300 for mental disease, drug addiction and alcoholism. These figures correspond to a mean density of 8.1 beds per 1,000 inhabitants, half in short-term departments thereby putting France near the European average.

Alternatives to conventional, full-blown hospitalisation in the system represent about 10% of total capacity, *i.e.* about 46,000 places (on January 1 2000). This breaks down between 7,000 places for outpatient surgery and anaesthesiology, 27,000 for daytime or night psychiatric hospitalisation, and 12,000 for similar modes of admission in non-psychiatric medicine.

Activities are quite different in the public and the private sector. As stipulated in the Quantified National Target (OQN, *Objectif quantifié national*), the private sector only accounts for 20% of overall admission capacity, and this is highly concentrated in the disciplines of surgery and obstetrics: 60% of surgical procedures, 50% of oncological treatment procedures, 40% of deliveries (for which the mother is hospitalised), 60% of courses of chemotherapy, and 90% of outpatient surgery. In contrast, the private sector administers little follow-up care or rehabilitation, and even less long term care and psychiatric treatment.

As in most other Western European countries, the density of conventional hospital beds has declined over the last twenty years under the dual influence of the curtailment of hospital stays and the increased potential of outpatient-based treatment modalities.

The reduction in the number of conventional, full admissions is also associated with increases in partial hospital admissions and outpatient surgery.

Table 2 **Some figures on hospital equipment and activity**

	1980	1985	1990	1995	1996	1997	1998
Total number of admissions							
Number of beds per 1,000 inhabitants	11.1	10.5	9.7	8.9	8.7	8.5	8.4
Occupancy rate (%)	81.4	81.8	80.4	80.7	80.9	81.6	81.8
Number of admissions per 1,000 inhabitants	193.0	210.0	232.0	228.0	228.0	230.0	229.0
Mean stay (days)	17.1	14.9	12.3	11.5	11.2	11.0	10.9
Short stays							
Number of beds per 1,000 inhabitants	6.2	5.7	5.2	4.6	4.5	4.3	4.2
Occupancy rate (%)	79.0	79.1	77.3	76.0	75.9	76.4	76.1
Number of admissions per 1,000 inhabitants	175.0	189.0	209.0	203.0	203.0	204.0	203.0
Mean stay (days)	10.2	8.6	7.0	6.2	6.1	5.9	5.8

Source: Drees, in Eco-santé France 2000.

Between 1988 and 1998, nearly 52,000 conventional beds disappeared in the private and public sectors combined. This major shift was largely inspired by the private sector in which capacity in this respect fell by 7% (as opposed to just 3% in the public sector) from 1995 to 1999. These cuts affected all disciplines apart from long-term care, but surgery and psychiatry were partic-

Health system resources: the current situation

ularly heavily touched (with one-third of all such beds disappearing in just ten years), both disciplines in which various different alternatives to conventional hospitalisation were developed during this period.

Major disparities in density are observed at both the regional and the departmental levels, *e.g.* for short-term care services, departmental densities vary from 2.5 to 6 beds per 1,000 inhabitants, not counting Paris were there are 9.8 beds per 1,000 inhabitants. Of course, the capacity to provide care is not dependent on bed numbers, the number of staff, their level of training, and equipment being all other key factors (table 2 and figure 3). These are particularly important when it comes to the ability of a hospital to provide outpatient care and cut down the duration of hospital stays, *i.e.* increase productivity and cut down on the need for beds.

Figure 3 **Density of short-stay beds in 1998**
(per 1,000 inhabitants)

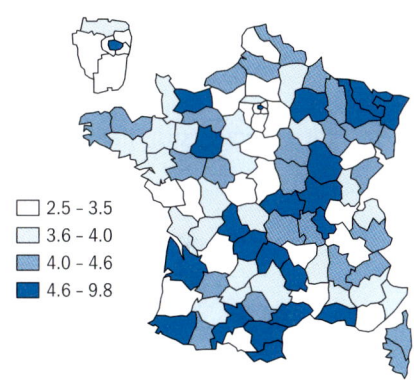

Source: Drees, Eco-santé régional 2000

Equipment Numerous new methods for the diagnosis and treatment of diseases have been developed through research in France and elsewhere. Many of these are associated with the need to buy new equipment.

Table 3 illustrates the spread of special machines (the pieces of equipment detailed being those for which authorisation has to be obtained prior to installation). Because of restrictive regulations, France has been slower than many other countries to accumulate high-technology equipment, especially new forms of imaging technology. Attention has been drawn to this lag by the relevant learned societies, and catching up with the levels of equipment in neighbouring countries has been identified as a priority.

Pharmaceuticals There are more than 4,417 different pharmaceutical products (2,326 of which can only be dispensed on prescription) on the market in France, corresponding to an annual turnover of 20.4 billion euros (1999).

Table 3 **Pieces of equipment which have to be approved prior to installation**

	1985	1990	1998	1999
CT scanners	128	379	531	562
MRI scanners		46	146	164
Scintiscanners		252	377	361
Telecobalt therapy machines	227	195	99	
Linear accelerators	94	146	263	337
Angiographs		438	521	670

Source: Drees, in Eco-santé France 2000.

The main pharmacotherapeutic classes to which reimbursed drugs belong correspond to the cardiovascular system, the central nervous system, the digestive tract and metabolism, the respiratory system, and general systemic anti-infectious agents. In contrast, the main classes of over-the-counter drug are pain-killers, anti-inflammatory drugs, antiseptics, laxatives and vitamins.

Measures recently implemented in the pharmaceutical sector – such as systematic evaluation of medical service rendered and use of the criterion of improvement as a basis for setting reimbursement levels – open perspectives of evaluation (evidence-based medicine) in other areas of care and treatment.

In general, the above review shows that changes in the very recent past have tended to bring an end to the general expansion in various areas of the preceding two decades with a reduction in care capacity due to falling numbers of both professional health care providers and hospital beds. However, these trends have been paralleled by expansion in the area of medical commodities.

How resources are estimated and allocated

Four broad principles underlie the allocation of public resources in society, namely equality, market factors, need and merit. These four enter into the allocation of resources to the health system to different extents.

It is the principle of need which is most often referred to but, given the difficulty of evaluation in this field, the idea of equality has been central in the organisation of certain screening campaigns. The idea of merit was evoked in the context of dental care in the plan proposed in 2000 by the Cnamts *(Caisse nationale de l'assurance maladie des travailleurs salariés)*. As to the market, its role is apparent in discussions of the group of reimbursed commodities and services which focuses on exactly those that need to be protected against market-based factors, *i.e.* those to which the "rich" should not have greater access simply by virtue of their superior spending power.

Three-quarters of the resources allocated each year to run the health system come from regulatory health insurance institutions, the rest coming from individuals, either in the form of direct payments to independent health care providers or organisations, or indirectly through the paying of contributions to mutual and private insurance societies. Obviously, the obligations of payers and the way in which sums due are calculated differ according to the type of organisation. Below, we will mainly be referring to health insurance, a collective payer which ensures some degree of redistribution of resources from the well to the ill. In accordance with its founding principle, the health insurance system only makes a small contribution to costs related to screening procedures and dependence.

Numerous parties are involved in the allocation of resources to the health system, including the State (the ultimate guarantor of public health), Parliament (since 1996), and finally patients themselves, either directly through their payments or indirectly through participation in political and social discussions of health-related issues.

If the means of production (resources) is to be matched to demand (insofar as it can be accurately estimated), the best possible combination of means of production needs to be identified since these means, far from being unlimited, are inferior to the theoretical technical needs in the vast majority of cases.

Combinations are subject to restrictions, sometimes serious restrictions associated with necessary complementarities and consistencies. Respecting complementarities is the primary condition for a system to be viable, useful and effective. Thus, the volume of hospital investment should not be dissociated from the number of personnel involved in operations, or nurse training capacity should be based on projections of the number of staff needed in the future.

The following sections deal with the ways in which financial resources are allocated each year to keep the health system working, in particular focusing on the National Health Insurance Expenditure Target (Ondam, *Objectif national des dépenses d'assurance maladie*), and how personnel and equipment are managed.

What should the level of health insurance funding be? The Ondam

Every December since 1996, Parliament has voted on the Government-proposed Social Security Funding Bill. Before the debate, members of Parliament review reports compiled by the High Committee on Public Health, the National Health Conference, and the Social Security Accounts Commission which tackle health problems and, in the last case, related financial matters.

The Funding Law contains provisions on resources and expenditure in three branches of the social security system and sets, in particular for the basic, mandatory forms of coverage, a national target for health insurance expenditure over the coming year – the Ondam – which is then broken down by the government between the various care sectors on the one hand, and between the regions on the other hand with respect to public hospital expenditure.

The Funding Law is accompanied by iteration of new provisions concerning resources, services and regulation of the system, which may have repercussions on the total and distribution of the mobilised moneys. These provisions are nevertheless inadequate in operational terms.

Apart from resources, the Social Security Funding Law (LFSS, *Loi de financement de la sécurité sociale*) fixes the totals available to cover health expenditure by the insurance system by setting (or modifying, if such is the case) the level of Generalised Social Contributions (CSG, *Contribution sociale généralisée*) or employers' contributions by imposing taxes (*e.g.* on tobacco or alcohol) or by including new provisions (*e.g.* exemption for the low-paid).

Apart from health insurance expenditure which corresponds to resources for the care sector, the LFSS contains a variety of other provisions, *e.g.* for improving reimbursement modalities for the self-employed in order to bring them into line with salaried employees, or, as in the 2001 LFSS, for the creation of specific funds to modernise health care establishments.

A "Report on directions in public health and social security policies and targets which determine the general conditions for financial balance" is appended to the Law. This summary reviews the State's priorities and directions in the light of the proposals of the Regional Health Conferences and the National Health Conference, and by opinions, recommendations and conclusions sub-

Setting the Ondam

mitted by the various bodies concerned with the field of public health. This Report has no dimension of opposability.

In compliance with the 1996 Rulings, in theory, total expenditure by health insurance organisations in the year "t" should result from the addition of an annual increment (percentage) to the previous year's Ondam. This mode of calculation was designed to forge a temporal link in expenditure in order to make the players responsible, in effect constituting a means of recovery should the target be exceeded.

In practice, the Ondam has been exceeded every year since 1998, so the Government decided, for the 2000 Law, to ignore the past and change the mode of calculation. The Ondam is now calculated by applying the rate of change not to the previous year's Ondam (which is merely a theoretical figure) but to a prediction of actual expenditure in the year "t-1" as made by the Social Security Accounts Commission in September of year "t-1", just before the Government submits the Social Security Funding Bill to Parliament.

This change effectively ratifies missing the target (usually overshooting) as long as the predicted figure is close to the true one. However, if it is wrong and actual expenditure in year "t-1" (which figure is known at the beginning of year "t") differs significantly from the September projection, adhering to the Ondam can mean that the "authorised" rate of increase in expenditure differs from that envisaged in the LFSS.

Table 4 summarises the targets set over recent years, the parameters on which they were calculated (baseline level and percentage increase), and actual corresponding expenditure. It can be seen that the gap between target and actual expenditure has been widening since 1998.

These differentials show: on the one hand that the Ondam is proving to be an established indicative figure without taking into account the parameters which contribute to the rise in health insurance expenditure (*i.e.* needs, the capacity of care provision and reimbursement rates); and on the other hand that, for both technical and political reasons, the instruments which are supposed to ensure adherence to the Ondam are not working.

Part three Resource allocation in the health system

Table 4 **The Ondam and health insurance expenditure (1997-2001)**

	1997	1998	1999	2000	2001
Target					
Value (billions of euros)	91.5	93.57	96.03	100.36	105.69
Base (billions of euros)	90.00	91.50	93.57	98.02	102.11
Increase (%)	1.70	2.27	2.62	2.50	3.50
Expenditure under Ondam					
September projection for the previous year (billions of euros)				98.02	102.11
Real (billions of euros)	91.39	95.06	97.75	103.11	
Differential between the target and actual expenditure					
Billions of euros	–0.11	1.49	1.72	2.74	
Percentage of target	–0.12	1.60	1.79	2.73	

Source: Social Security Accounts Commission

ONDAM CASE ON 2001

The National Health Insurance Expenditure Target (Ondam, *Objectif national des dépenses d'assurance maladie*) for 2001 has been fixed at 105.7 billion euros. This corresponds to a 3.5% increase over the estimated expenditure in 2000 (102.1 billion euros). However, it represents a 5.3% increase over the Ondam for that year (which was 100.4 billion euros). Since the real expenditure in 2000 was greater than the figure estimated in September (103.1 as opposed to 102.1 billion euros), if the Ondam stipulated in the law passed by Parliament is to be adhered to, health expenditure would have to actually increase by a factor of only 2.5%, not 3.5%.

Components of the overall Ondam

Once the Ondam has been fixed, it is up to the Government to break it down into four different components which correspond to sector-based targets:
– The independent care sector, including the salaries of all independently practising professional health care providers (doctors, dentists, nurses, medical laboratory staff, etc.) and prescriptions dispensed in high street pharmacies plus sick leave costs.
– Public and affiliated health care establishments.
– Private clinics (not including salaries).
– The medico-social sector: institutions for the elderly and disabled.

The totals allocated to the four components are supposed to be stipulated within two weeks of publication of the Funding Law.

For 2001, the overall target of + 3.5% breaks down to + 3% for independent care, + 3.4% for public hospitals, + 3.48% for private establishments (an overall figure although the actual increase varies from discipline to discipline), and + 5.8% for the medico-social sector. The leeway left to the government to vary the percentage increase is relatively small but its choices are partly made on the basis of priorities in that different increases are allowed in different sectors. However – and these points will be discussed further on – restrictions related to production functions (notably personnel costs) and to the competition or complementarity of different sectors mean in the final analysis that the increases in all the different areas are fairly similar.

Hospital sector resources

The Government intervenes at two distinct levels when it comes to allocating resources to hospitals.

Firstly, it sets separate target increases for public sector and private sector establishments, and then it breaks down the public sector target at the regional level.

Public hospital sector (included affiliated private establishments)

In the context of the Ondam, the Government can attribute different sums to public hospitals to concretise public health policy targets such as reducing regional inequalities in health status and health care. This flexibility also makes it possible to focus on other priorities in public health and organisation of the health care system.

The amounts to be allocated to the different Regions are calculated in a two-step process in which first a target sum is worked out and then a convergence method is used to arrive at this figure.

Calculation of the target sum has been refined in recent years and is based on an estimate of a Region's theoretical needs in medicine, surgery and obstetrics, and long-term care, and on the calculation of an efficiency index. Three indicators are taken into account when calculating the needs:
– an indicator of health needs in the form of an index based on the ratio of mortality in the Region to the national average,
– an indicator of hospital needs based on a target of equal resources to meet needs, calculated by counterbalancing mean national admission rates according to the Region's demographic structure,
– a review of expenditure related to the movements of patients (in medical, surgical and obstetrical services) between different Regions.

The indicator of economic efficiency – which measures regional productivity – is derived by means of the spot mean value of the Compound Activity Index of the Region (calculated from PMSI data) and comparing it to the spot mean national figure (regional productivity).

One objective of the process of allocating resources to the Regions is to – on the basis of a series of criteria – bring the real

observed sums in line with the target sum. The convergence method used by the Government involves:
– to bring the three least well-endowed Regions (Poitou-Charentes, Picardie, Nord-Pas-de-Calais) up to the level of the fourth Region (Alsace) in the order of increasing target endowment, within five years;
– to ensure the steady convergence of moderately under-endowed Regions (Bourgogne, Centre, etc.) towards the target endowment level;
– to require no more than a bearable effort for the best-endowed Regions.

The resources devoted to public health priorities and care logistics constitute an immutable endowment which must be exclusively dedicated to their implementation or to measures aimed at enforcing safety norms. The Regional Hospital Agencies are free to attribute their public health and organisation endowment according to regional priorities although preventing the transmission of infectious diseases, developing palliative care and the "transplant plan" must be dealt with first.

Private hospital sector (non-affiliated establishments)

For unaffiliated private establishments, the total Quantified National Target (OQN, *Objectif quantifié national*) is now set by the Government according to the Ondam, being stipulated every year in the context of the Social Security Funding Law. Every year, a bilateral agreement is reached at the national level between the State and the federations of clinics (the health insurance system originally included in this agreement was removed in 2000) to fix on the one hand the mean national increase and the mean increase in each region in charges, and on the other hand maximum and minimum variations in the rates of increase which can be attributed to the establishments by the Regional Hospital Agencies. Regional agreement can also fix the rate of increase of the charges in different establishments on the basis of medical activities (disciplines).

It should be noted that, in contrast to the situation of affiliated establishments, the adjustment mechanism is exclusively based on the spot Compound Activity Index without any consideration of indicators of health status or needs.

Otherwise, the procedure-based pricing system needs in some cases to be complemented when an establishment is assigned a specific task (which is not catered to by the public hospital system) in the organisation of regional care in the context of the Regional Health Organisation Scheme (Sros, *Schéma régional d'organisation sanitaire*). In this event, the private establishment may be the only one offering a particular form of care even though the volume of patients does not justify the activity in economic terms.

This is why a new mode of funding for private clinics was created in the 2001 Social Security Funding Law for the special case of emergency services. Thus sites with Sros-approved emergency services authorisation (Upatu, Satu, Posu) will receive a fixed, annual endowment to cover operating costs plus a fixed per capita rate for every patient seen for an emergency who was not subsequently admitted into the clinic.

Finally, in order to improve monitoring of the OQN, the Social Security Funding Law for 2000 also provided for the establishment of a single fund to pay the clinics that fraction of the hospital costs reimbursed by the health insurance system. This instrument came into force on January 1 2001 for salaried employees and will be gradually expanded to cover all insurees.

Independent practice

Since 2000, a separate Delegated Expenditure Target (ODD, *Objectif de dépenses déléguées*) has covered the fees of independent professionals (ten professions) and health-related transport costs. This target does not concern drugs or orthopaedic and ophtalmologic devices prescribed by independent practitioners.

The ODD is managed by the health insurance agencies which are obliged to adhere to it. Thus, the agencies are responsible for negotiating expenditure targets with health professionals for each profession, and negotiating prices and any measures intended to ensure that these targets are adhered to. In this context, prices may be raised or lowered. Twice a year, collaborating with the professionals, the agencies monitor expenditure and compile a balance report which is submitted to the Government. If agreement cannot be reached with the professionals, the agencies make unilateral proposals to the Government to ensure that the targets are met.

The agencies can also set up experimental target/means contracts, *e.g.* in the fields of prevention or dental care.

It is in the field of independent practice in which the French health care system is characterised by freedom of access to care on the part of patients, free prescription by doctors, and procedure-based payment of professionals – that adhering to the stipulated budget is most difficult to guarantee. In 2000, considering all the care which comes under the Ondam, expenditure was 47.1 billion euros, 2.6 billion euros higher than the target. The 22.2 billion spent in the context of the ODD alone was 0.8 billion euros over the target. This illustrates the fact that the financial resources absorbed by expenditure on independent practice substantially exceed Government targets.

Part three — Resource allocation in the health system

Drugs — Since 2000, no specific target has been set for expenditure on drugs in the context of either the Ondam or the ODD. The regulatory instrument in this area – intended to restrict the resources consumed by the reimbursement of drugs – depends on the underlying hypothesis that the pharmaceutical industry, through its interventions, can affect the rate of prescription by doctors, of expenditure on drugs by patients, and therefore the level of funding by the health insurance system. The instrument managed by the Economic Health Products Committee provides for the payment of discounts by pharmaceutical companies as soon as their turnover exceeds the growth rate of the independent practice target, in such a way as to recover 70% of the excess. Here again, there was a clear failure to meet initial targets in 2000: pharmacy reimbursement rose by 9.8%, *i.e.* far in excess of the independent practice target (+ 2.5%).

Funding of general and specific measures — The sum of its parts (independent practice, public hospitals, private clinics and the medico-social sector) is not equivalent to the overall Ondam voted by Parliament. Therefore, the Government has room for manœuvre corresponding to the difference to fund any special measures devised during the year. In 2000, the margin was of 122 million euros on an overall Ondam of 100.4 billion. Some of this was used on campaigns to prevent violence, to promote emergency services, to upgrade treatments by hospital practitioners, and to fund technological progress (new drugs and devices).

Human resources
Physician numbers — Because of the length of the training process, the number of physicians practising at any time is determined by decisions taken with respect to medical schools ten or more years previously. Similarly, decisions taken in this area today will only begin to affect overall numbers as of 2010, and will not correct any deficit in the shorter term.

Other measures may be able to increase care provision in the short term and correct certain forms of geographical inequality, namely the recruitment of doctors trained abroad, incentives in the form of enhanced remuneration, continuing training, retirement age, Good Practices guidelines, and the organisation and distribution of care provision.

Note should first be taken of the procedures applying to the initial training of physicians.

Since 1971, admission into second-year medical studies has depended on success in an examination, the number to be passed (the *"numerus clausus"*) being set by Decree each year. Various opinions are voiced when this number is being fixed: the learned medical societies tend to propose a low number in order to restrict competition; the health insurance system, for economic reasons, thinks that having more physicians will tend to increase care consumption and therefore expenditure; and finally the University Faculty heads who worry about whether they will have enough students to keep their hospital services running properly. Taking needs into account remains a theoretical idea when it comes to setting the *numerus clausus* because short-term exigencies tend to weigh more heavily than long-term projections of uncertain reliability.

Thus, against a background in which the number of physicians is generally seen as excessive, the *numerus clausus* has been steadily dropping for more than twenty years, from 8,588 in 1971 to just 3,500 in 1992. Since that low, it has risen slightly back up to reach 4,100 in 2000.

Apart from the *numerus clausus*, the regulatory instrument controlling physician numbers also includes the setting of the number of posts offered in the competitive process at the end of internship (the sixth year of medical training). Passing this examination is an absolute requirement for those wishing to specialise. The number of posts is fixed each year (at 1,847 in 2000) for each discipline and each medical school. In the future, according to a Bill currently being debated in Parliament, all students will have to do an internship and both general medicine and specialisation will be decided in a single, competitive examination.

Independent physicians are entirely free to choose where they practise whereas numbers in public hospitals are determined by the authorities, doctors being recruited in competitive processes or employed on a contractual basis to fill vacant positions. It should be noted that, despite very different modalities with respect to installation and recruitment, regional inequality and a failure to match care provision to needs affects both the independent and hospital sectors.

Recruiting foreign physicians has been one way of filling some of the gaps, especially in the 1990's. This includes European doctors who qualified in Europe, foreign (or French) doctors who qualified elsewhere, who are authorised to practice exclusively in hospitals (the PACs) or in independent practice. There is a total of 7,500 foreign-qualified doctors working in French hospitals (many of them for a long time): 4,357 are Ministry-registered PACs, and 2,958 are authorised to practise anywhere in France (in a process which involves assessment by a panel of physicians and administrators).

Part three — Resource allocation in the health system

Other professional health care providers

The same is true for other paramedical professions – nursing, physical therapy, etc. Numbers are subject to a degree of inertia in the balance between the number of newly-qualified personnel and the number retiring.

The only means of controlling numbers is the *numerus clausus* for training institutions which is set by the authorities for all the various professions (apart from orthoptics).

In order to match provision to needs, by raising or lowering the *numerus clausus*, the number of practising professionals can be controlled. Since paramedical training is usually shorter than medical training, there is less lag in the system, so a change in the *numerus clausus* can mediate an effect within four years. However, questions of training capacity restrict the magnitude of change possible in the short term.

Independent paramedical practitioners are free to choose where they practice, like their medical counterparts.

Numbers compatible with provision

Staff numbers are a good indicator of the resources available to meet care consumption, but they are not the only one. With constant numbers, other factors may affect productivity, in particular quality, hourly productivity, and working time (at the daily, weekly, annual or career-long scale).

Remuneration modalities – be they procedure-based, a salary or per capita – all entail theoretical incentives which affect the behaviour of medical staff. The role of these incentives is often overestimated, in particular the tendency of procedure-based compensation to increase care consumption. In fact, the level of unitary remuneration, the size of the demand, the numbers and the competition are all equally important factors.

The pricing of procedures (in formal lists and attributed agreed charges) entails incentives to either promote or withdraw certain procedures insofar as they do not reflect the relative scale of production costs (time, intermediate consumption, etc.). In this context, cautious mention could be made of the reduction in the number of home visits by General Practitioners, and the sharp rise in the frequency with which certain technical procedures are performed.

In the 1990's, improving the quality of care became a major theme in the reform of the distribution and organisation of the care system. In this perspective, the National Agency for Health Accreditation and Evaluation (Anaes, *Agence nationale d'accréditation et d'évaluation en santé*) is responsible for compiling and diffusing guidelines and references for Good Practices. Good Clinical Practices (GPC) and Opposable Medical References (RMO, *Références médicales opposables*) are used to define the resources necessary to caring for a type of patient and can thus constitute a tool when in the endeavour of resource allocation.

Thirty recommendations on clinical practice concerning the diagnosis, treatment and monitoring of certain diseases have been diffused to all physicians. The RMO's – 200 for generalists and 250 for specialists – mainly concern drug prescription and to a lesser extent, the ordering of tests. The financial sanctions for non-respect of the RMOs were cancelled by the State Council in 1999 but these instruments have considerably cut down redundancy in drug prescription (*i.e.* the prescription of more than one drug of the same family with identical mechanisms of action).

Ongoing medical training is another means of improving the quality of care. The 1996 Rulings re-affirmed the importance of continuous training and made it obligatory for both independent and hospital practitioners who must obtain an attestation that they have fulfilled this obligation every five years. However, difficulties in establishing an effective system have meant that there has been little improvement in continuous medical training for physicians.

Other provisions contribute to providing professionals with information, *e.g.* transparency sheets which compare the costs of different drugs used to treat the same condition and are compiled by the Transparency Commission with a view to promoting the prescription of generic drugs. In a similar vein is the recently created Medical and Medico-Social Information Fund, the remit of which is to provide professional health care providers with objective information about reimbursed medical products.

Finally, measures touching on the organisation and distribution of care can promote a more rational exploitation of resources by improving the matching of supply to demand and by re-defining the roles of the various professionals. For the moment, the vital question of how resources can be distributed to correct geographical imbalances has not been addressed by specific incentives. With respect to complementarity and substitution in care distribution, a number of points need to be made:
– a set of factors has contributed to the decrease in the length of the average hospital stay, and to the partial transfer of treatment and monitoring functions from hospital to independent practitioners (medical test laboratories, independent physicians, auxiliaries);
– the "referring physician" instrument will expand the responsibilities of General Practitioners and reduce those of specialists. Up until now, few doctors (10%) and even fewer patients (1%) have made use of this instrument;
– computerisation of the health professions with the support of the health insurance agencies should result in improved medical practice, not only in the organisation of activities but also in patient monitoring and in the ability of the system to circulate important information.

The hospital sector

The number of hospital beds is heavily dependent on past building and modernisation policy but a series of provisions are designed to effect changes, especially at the regional level.

The Directors of the Regional Hospital Agencies (ARH) are responsible for authorising or rejecting the creation or change of establishments, the installation of expensive technical equipment and certain activities related to the health map and the Regional Health Organisation Scheme (Sros).

The health map breaks every region down into sectors based on physical or mental health, for which the Director of the ARH fixes quantitative norms in the form of ratios of the number of beds to population size in each discipline – medicine, surgery, obstetrics, psychiatry, follow-up care, rehabilitation and long term care – and equipment/population ratios for dialysis machines, radiotherapy equipment, magnetic resonance imaging units, CT scanners, and lithotriptoscopes.

In practice, there is now judged to be an excess of beds in almost all areas, and the authorisations mainly affect operations involving restructuring, reconversion and merging.

Over the last ten years, against a more qualitative and medically oriented planning background, certain care procedures must also be approved, including organ transplants, the treatment of serious burns, heart surgery, neurosurgery, medically assisted reproduction, emergency services, intensive care and radiotherapy.

The Regional Health Organisation Scheme is the main instrument in this approach. This sets five-year targets for regional changes by proposing operations involving re-deployment, restructuring and co-operation. For the ARH, it constitutes a reference to deliver authorisation, approve establishments' projects and draw up with them agreements on targets and resources.

One recent striking direction is the wish of the authorities to encourage establishments to work together in networks in which each takes care of patients in line with its own technical expertise, with other establishments take caring of both the more and the less demanding cases. This type of functioning corresponds to a major change in habits. It is already specified in texts on perinatal care and emergency services.

Thus, establishments which specialise in obstetrics and neonatology are classified into one of four classes on a technical basis (from the neighbourhood centre where pre- and post-natal consultations are organised up to the specialised care centre capable of full-blown neonatal intensive care). For emergency services, reception must be organised according to the seriousness of the case in a nearby unit or in a service capable of caring for more serious cases, all the structures being bound by contract with notably the possibility of personnel rotation at less busy sites.

The 1990's marked a boom in the promotion and evaluation of care in health establishments. Thus, improvements in safety and general quality are dealt with in provisions (and are therefore funded) within establishments and when hospital care is being restructured: the fight against nosocomial infection with the CLIN since 1998, Anaes accreditation.

The pharmaceutical sector

When it comes to drugs, the available resources are associated with several procedures: Marketing Authorisation (MA), the evaluation of medical service rendered by the Transparency Commission which assesses new drugs' therapeutic efficacy and cost, and the decisions of the Health products Economic Committee which fixes prices and reimbursement rates for products.

The recent trend toward better resource allocation in the area of pharmaceuticals has led to an attempt to encourage the use of cheaper generic drugs (substitution by pharmacists, incentives to prescribing physicians) and negotiate prices in the light of expected prescription rates.

Clinical research

We have chosen to focus on clinical research because since 1993 this has benefited from special funding by the Directorate for Hospitalisation and Care Logistics (DHOS, *Direction de l'hospitalisation et de l'organisation de soins*) of the Employment Ministry. The hospital-based clinical research programme was launched by Bernard Kouchner in an Official Statement of November 19 1992. The clearly stipulated objective was to finance clinical research applied to sick humans in hospitals and carried out by hospital practitioners attached *"in priority to teams with no status as institutional research teams"*. The clinical research should *"follow on from fundamental research"*. The objective was to bring into existence in hospitals *"teams capable of carrying out their care functions on a research context"*, especially in multi-centre clinical trials. The Official Statement announced *"retrospective evaluation, based on an obligation of outcome"* (*i.e.* publication in *"peer-reviewed international journals"*). The funding mechanism chosen was to attribute to the PHRC an amount of credit corresponding to 0.05% of the main rate notified for several years (initially 4 but 3 for a number of years now). This credit appearing in the baseline hospital budget should be (and has been) reattributed then to new projects after the end of the projects chosen in 1993. The funding mechanism is a "sliding" one in the context of a sustained budget. There has been steady annual erosion of the credit attributed to the PHRC. 32 billion euros should have remained as an annual base whereas the budgets were reduced to 26 to 27 billion euros. This funding represents a major incentive to carry out projects for which no private sector sponsor can be found (*e.g.* research outside of the field of therapy, research into traditionally orphan areas, or comparisons of drugs which already have MA). Moreover, it is highly improbable that the 13% rebate of the spot Teaching Hospital value (and in cancer units) will correspond to the expenditure excess due to the care of patients participating in clinical trials. No study has been conducted to investigate this excess expenditure. The financial amounts considered (13% of the MCO budget of teaching hospitals and cancer centres) more than compensate for the excess costs (direct and indirect) related to clinical trials.

Attention is drawn to the importance of ensuring the public funding of research teams by the observation that, in certain fields, a large fraction of medical understanding derives from trials sponsored by the pharmaceutical industry. As a result, the research questions asked necessarily reflect the priorities of the companies; other questions need to be asked, outside of the realm of drugs and medical devices.

The role of crises in implicit and explicit decisions pertaining to resource allocation

So-called crises demonstrate the limitations of rational cost-efficacy criteria when it comes to political decision-making. A given explanation for the apparent inconsistency of certain decisions is firstly a difference between patients as statistical units and physically identified patients. Measures which are intended to prevent the development of diseases with an identified causal relationship are far more expensive than prevention in statistical patients. An illustration can be provided in the form of a comparison of the cost and efficacy of two types of measure, one in which the victims and beneficiaries are statistical and another in which the victims are identifiable. A study of the relationship between death resulting from iatrogenic complications and hospital expenditure in the United States concluded that an increase of 1.34% in hospital expenditure (assuming constant patient numbers and casemix, and making the relevant price adjustments) would reduce iatrogenic mortality by 1%[1]. In France, this would come down to saying an increase of 1.34% (*i.e.* about 762 billion euros) would save 3,500 lives, *i.e.* a cost of 153,000 euros per death prevented. This cost is well below that attributed for prevention of HCV transmission by transfusion which is estimated at over 152 million euros per life saved.

---

1. Morey R., Fine D., Loree S., Retzlaff-Roberts D., Tsubakinatini S. "The trade-off between hospital cost and quality of care". *Med Care*, 1992, 30: 677-98.

The new role of patients in resource allocation in the health care system: from informed consent to shared decision-making

In recent years, how to pay more attention to users' expectations in the running of the health care system has been a central topic for public discussion. The activities of certain patient support groups has been one of the main driving forces behind this change, and the AIDS epidemic has changed how the non-profit-making sector is involved in the field of health. Such organisations no longer limit their activities to patient support and collecting funds for research into specific areas. They are now beginning to influence policy in the matter of identifying public health priorities and safety issues, *i.e.* they are seeking to get involved in questions of resource allocation within the system. This corresponds to a new model for the patient, that of a player in his or her own health.

The Bill on modernisation of the health system currently before Parliament embodies these changes. As is already the case in the United States, the situation in France could evolve toward better patient information in order to bring them into the medical decision-making process. Experiments in shared medical decision-making have already been conducted in the context of post-menopausal hormone replacement therapy, and of whether or not to undertake surgical treatment for benign prostatic hyperplasia and breast cancer. Other studies bearing on heart disease, ulcers and diabetes have also shown that, when patients are involved in their own treatment, they tend to recover more quickly and attain a generally better state of health.

Discussion

Having concluded this review of resources in the health system, including a look at the limitations of the resource allocation mechanisms and the inconsistency between the various instruments, we will now propose four topics for consideration and discussion:
– the level of resources,
– the demographics of professional health care providers,
– resource allocation,
– the monitoring of the use of resources.

On each of these points, recommendations are made, qualified by their urgency or their feasibility in the short, medium or long term.

Health expenditure

Two indicators are usually used to compare health expenditure in France with that in other countries, namely per capita expenditure and the fraction of the Gross National Product (GNP) devoted to health.

Part three   Resource allocation in the health system

In terms of per capita expenditure, France ranks 11th among the 29 OECD countries (9th in the OECD-Europe group, see figure 4). According to the fraction of the GNP devoted to health, France ranks 4th. Depending on which parameter is used, France is either near the middle or among the highest spenders on health.

In both cases, no conclusions can be drawn about whether France is spending too much or too little unless answers are found to a number of questions: What is the relationship between expenditure, the amount of care provided, and its cost? Or between increased health expenditure and improved health status? Or between health expenditure, the country's economic state and social cohesion?

Figure 4   **Per capita expenditure on health (1998) ($)**
(equal buying power-adjusted OECD-Europe figures)

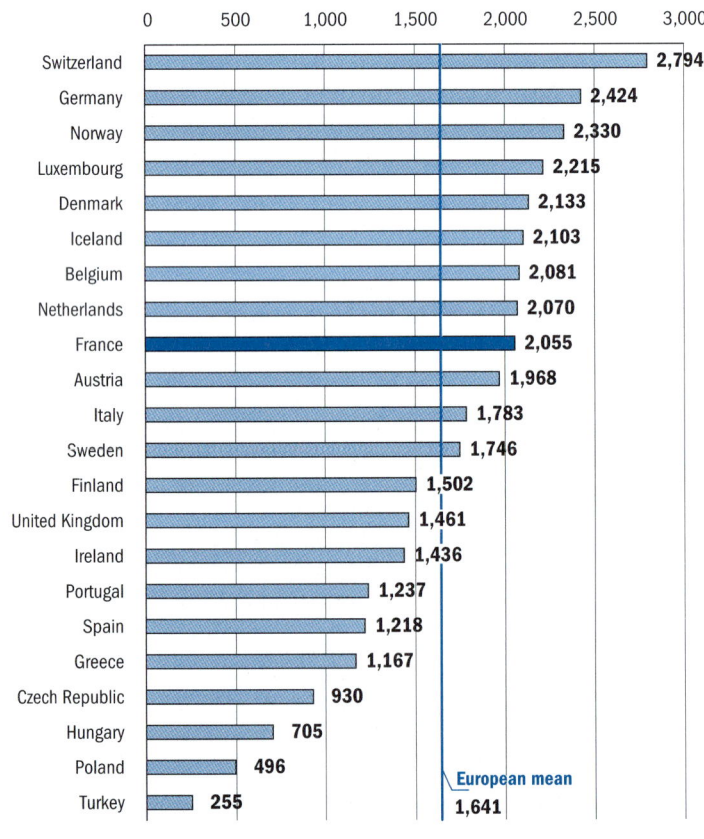

Source: Eco-santé 2000, OECD.

Discussion

The answers to these questions are often no more than extrapolations from very limited data which are not conducive to the setting of norms. The fact that France falls above the regression curve describing the mean relationship between a country's wealth (OECD countries) and their per capita health expenditure does not mean that it is spending too much but rather reflects – retrospectively – that health has been made something of a priority in the division of the country's resources.

The ratio of health expenditure to GNP is a non-robust indicator which changes according to both the numerator (health expenditure) and the denominator (national wealth).

Currently, the health accounts do not make it possible to break down available resources, either at the regional level or at smaller scales, nor even by disease. And this despite the fact that these data would be extremely valuable for planners who wish to divert resources in favour of those Regions or diseases where the need is greatest.

With the ageing of the population, rising expectations with respect to longevity and quality of life, and the introduction of new diagnostic and therapeutic modalities, it is likely that the demand for care is going to rise significantly in the near future. This increased demand will manifest as increased solicitation of the health care system and, as a result, increased health expenditure.

Rather than merely representing improvements on older therapies, most of the recent, innovative treatment modalities make it possible to treat patients in a poor overall condition in a more proactive fashion – in ways which just did not exist in the past. The new modalities (which tend to be less invasive and initiated at an earlier stage of the disease process) improve patients' quality of life but which, in the shorter or longer term, are succeeded by more invasive modalities when their therapeutic potential is exhausted. Thus, increased life expectancy entails more consumption of care.

Both the wish to expand preventive medicine and the principle of precaution established as a result of recent crises and "scandals" are no doubt going to lead to further increases in health expenditure, at least in the short term, by broadening the basis of intervention of health care professionals to individuals.

The increase and diversification of the demand for care will have an impact – through a complex political and social process – on change in health care system resources and on their attribution to different sectors (prevention, care, etc.).

The model in which health expenditure changes to match a stipulated target has proven unrealistic, as illustrated by the regular failure to respect the Ondam. Therefore, decision-makers are going to have to take real health needs into account and prepare to release the funds necessary to address these needs in the medium term.

At what level should decisions be taken, and who should be supervising health programmes?

Priorities should be identified and ranked in a political process. The method should involve defining the medical dimension of each priority, establishing Good Practices and acceptable degrees of deviation, defining the resources necessary for these practices taking into account areas of overlap between both hospital and independent practice and between different types of professional health care provider, and planning resource allocation in time and space. Implementing a health programme necessitates stipulating a temporal schedule (what resources, when, in what order, etc.) to arrive at the desired result.

The key issue here is to find appropriate instruments to ensure the consistency of political directions and the allocation of resources to both curative and preventive medicine. These include but are not confined to legislative instruments.

Resource allocation to the health system cannot be reduced to an annual target expenditure, but must be an integrated budget, formulated on a time scale longer than one year, if necessary. Exploitation of this budget in the medical field can be monitored because numerous indicators exist or can be devised to construct links between the use of resources and care processes. From knowledge about care processes, it is often possible to extrapolate the impact on the population's health status. Existing instruments for allocating special sums for medical advances may offer a model for this type of monitoring, as long as procedures and results are evaluated.

Hospitals

The data presented in the review of the situation in short-stay hospitals reveal a worrying picture. Over the last five years, the number of beds has dropped by a factor of 9% without any change in either occupancy or admission rate. This suggests that this decrease coupled with improved long-term care provision has not had any impact on global access to health care. On the other hand, the intensity of hospital activity – as measured by the reduction in the length of stays – has increased. The numbers of physicians and other professional care providers have not increased in parallel to this increase in activity, neither quantitatively nor qualitatively.

Without going back on the closure of beds which seems to be a fait accompli, the options to be explored are increasing the

Discussion

Care providers

numbers of professional care providers or developing new forms of qualification for both doctors and nurses.

There are currently 3 doctors for every 1,000 inhabitants. Is this too many, about right, or not enough? There is no clear-cut answer to this question for a number of reasons: because the density of physicians varies throughout the country; because the picture depends on the specialism under consideration; because morbidity at the local level is poorly understood; and because we are not very good at forging links between the health needs and care needs.

It is even more difficult to answer the question "How many doctors are we going to need in the future?" In practice, changes in medical techniques and in the way care is funded and distributed, may have a significant impact on the nature of the population's needs in the future, on its feasible demand, and on the activities of various types of care provider.

On the one hand, certain factors such as growth in preventive medicine and patient information and/or improved reimbursement may tend to increase the level of medical activity. But on the other hand, innovations in diagnosis and treatment, and the development of new forms of organisation such as networks might help enhance efficiency in the health sector as a whole, in particular by redefining the jobs and remits of various professionals and health care establishments. Equivalent health outcomes could then be obtained with less resource, or alternatively, the same amount of resources could give better outcomes.

Finally, regulatory measures concerning access to care and care processes might encourage more economical behaviour patterns among both consumers and care producers.

Table 5 **Projected number of physicians in 2024 according to 2000 age brackets**

	Number	Years from retirement (at 65)	Turnover (based on the current rate)	Shortfall
50-54 ages	35,054	2010-2014	20,400	–15,000
45-49 ages	43,749	2015-2019	20,400	–23,200
40-44 ages	37,560	2020-2024	20,400	–17,000

Source: "Medical demographics: the current situation and projections" National Council of the Order of Physicians, Public Health Division, 2001.

In the years to come, these points will have to be more deeply investigated, in particular by comparisons with foreign countries, and by launching new experimental systems and evaluating them in both medical and economic terms. However, it would be dangerous to base projections of the number of professionals needed on schemes which experience has shown are difficult to implement and of which the overall effects only become evident relatively slowly over and after a long time.

As was discussed above, France is below the European average in the matter of medical demographics. According to current projections (table 5), the overall number of physicians should start to drop in 2006, falling to about 225 doctors per 100,000 inhabitants by 2020.

This downward trend could have been predicted ten years ago when the ageing of the medical community first became apparent. Nevertheless, it is only recently that discussion of the "excess" of physicians gave way to worries – justified or not – about insufficient numbers to cope with needs in the near future unless there is significant improvement in the way care distribution is organised. It should be pointed out that there is already a lack in a number of disciplines (anaesthesiology, intensive care, paediatrics, gynaecology and obstetrics, ophthalmology, general surgery and internal surgery) and certain geographical areas (the Nord and rural areas in general). Despite extensive recruitment of foreign doctors, about 3,000 hospital posts remain vacant.

The *numerus clausus* (the number of students admitted into medical school) and the number of internships are set by the public authorities and could eventually be used to remedy this problem but the long lag between the commencement of medical training and qualification means that any policy in this area would not bear fruit for at least ten years.

In the meantime, the question of possible increases in productivity through new logistical structures (*e.g.* networks) and the transfer of tasks from physicians to other professional care providers is becoming an urgent one.

It seems likely that specific resources could be allocated to accelerate changes judged desirable in the matter of the continuity of care and complementarity between different professionals. But how can these points be objectively integrated into projected needs for doctors, and how can growth be sustained in the areas of prevention and patient information? And this without being obliged to have a desired target to aim at rather than being able to rely on objective results from relevant surveys?

Would other professionals be able to compensate for a shortfall in physicians?

In some European countries, non-medical staff are entrusted with procedures which in France are the exclusive domain of qualified physicians. In this country, the division of labour between medical and paramedical personnel is stipulated in regulatory texts pertaining to medical procedures and professional qualifications, and also in the provisions of the future Common Classification of Medical Procedures (CCAM, *Classification commune des actes médicaux*).

Whatever individual opinions are on this subject, it seems essential to conduct a serious study to define areas of activity, ascertain the advantages which might accrue, and identify any possible dangers. Such a study should address a number of topics, including quality and safety, obligations, incidence on the content of studies, expected economic impact, etc.

No-one can now predict the extent to which members of the medical community and paramedical staff will co-operate with such an initiative. Many acts require a certain level of skill, and may affect the diagnosis and treatment of the patient concerned, for which the doctor alone remains ultimately responsible.

Care networks represent an opportunity to experiment with different modes of sharing tasks between physicians and nurses, including menial tasks as well as less menial ones.

Recommendations

Resource levels
Short-term

Research into the evaluation of needs should be undertaken with a view to establishing a plan for future needs and designing ways of matching care provision to identified needs. This concerns conventional medical needs associated with any of the classic major classes of problem such as cardiovascular, haemato-oncological and infectious disease, or more recent problems associated with ageing and dependence. In the case of chronic disease, areas of overlap need to be found between the health care sector and other players.

The funding of care provision, be it for drugs, medical devices or hospital and outpatient medical and nursing services, cannot uniformly obey an annual logic. The medical progress budgets represent a first response, but an incomplete one because, whereas a fraction of the supply is to be attributed on a longer term (several years) basis, the rest is to be decided every six months.

It would also be desirable to provide for mechanisms to set up pluriannual budgets to deal with technical and economic developments (*e.g.* new treatment modalities or price changes).

Demographics of care providers

Needs for physicians over the next few years will depend on measures taken in the area of the organisation and distribution of care. To attain a given target density, action needs to be taken now at the level of the number of students being trained.

Ignoring future needs which are difficult to predict, the National Council of the Order of Physicians has calculated that, in order to replace those who will be retiring around the year 2010, the *numerus clausus* (currently 4,100) will have to be raised to 7,000, a major increase although this is indeed the level to guarantee a medical density equivalent to that today. Short of concluding that the current density is too high or counting on reduced needs by virtue of increased productivity resulting from logistical changes implemented in the care system in the next ten years, this is the annual number of students required to sustain physician numbers through 2010.

A total of 1,843 posts have been offered in the competitive internship process in the last two years. This needs to be increased in the absence of more profound reform, and this instead of adjusting internal distribution which tends to lead to destabilisation in disciplines which were not previously under-subscribed.

In parallel, the expansion of nursing expertise may allow for substitution and affect the total number of physicians needed in various disciplines.

For nurses, retrospective national studies (distinguishing between people who graduated at different times and who have had diverse career tracks) conducted over the last ten years have revealed certain costly consequences of changed behaviour patterns in the matter of part-time working, career planning (including premature departure from the profession) and retirement. These studies would be of enormous use later for analysing the impact of bringing the working week down to 35 hours.

Substitution is also possible within health professions, including in hospitals. Note should be made of the absence of any system to reimburse the interventions of independent medical auxiliaries.

Research into authority, responsibility and economic incentives should be undertaken.

Recommendations

Medium-term

Link the level and the attribution of the various resources to health targets

This is a very difficult exercise insofar as the various resources are used to produce a variety of commodities and services without any idea of how the two different dimensions correspond. Nevertheless, attempts to establish input/output matrices associated with hypotheses might show that certain resources are being under-exploited or that seeking to attain certain targets is unrealistic given the immediately available resources.

Repeating the exercise at regular intervals (or in different Regions) may refine our understanding of the relationship between resources and targets, and therefore improve resource allocation.

Studying links cannot be confined to a single direction: it is also important to ask questions about the health consequences of the failure to attribute resources.

With equity in mind, it would be desirable to obtain a better distribution of numbers of the various disciplines throughout the territory.

The restocking of rural areas with doctors depends on a strategy likely to be at the expense of the big cities, by encouraging new doctors to install in the countryside by means of incentives, notably economic and/or organisational incentives.

In order to improve access for populations to comprehensive care provision, one option is establishing group practices and improving patient transport facilities, or making it possible for single physicians to exercise in more than one practice. This latter option is particularly applicable to specialists.

When choosing to adopt one formula rather than another, local conditions must always be taken into account. This pre-supposes that health care system logistics will be decentralised and that specific resources will be available at least at the regional level.

Adequate provision is also necessary in hospitals as well as in independent practice. Questions can be asked about the lack of appeal of certain specialisations, about the quality of the service rendered when there are insufficient doctors, and even about the ability to maintain understaffed structures in operation. If they correspond to needs, they should be provided with the appropriate resources.

Short-term measures for long-term effects

Innovations which accompany medical advances have major consequences on various aspects of care distribution. The activity in some current specialties will probably fall off or even disappear, thus necessitating the re-dedication of personnel and facilities.

The way medical training is currently organised tends to mean that doctors are only equipped to practice in a certain, more or less specific field throughout their career. It seems desirable to establish regulatory instruments and the necessary training modalities to make it possible for them to change direction in mid-career (bridges between hospital and independent practice, between general medicine and specialisation, between different specialisms). The profession seems to accept the necessity for such instruments.

Resource allocation

The Social Security Funding Law (LFSS), like other financial mechanisms which govern the health sector, does not fully meet the objective of optimal resource allocation to match identified health needs. The main weaknesses are the following: a lack of data which compromises the evaluation of resource allocation in the light of needs; a lack of organisation and co-ordination; a lack of monitoring and therefore of global rationality. There exist responses for each of these lacks: some of these responses are being made, some are being discussed, and some have been no more than alluded to.

A first improvement is provided for in the Bill on modernisation of the health system, in the form of instigating discussion of public health priorities in the Parliamentary debate prior to the vote on the LFSS. The priorities identified must be ranked and scheduled.

Short-term

In the quest for improved ways of matching resources to health needs, establishing a formalised list of procedures represents a step.

The current information-gathering system for hospital and independent practice can be criticised for being almost exclusively based on financial parameters, sometimes detailed but nevertheless incomplete. Although the resultant data give a general idea of how resources are attributed to the different sectors of care production, there is no way of putting the available information into the context of estimated needs or health outcomes.

The Common Classification of Medical Procedures (CCAM, *Classification commune des actes médicaux*) should provide a common framework for independent and hospital practice, and should also result in the reformulation of medical tariffs to establish a consistent, "neutral" pricing system. Such a system is already in place for medical tests and drugs. The CCAM is now in the finalisation stage. The existence of such a coding system for procedures will make it possible to follow the activity of the medical profession and could later be extended to include paramedical care providers and non-technical procedures.

It is important to continue and evaluate the work begun in 2000 to test new modes of funding public and private establishments on the basis of a disease-specific pricing system. This work is an essential component in the medium-term objective of matching care provision to the population's needs.

Short-term measures for medium-term effects

With a view to improving logistics and enhancing co-ordination between professionals and between professionals and users, remuneration systems should be reviewed in order to make the most of the associated incentives.

The preliminaries to re-organising how professionals are compensated for their work include establishing and validating a medical information system to integrate data and allow for the compilation of accounts on a disease-specific basis.

Assuming that the CCAM improves matching between a given medical procedure and its level of compensation, the next issue to be addressed is how to forge a better relationship between expressed health needs and the response of the care system. Freedom – free access, free prescription – is a founding principle in the French care system and means of improving efficiency now need to be found, *i.e.* ways of matching the demand for care to the system's response at the lowest price.

With respect to improved logistics, the network solution seems to be a promising way of overcoming the present compartmentalisation problem. One immediately thinks of regulated networks based on a single disease which bring together hospitals and independent practitioners. But many other possibilities exist: above and beyond networks built up around a reference theme, organisations could collaborate with a range of partners (users' groups, physicians, etc.). Most existing networks are based on a specific disease (*e.g.* HIV, HCV, diabetes, cancer, etc.).

The concomitant definition of a disease-based pricing system and better co-ordination of the development of care should lead to genuine improvement in the quality of treatment. Experiments – more flexible and larger-scale than the "Soubie" networks – should be undertaken, and should include testing of the effect of financial incentives on productivity in the system. Regionalisation would seem to be a first step in this direction.

New modes of remuneration could also be applied to drugs if evaluation of current experimental price-volume contracts shows them to be a useful instrument.

Short-term measures for long-term effects

Valuable results can be expected from a number of projects investigating various aspects: the impact of organisational changes; the efficacy of financial incentives for the various players; the restrictions with respect to centralised patient monitoring which result from the obligation to respect confidentiality; and remuneration paid on a per-patient basis. The logic of such a remuneration mechanism for a given time interval and dissociated from the volume of care activity is that it would encourage professionals to emphasise prevention as well as care. Nevertheless, this idealistic plan will have to be reconciled with the reality of the temporal lag between expenditure on preventive medicine and reduced treatment costs.

This instrument will have to be co-ordinated with that defining a set of commodities and services which must at all times be accessible to the entire population. However, certain services may be concentrated between a few reference centres without necessarily having to be provided throughout the country.

These measures must be coupled with the provision of information to users about how best to exploit the available resources: maintenance of freedom of choice, but responsibility for safety aspects. In practice, the ultimate purpose of bringing different forms of high technology care under the same roof is enhanced safety. In the case of modalities for which the expertise of the operator is a key factor in the outcome, it is logical to limit the number of reference centres according to the number of procedures carried out and results. This fulfils the safety requirement for treatment but not that of either proximity or access. Great distance between the home and the treatment centre can create genuine difficulty for patients and their families, especially in the case of long-term, serious disease. Thus, concentrating care provision should be coupled with measures to improve transportation and accommodation.

At what level should resource allocation decisions be made?

Thought should be given as to the level at which health care policy is made, taking into account the European dimension: Europe, nation State, region, department? Consideration could be broken down on a disease-specific basis, and also between the different sectors of preventive and curative medicine.

Monitoring the use of resources

Short-term

It has been seen that trying to determine the level of health system resources needed before the fact is fraught with problems. Health accounts and one-off studies provide retrospective data for the analysis of funding decisions and their consequences, *e.g.* "What fraction of resources is attributed to preventive medicine as opposed to treatment?"

Other information can be obtained from the health accounts or parallel sources to evaluate the results and consequences of decisions concerning resource allocation.

Price changes and changes in the volume of expenditure on care are well described in the accounts. On the other hand, the way in

Recommendations

which price and volume are divided – which is imperfect and could be improved – could be discussed. In a more limited context, since prices are negotiated by the hospitals, price differences do not necessarily demonstrate inequalities but rather logistical differences between different institutions.

The purpose of the health accounts is to describe, as accurately and as comprehensively as possible, all expenditure on health. Interpreting changes as revealed in the accounts is another matter. In order to guarantee neutrality and thereby preserve the credibility of the health accounts, it is important to make a clear distinction between these two approaches. The data in the accounts are public and available in detail, and researchers and any other observers can use them to carry out any studies or analyses they want, including analysis of why the Ondam is rarely respected. For this exercise in particular, it is probably technically simpler to rely on a direct comparison of the predicted and actual figures contained in the Ondam.

Complementary analyses should reveal the factors underlying the discrepancy between the Ondam and expenditure observed at care facilities, these factors being associated with either supply (in particular, technical progress) or demand (*e.g.* morbidity or changes in habits vis-à-vis the seeking of medical advice).

This type of analysis could help explain why the Ondam has only ever been respected once, and may contribute to fixing it in a more realistic way in the future.

In order to establish a link between health policy and resource allocation, it will be necessary to improve co-ordination between different Ministries. If necessary, a General Secretariat will have to be created to formalise the information on resource allocation to be provided to politicians. Answers have to be found to an increasing number of questions about links between health policy priorities and directions for reimbursement of care emanating from the National Health Conference. In particular, the extent to which the Ondam voted by Parliament will be able to cover treatment deemed necessary – the needs as estimated by the National Health Conference.

Medium-term The annual publication of the health accounts is an ideal moment to define the role of crises and public opinion in resource allocation decisions, to provide information on costs and the consequences of decisions, and to assess the overall results of these decisions. The purpose of providing *post facto* information about resource allocation in this context would be to enlighten decision-makers and the general public about the preferences implicit in these choices. Critical analysis – removed in time from the crisis or scandal – of past policies and the medium and long-term consequences of decisions taken at a time of uncertainty is an academic exercise which is common in fields other than health. Such instruments could profitably be applied to the evaluation of certain decisions such as those to use erythropoietin to treat kidney failure, immunisation against Hepatitis B, and the screening of blood for transfusion for HCV.

In order to monitor the application of policies and their critical analysis, indicators have to be found that establish a relationship between a particular instance of expenditure and the corresponding health outcome, and to modify the list of registered medical services to take into account diverse preventive measures by dissociating them from common diagnostic and therapeutic procedures.

It would be possible to begin with simple cases in which it suffices, for example, to know the activity to be able to deduce the health outcome (this applies to all situations in which there is a direct and known relationship between a procedure and an outcome) such as immunisation, or thrombolysis during acute myocardial infarction, etc.

Screening, preventive medicine and overlapping activities performed by a physician are more complicated. Nevertheless, public health measures such as immunisation or preventive campaigns must always be evaluated. Such an evaluation instrument could be overseen by the High Committee on Public Health.

In order to obtain quantitative and qualitative data (qualifications, working hours, modes of production, technical environment), steering instruments will have to be devised, and markers will have to be developed to make it possible to follow the spread of innovation in the French health system.

Long-term Efforts to improve medical information systems by means of the PMSI and to introduce different classification and pricing systems (*e.g.* for drugs and medical tests) in the health insurance system (which would make it possible to break down the accounts on a disease-specific basis) should be continued. The objective here is to understand how health expenditure breaks down according to diagnostic category and risk factor, to evaluate the fraction of resources devoted to preventive medicine and the monitoring of health status, to evaluate temporal distortions in expenditure with respect to changes in disease profiles, and to follow the spread of innovation.

PART FOUR

The user, a player in the health care system

Part four The user, a player in the health care system

Composition of the Working Group

President Pierre Guillet, High Committee on Public Health

Rapporteur Bernard Cassou, René-Descartes University, Paris 5

Members Étienne Caniard, the French Mutual Insurance System
Michel Depinoy, French Committee on Health Education
Véronique Ghadi, the Development, Innovation, Evaluation, Health company
Danièle Mischlich, Directorate for Hospitalisation and Care Logistics, Ministry of Employment and Solidarity
Michel Naiditch, Image group, National School of Public Health
Bertrand Sachs, General Health Directorate, Ministry of Employment and Solidarity
Annie Serfaty, General Health Directorate, Ministry of Employment and Solidarity

Co-ordination Claudine Le Grand, General Secretariat of the High Committee on Public Health

The Working Group wishes to thank for their contributions Dominique Baubeau, Directorate of Research, Studies, Evaluation and Statistics, Ministry of Employment and Solidarity
Maryvonne Bitaud-Thépaut, High Committee on Public Health
Nicolas Brun, National Union of Family Associations
Alain Coulomb, High Committee on Public Health
Daniel Defert, High Committee on Public Health
Pierre Lascoumes, Interassociation Health Collective
Thérèse Lecomte, Association for Socioeconomic Questions and Health
Isabelle Manzi, Directorate for Hospitalisation and Care Logistics, Ministry of Employment and Solidarity
Norbert Nabet, Public Health Intern
Jean-Jacques Nansot, General Health Directorate, Ministry of Employment and Solidarity
Laurent Dubois-Mazeyrie, General Health Directorate, Ministry of Employment and Solidarity

Introduction

Involving patients to a greater extent in the health-related decisions that affect them is an idea that is gaining ground, since it is the patient – and, more globally, the citizen – who is the user in any health care system. It is however an idea that presupposes profound changes in the status and attitude of all involved in health care. Such changes will have an impact at a number of different levels: that of the patient who is asking for help; that of the user who wants the health care system to take care of his or her problems; and that of the citizen who wants to play a part in the formulation of the public health policy. These are the three faces of *Homo sanus* that will emerge in everyone at some point in life.

In this report, we are interested in contributing to the dialogue which is taking form in society about how to promote the involvement of the user in the health care-related decision-making process. The processes of education, consultation, dialogue and decision-making all need to be rethought with a view to:
– involving members of the general public in decisions concerning public health issues,
– bringing the user into the governance of health care and social institutions in order to get a better idea of their expectations and address them more effectively,
– according the patient a more important place in the making of diagnostic and therapeutic decisions.

For easier reading, we intend to use the word user without distinction whether we are talking about the patient in the health care system, a citizen involved in health or, of course, the user of health care services. However, we are not unaware of the divergent meanings and issues underlying these semantic subtleties *(see box)*.

Part four — The user, a player in the health care system

SOME SEMANTICS

Many different terms are used to describe the user of the health care system although each has its own particular meaning and implications. Following are some definitions:
- **Subject:** refers to an individual with a specific history who can act independently.
- **Sick:** a sick person is someone whose *"state of health is compromised"*, who is unhealthy, *i.e.* the term is defined first and foremost by health status. A relatively neutral word which is commonly used by sufferers themselves.
- **Patient:** someone who is undergoing or to undergo some form of medical examination or treatment. Primarily defined by the fact that care is being provided. The passivity of the position of the patient, and his or her dependence on the care provider is betrayed by the word "undergo" in the definition. A term often used by health care professionals.
- **User:** he or she who has a right to use or who actually uses a public service. This term therefore contains ideas of both rights and public service. Often used by patient support groups and other non-profit-making organisations who defend patients' rights as well as by public authorities who are responsible for guaranteeing equitable access to public services.
- **Consumer:** he or she who uses commodities or resources to satisfy a need. This is above all an economic term. In this context, health is seen as a consumer good like any other. In France – with its highly administered health care system – the word is only really used by consumer groups, whereas in the context of the free market-based health care system in the United States, it is common in health-related literature: users are equivalent to consumers. The risk of this philosophy is to make of the doctor a technical adviser on illness or, at the worst, somebody who is there to cater to the consumer's own wishes.
- The term **customer** is used by administrators running their establishments on the lines of a business, with the purpose of encouraging staff to satisfy the customer's expectations. It implies a two-way relationship, between he who is paying and he who is providing the service.
- **Beneficiary:** he or she who benefits from advantages to which they are eligible, *e.g.* those receiving social security payments.
- **Citizen:** a member of the community. Defined by a person's responsibilities, obligations and rights vis-à-vis that community. Primarily a political concept which defines the individual in the context of society rather than as a user of services.

Making the user a player in the health care system amounts to a democratic obligation, from which enhanced efficacy and efficiency can be expected to result [186]. But this advance will only be possible unless, at the same time as we are reviewing the rights and responsibilities of users together with those of the State and those of the authorities responsible for monitoring and management, we take into account professional health care providers, pharmaceutical companies and the suppliers of medical services. Building new relationships between all these players seems to us a key element if the changes currently being made in the way the health care system is run are to have a successful outcome.

These changes are intended to bring about improved patient care and, more generally, better management of public health problems by society. They may also result in taking care of the financial shortfall by transferring part of the burden onto the user. Underpinning the way these changes are to be implemented are two concepts which are relatively new in the field of health care, namely citizenship and democracy.

Citizenship and democracy in health

What does "citizenship in health" mean? The word citizen is used more and more these days – it is impossible to count all the programmes, forums and public institutions which make reference to the word and the idea is commonly used in many different disciplines, most obviously the law but also sociology, political philosophy, anthropology and history [155], with a more or less different signification in each. In legal parlance, citizenship is a personal status, the granting and withdrawal of which is up to national and international law: upon this status depends a whole set of rights and duties.

In sociology and anthropology, the emphasis is on citizenship as a relationship between human beings, as confirmation that one belongs to a certain community and affirmation of a specific identity. Citizenship transcends differences – be they occupational, cultural or social – in order to ensure the participation of the members of a community in its affairs. In this sense of the word, a "citizen" in the field of health would want to bring out into the open questions which, hitherto, have been dealt with on a procedural basis in a way that is highly dependent on professional expertise [159].

One might also ask what "democracy in health" means. The word democracy usually refers to a particular structuring of social relationships in the political process and a way of putting the wish of the majority to the fore. It suggests discussion, deliberation, representation and taking responsibility. But in health-related issues, the opinion of the majority does not necessarily correspond to that which is the most valid and, apart from that, it is not a useful idea from a practical point of view. It seems to us that the term "democracy in health" is comparable to the terms "social democracy" and "wage democracy", the former came into widespread use in France at the time of liberation at the end of the Second World War and the scope of the latter widely spread from this period.

Part four   The user, a player in the health care system

The idea of social democracy underpins the post-war French social security system. Rather than establishing a British-style social security system entirely managed by the State, the French Government and parliament of the time opted for a social security system to be managed by the insurees (represented by the Trade Unions) and their employers, with the State playing a purely supervisory role [184]. Certain commentators hold that, when it comes to social security, "social democracy" was never really achieved, largely because of problems concerning the sharing of responsibilities between those actually managing the system and the State. The idea must however be given some credit for having extended the formal mores of political democracy and for making it possible for the first time for a large fraction of the population to develop personal strategies, an end achieved by enhancing the protection offered with respect to the right to work and social rights. In this light, the term democracy in health would refer to the implementation of new ways of ensuring the collective participation of all citizens in the design of the health care system.

In conclusion, the question is whether these ideas – "citizenship" and "democracy" – have any concrete relevance in the field of health care or whether they are simply words signifying a desire for a change in the relationships between the various parties involved, *i.e.* the State, professional health care providers and users. In order to fully appreciate the scope of the rethinking implied by meaningful use of these two ideas, it will be necessary to review the movement to recognise users as players in the health care system in their own right, and to accord them their proper role in the changes currently being undertaken.

A changing health care system

Up until relatively recently, good health care seemed to be guaranteed by a synergistic interaction between generous social coverage (which ensured access to treatment and reimbursement) and biomedical progress. This synergy sufficed to keep the image of the system broadly positive. The fact that the evaluation of medical practices and services was left up to health care professionals themselves with barely any input from other sources reflects not only the strength of the social contract between those professionals and the State, but also the confidence of the users in both the ethics of the profession and the merit of scientific progress. Most of those involved seemed to be happy with the situation. It resulted in democratisation of medical consumption which was destined to be sustained as long as economic considerations were not perceived as a great problem, which was the case up until the beginning of the 1970s. However, consistent growth in access to medical services never succeeded in eliminating inequality in health care. Similarly, the way the health care system works does not make it possible to respond to dissatisfaction – sometimes expressed, sometimes not – on the part of any of those involved.

Four issues seem to us to underlie the questions about the status and role of players in the health care system:
- the crisis in the public decision-making process which is also a crisis of expertise since it raises the question of the legitimacy of the State taking decisions with consultation confined to experts [170]. This crisis became apparent in the media as a result of the "HIV-Contaminated Blood Affair" [182], and the scandals associated with asbestos and bovine spongiform encephalopathy;
- there is increased consciousness of the possibility of progress in biotechnology having an adverse impact on human health, as evidenced by the reluctance of the general public to embrace genetically modified organisms. In the same vein, the part played by the health care system in the overall improvement in the health of the French people has been placed in doubt with the publication of a large number of studies which recommend diverting funds to other types of collective programme which also have strong beneficial effects on health [150];
- increasing individualism – in evidence at all levels of society with ever-expanding overlap between the private and public sectors – has had a corollary effect in the form of growing mistrust as to how the care system works in that it does not allow its users to make choices informed by a full knowledge of either the issues involved or the consequences associated with the various options. The increasing influence of patient support groups which represent the interests and relay the concerns of patients and their close ones has been and is continuing to be a key factor in determining how the health care system is perceived by users;
- finally, with chronic disease becoming more and more widespread, professional health care providers are having to rethink their role vis-à-vis patients who are better informed than previously, and who want to become more involved in their own treatment. Medical professionals today often find themselves the object of criticism – often contradictory criticisms – from diverse sources, *e.g.* legal, governmental and political bodies, and also patient support groups and users' associations: this experience can be very dramatic for them.

All these trends explain the changes which have occurred over recent years in terms of the status and behaviour patterns of those involved in health care. The patient is becoming a consumer in a health care marketplace, a trend which is being fostered by the pharmaceutical companies and other health-related industries. The users, while still having great expectations of professional health care providers, are all the more ready to question their opinions and blame them for setbacks. The status of many physicians has evolved from that of "craftsman" to one of a simple link in a chain of industrial-style care, a mode of functioning which is taking over and of which one of the signs is the widespread standardisation of protocols. And public service providers, under an obligation to enhance efficacy and efficiency, are tending to operate more like private companies with public service provision becoming a "strategy" and the managers becoming "Project Leaders" [146].

The user, a player in the health care system

It is against this dynamic background that it is necessary to consider consolidating the rights of the user who, it is important to remember, has a legal status *(see box)*. This should be reinforced by the legislation pertaining to modernisation of the health care system *(see box)*. In this respect, it is worth noting that society has always changed the way it looks on the sick according to its attitude to its members: charitable in the Middle Ages, then humanists in the following centuries, and finally utilitarian with the advent of the Industrial Revolution. In our time, it is an attitude based on the rights of the individual and democracy that dominates. However, it is important not to confuse the rights of the individual with human rights, as is often done in politics [164]. The concept of individual rights makes it possible to establish a set of diverse rights re-focused on the single person without any consequences on the ideas of citizenship or membership of the social system. But, as pointed out by M. Setbon [181], physicians as well as patients are members of society, and any changes in the relationship between the two is a social phenomenon, one which today is characterised by extension of the scope of the ideas of human liberty and democracy. The new attitude to users must be considered in the increasing individualism which, in principle at least, makes of the user an independent, free player, a rational being who operates within the logistical health care structure without any kind of conflict of interest. The reality of how the health care system actually works is far from this ideal.

In this chapter, we are particularly interested in conditions which will enable the user to participate more fully in the health care system. Ideally, this involvement would be so structured as to result in increased responsibility of the individual in his or her own health, and in public health in general. It needs to lead to consolidation of the mutual confidence of the all various groups of players with their diverse priorities, including State institutions, professional health care providers, administrators, users and commercial organisations.

These goals will not be easy to achieve because such changes necessarily depend on significant cultural transformations. And it is important not to under-estimate the deep rifts which have

Introduction

SOME LEGISLATIVE AND REGULATORY LANDMARKS

Many different pieces of legislation and regulatory texts pertain to health care system users' rights. They are contained in various codes, *e.g.* the Public Health Code (CSP, *Code de la santé publique*), the Social Security Code (CSS, *Code de la sécurité sociale*), the Civil Code (CC, *Code civil*), and the Code of Medical Ethics. The following is not an exhaustive list but rather focuses on the rights of hospital patients (in which area, much legislation has been passed).

Declaration of the Rights of Man and Citizens (August 26 1789)

Article 15: *"Society has the right to require any public agent to provide an account of his administration."*

Preamble to the Constitution (October 27 1946)

Article 11: *"[The Nation] undertakes to protect the health of all, particularly the young, mothers and old workers."*

Respect of the human body

(Chapter II of the Civil Code)

Article 16, Paragraphs 1 to 9 (Law n° 75-596 of July 9 1975 Art. 6, *Journal officiel* of July 10 1975, inserted by Law n° 94-653 of July 29 1994 Art. 1 I, II, Art. 2, *Journal officiel* of July 30 1994). *"The Law establishes the primacy of the individual, prohibits any attack on individual dignity, and guarantees the respect of the human being as of birth."*

Code of Medical Ethics

Decree n° 95-1000 of September 6 1995 which defines the ethical obligations of the medical profession vis-à-vis patients.

User representation on the administrative councils of public hospitals

Article L. 714-2 of the Public Health Code, Paragraphs 1, 25, 27 (Order n° 96-346 of April 24 1996): *"The administrative councils of public heath care establishments are to include six categories of members [including] representatives of users."*

Admission Booklet

Article L, 710-1-1 of the Public Health Code (Order n° 96-346 of April 24 1996): *"High quality patient care is a primary objective of any health care establishment. This must include regular evaluation of patient satisfaction, notably with respect to admission procedures and the period of hospitalisation. The results of such evaluation procedures will be taken into account in the process of accreditation provided for in Article L. 710-5."*

The Ruling of January 7 1997: *"Every establishment must provide the patient on admission with an Admission Booklet containing the Hospital Patient's Charter in accordance with the model stipulated by the Health Ministry."*

Hospital Patient's Charter

Article L. 710-1-1 of the Public Health Code (Order n° 96-346 of April 24 1996) and appended to Ministerial Circular Letter n° 95-22 of May 6 1995, which reproduces the Charter.

Satisfaction surveys

Article L. 710-1-1 of the Public Health Code (Order n° 96-346 of April 24 1996).

Conciliation Commission

Article L. 710-1-1 of the Public Health Code (Order n° 96-346 of April 24 1996).
Articles R. 710-1-1 to 10 of the Public Health Code, Decree n° 98-1001 of November 2 1998 (*JO* of November 7 1998).
Circular Letter DH/AF1/99 N° 317 of June 1 1999.

Medical records

Article R. 710-2-1 to R. 710-2-10 of the Public Health Code, in particular Article R. 710-2-1 for the content of medical records, Decree n° 92-329 of March 30 1992.
Decree n° 94-68 of January 24 1994 concerning blood transfusion procedures.

Health Care Access Offices (Pass, *Permanence d'accès aux soins de santé*)

Articles L. 711-3 and 711-7-1 of the Public Health Code (Law n° 98-657 of July 29 1998 pertaining to measures to reduce social exclusion) which entrusts the public hospital system with a novel responsibility, namely to actively participate in *"the fight against social exclusion, in a dynamic, collaborative network with other relevant professions and institutions, and with non-profit-making organisations which are active in the fight against social exclusion"*.
Circular Letter n° DH/AF1/DGS/SP2/DAS/RV3/98/736 of December 17 1998.

Public meetings of the Administrative Councils of National Health Insurance Agencies

Article L. 231-8-1 of the Social Security Code (Order n° 96-344 of April 24 1996 specifying measures pertaining to the organisation of the Social Security system):
"[The] *reports* [submitted to the Director of the Agency's Administrative Council] *should include at least one report on relations with users [...] At least one annual meeting of the Administrative Council is to be devoted to relations with users and this session is to be public."*

Access to administrative records

The Law of July 17 1978; notably creating the Commission for Access to Administrative records (Cada, *Commission d'accès aux documents administratifs*).

Source: [165].

Introduction

developed between different key players in recent years. The field of health is full of conflicts, between the medical and the scientific community on the one hand and financial and commercial interests on the other. This goes part of the way to explaining why it has been so difficult to implement long-standing legislation pertaining to patient information and personal access to medical records. It is also important to keep in mind the fact that health care is a special field in that it concerns people who are unwell and therefore vulnerable. Nevertheless, it is an economic sector in which the regulatory mechanisms whereby the market ensures the quality of products (in this case, the efficacy of diagnosis, treatment and prophylaxis) must be more complicated than in other economic sectors. It is vital to avoid the pitfalls which are inherent to this difficult situation, such as the compartmentalisation of different categories of "customer", or supply-side fostering of demand [169]. Finally, over-restrictive regulation of the health care system by state authorities and administrators risks leaving little room for manœuvre for either users or professionals who are interested in changing the system. (Yes, there exist professional health care providers interested in this!)

Keeping users informed: a vital public health issue

We have made a distinction between three different areas in which users can participate in the health care system:
– the formulation of public health care policy;
– the general working of health care and societal institutions;
– in the context of care provision.

These three separate questions will now be addressed, beginning with the idea of the citizen user. We believe that converting the user into a genuine player in the health care system will primarily constitute a political initiative. In some way, this is already recognised by the public sector authorities in that they are seeking to base future public health policy on the concept of "democracy in health".

First of all, we will examine conditions that might let citizen users participate meaningfully in the formulation of health care policy. Many health-related parameters are regularly evaluated, including occupational and environmental health issues, safety, how the care system is organised and health care priorities. In the light of the complexity of all these questions, the authorities have constructed an evaluation instrument based on scientific and/or medical experts. However, public health has economic, social and ethical components, as well as scientific and medical ones, so the question is "How can the citizen user be brought into the decision-making process?"

Then we will analyse how to involve the user in the management of institutions. It is not irrelevant to point out here that, up until

Part four The user, a player in the health care system

1941, the internal rules applicable in hospitals still included provisions on "order and discipline" on the part of patients. Since and especially over the last thirty years, a succession of acts and laws have been passed to consolidate patients' rights, but now more needs to be done to recognise the rightful place of users and patients in the organisation and running of institutions. What conditions are necessary to achieve this?

Finally, we will address the question of the relationship between patient and physician, in which major changes are currently taking place. Among other things, with respect to the previously paternalistic nature of this relationship in which the doctor made all the choices in terms of the examinations to be conducted or ordered, and the treatments to be prescribed. This needs to be re-orientated to a model in which the patient is an active participant in the treatment process so that the ultimate decision concerning which examinations are to be carried out and what treatment instigated results from a collaborative approach. How are the knowledge and opinions of patients to be taken into account in this process?

All these questions need to be addressed by society as a whole. Certain aspects of all these questions are a source of disagreement between the various different parties interested in the health care system, notably when it comes to medical records, access to high-quality care, and users' claims in health care establishments. These will be tackled briefly in the second and third sections because we have not focused on these problems. In fact, we think that recognition of the rightful place of the user within the health care system will soon lead to a global reappraisal of the modalities of both treatment and patient information. Such recognition is one of the necessary first steps towards real implementation of both the rights and the obligations of the user. Most disagreements (which are actually relatively rare) between care providers and patients these days can be attributed to a failure to keep the patient sufficiently (or comprehensibly) informed: information on his or her state of health, on the treatment modality implemented, on the associated risks, or on doubts and uncertainties in the minds of the care providers.

Information is at the heart of the dialogue about democracy in health, constituting a key issue in the matter of how care provision will be affected by changes in both the ways in which the relevant institutions operate, and how public health care policy is formulated. This is why we have placed information at the very centre of our approach.

With regard to involving users in the working of the health care system, certain people have found that the authorities are trying to block progress by regularly referring the law on modernisation back to Parliament for further discussion, an opinion that has led to some users' groups boycotting official meetings on health care. This resulted, early in 2001, in the representatives of users' groups quitting this working group appointed by the High Committee on Public Health in the framework of the 2002 Health in France Report. The other members of the group-researchers, professional health care providers, and representatives of the Government and of the High Committee on Public Health, continued the work but in conditions far from ideal, given that the topic under review is exactly how to promote the participation (!) of users in the decision-making process in the health care system.

THE BILL ON MODERNISATION OF THE HEALTH CARE SYSTEM

The Bill on modernisation of the health care system has been drawn up in response to strong demand for re-equilibration of the relationships between patients and professional care providers, between the health care system and its users. This demand was prominently expressed at the 1998-1999 Constitutive Assembly on Health. Developing and consolidating the idea of democracy in health is one of the focuses of this Bill.

Recognising and specifying fundamental rights

The Bill contains a summary of the current legal context. For readability, it brings together in a single text a review of the relevant jurisprudence and of all the provisions pertaining to people's rights in their relationships with the health care system, including health professionals, health care establishments and networks, and any other organisation involved in prevention or care provision:
- Respect of dignity, of protection of the corporeal integrity of sick people.
- Non-discrimination in access to care and prevention.
- Respect of privacy and confidentiality in the matter of health-related information.
- Principle of proportionality between therapeutic benefits and risks.
- Right to pain management, in the respect of the dignity of people at the end of their life.

Defining the responsibilities of users of the health care system and ensuring their participation in its workings

The Bill specifies the conditions necessary to involve the sick person in the care provision process. It reviews, specifies and updates the rules pertaining to patient information and consent, and access to personal medical records. It institutes a direct access procedure and provides for ways of helping patients obtain information. It restructures hospital Conciliation Commissions and re-organises professional orders.
It organises user representation in the health care system by providing for an accreditation procedure for users' groups and establishing the conditions necessary for effective representation.

Directorate for Hospitalisation and Care Logistics (DHOS, Direction de l'hospitalisation et de l'organisation des soins).

Participation in the formulation of public health policy

In public health as in all other areas, making decisions necessarily entails making choices. These do not only concern technical and concrete facts, but also value judgements about questions of health, disease, human beings and society, all the more so since the central issue is the preservation or restoration of the good health of individuals and populations. This is why we consider that the extent to which citizens are involved in the health-related decision-making process can be taken as a measure of a country's democratic development.

Since the 1970's in France, public action in a number of non-medical areas has been guided by a more consultative framework [153] as a result of pressure from motivated users. In the matter of health, the public decision-making process has been influenced by patient support groups. Thus, an overall change has taken place as a result of, on the one hand, general changes in the way public decisions are made following on from new forms of democratic expression and, on the other hand, the impetus provided by users of the system who are seeking more interaction with the other parties concerned [174].

In 1996, the right of the citizen to participate in health care was recognised institutionally by the inclusion of two provisions in the political agenda: the first was to create Regional Health Conferences to define priorities in the field of health; and the second was to appoint users to the administrative councils that run hospitals. In 1998-1999, public debate on health-related questions was promoted by the Consultative Assembly on Health. And then in February 2000, a Council of Europe directive recommended that structures be established to foster the participation of users and patients in the making of decisions related to health care[1].

But what are the essential conditions to promote the participation of citizens in the formulation of public health policy? It is not enough for the authorities to pass laws to establish and enforce patients' or users' rights. They need also to make sure that citizen users can make an effective contribution to the democratic dialogue on health, and participate in the process of making decisions about their own health. Thus, a forum for such a democratic dialogue has to be put in place, one which will help citizen users play a role in the evaluation of public health parameters according to procedures which are yet to be defined. How is such a dialogue to be fostered? And what exactly are the procedures

---

1. Recommendation N° R (2002) 5 of the Committee of Ministers to the Member States.

to be established to involve citizens in the formulation of public health policy? We will address these questions by reviewing the details of a few recently established structures and experiences in this area.

Discussion forums: under construction

Two kinds of deliberative body have a major role in determining priorities in the field of health: the Regional Health Conferences and the National Health Conference, both established by the April 1996 Ruling on the regulation of medical expenditure. Each of these bodies is attempting in its own way to establish a minimum of mutual consultation and dialogue between the various interested parties, each of which has a different logic.

Half of the delegates to the National Health Conference (CNS, *Conférence nationale de santé*) are professional health care providers, and the other half work for health-related institutions, so users as such are not represented. In contrast, State services, health care establishments, independent professionals and patient support groups are all represented in the Regional Health Conferences (CRS, *Conférences régionales de santé*). A committee appointed from among these representatives is responsible for drawing conclusions and compiling recommendations in the form of a report [160], in which specific actions can be suggested, *e.g.* Regional Health Action Programmes *(Programmes régionaux d'actions de santé)*. Although providing forums for contact and dialogue between the various players in the health care system is a step in the right direction, how such forums actually work is currently presenting problems at a number of different levels.

The composition of these bodies, especially that of the CNS, seems to reflect a strategy to concentrate on the opinions of the concerned professionals (no doubt following the precedent established Conferences for other professional structures such as the Agricultural Conference). Such a strategy is inevitably going to limit the range of the dialogue and leave users little room to express their views. And even when users are invited to participate at the policy-making level, as in the case of the CRSs, there are questions about the way in which certain people are selected to represent the users (who are not actually represented as such, even if certain members of the Conference are taken from the community as a whole) and the weight these delegates have in the Conference's deliberations. In particular, one wonders about the extent to which they are involved in identification of the problems to be addressed, in fixing the basis on which the questions to be discussed are selected, and in establishing modalities to rank different health care for the purpose of setting priorities when it comes to the allocation of resources. As will be expanded upon later, all these issues are central if citizen users are to be brought into the determination of health policy in a real way.

The Consultative Assembly on Health has a different way of organising and staging public dialogue on health questions [160]. Although the process is not one in which the idea of "democracy in health" can be implemented at a regular rhythm, it has the merit of focusing the spotlight on users' requirements and needs for information and recognition of their rights in this area. The establishment of committees composed of members of the community under the aegis of the Consultative Assembly represents a progressive formal structure in the context of which users can become directly and collectively involved in health and health care. These committees were established on the basis of certain parameters to do with both science and technology which first emerged in the United States, Germany and Denmark about thirty years ago [156].

These ways of promoting dialogue have two points in common: firstly, they make for better decisions on matters in which at least some of the choices involved potentially have major social impact and may have serious repercussions on public health; and secondly, the dialogue is so structured that the private citizen is brought in early in the decision-making process, when the bare bones of projects are still being formulated.

From the point of view of the public authorities, distinction can be made between four different objectives associated with these instruments: to stimulate public dialogue about questions which involve multiple issues (*e.g.* economic, political, social, philosophical and ethical issues); to cut down the risk of rejection of projects being defined in too unilateral a fashion; to promote scientific, technical, social and economic arguments in the public at large; and to confer a greater degree of legitimacy on projects by virtue of expanding their base [162]. This is the type of approach undertaken in the Citizens' Conference on genetically modified organisms set up in July 1998 under the aegis of the Parliamentary Office for the Evaluation of Scientific and Technological Options.

P. Lascoumes [166], analysing such new consultative modalities, points out the importance of making a distinction between the various different structures. He positions them in a continuum between those set up as "means of communicating" (intended to take responsibility for decisions that have already been made) and those which "generate a decision" (or contribute to the prior deliberation). He proposes four criteria which can be used to differentiate between these different forms of forum: how the delegates are appointed (whether it be by the Government or on an *ad hoc* basis); the nature of the conclusions (whether they be simply presented or generated as a result of dialogue); the amount of interaction that takes place between the representatives (whether a minimum consensus position is sought or whether areas of agreement and disagreement are explicitly detailed); and the role therein of users' representatives (whether they are just present or actually contribute to the discussion with, among other features, the ability to re-formulate the questions to be addressed). On the basis of these criteria, most of the structures put in place by the public authorities up until now appear to him as little more than "talking shops", intended to justify decisions that are *faits accomplis* rather than agencies designed to "generate a decision" or contribute to the decision-making process.

This being the case, the value of these citizen committees – above and beyond having provided a medium for several fruitful debates – is that they have been living laboratories for the formulation of a response to the following central question, "How can the selected representatives be endowed with the capacity to arbitrate in possible conflicts between different experts?" This presupposes that the citizens' representatives have a sufficient understanding of the facts to become a sort of "cultural hybrid" half way between the experts and the layman. In other words, "What are the conditions necessary to a 'non-expert' expertise which is capable of making a constructive contribution in this field at the same time as being democratic?"

These forum for public debate raise certain key questions:
– What is the place of the private citizen in this type of structure?
– How can they participate in a meaningful way?
– How are such agencies to interact with other forums for public dialogue?

The place of the citizen in discussion forums

As already discussed, the idea of user covers patient, customer, citizen and beneficiary, according to the circumstances. Each views the question of health from a different perspective. Who is to be represented in discussion forums? The user of health care services? Patient support or consumers' groups? Special interest, family-based groups? Or simple citizens whose legal status confers the right to vote and therefore influence public policy? The ability of all social groups to make themselves heard in the field of public health is not equivalent. The increasing complexity of the system, and the resultant inequalities and injustices can incite incomprehension among the less privileged, and in some cases resignation, anger and even rejection of the system in the more volatile.

For this reason, the idea of "democracy in health" can only concern and interest people according to their position and status

Part four The user, a player in the health care system

THE DEMOCRACY IN HEALTH OFFICE OF THE GENERAL HEALTH DIRECTORATE- EMPLOYMENT MINISTRY

How to encourage user and patient participation is going to represent a major challenge for tomorrow's public health policy and health care system. There is an ever-increasing collective consciousness of the place of the citizen in the evaluation of medical, psychological and social needs, of the expectations of users, and of their participation in the definition and implementation of public health policy, a consciousness which is embodied in the July 21 2000 Ruling on reorganisation of the General Health Directorate into services and sub-departments with the following missions:
– developing the participation of populations and non-profit-making organisations in the definition of public health policies and designing programmes to implement them;
– stipulating measures pertaining to the rights of patients and users of the health care system.

A Health in Democracy office was created at the Ministry of Employment and Solidarity in September 2000. The challenges for the General Health Directorate are:
- Involving users as players in the public health decision-making process.
- Promoting recognition of the person as a player in the care process.
- Promoting and safeguarding the organisation of democratic debate on questions of public health policy.

The Bill pertaining to modernisation of the health care system is an important component in consolidation of the democratic discussion of health and health care. In this field, the Democracy in Health office of the General Health Directorate is pursuing the following objectives:
- Making sure that priorities in health policies and programmes are understood and shared with and by concerned users and non-profit-making organisations.
- Consolidating the rights of individual patients in the fields of care, prevention and health education.
- Reinforcing the collective expression of users in the health care system.
- Developing a culture of "democracy in health": an approach in which public health policy is formulated and implemented on the basis of principles and values, notably those of equitable access to care, equitable access to information, the principle of reliable information delivered and received, of advice on prevention and care, all in the context of an overall imperative of safety.

within the system, which ultimately depends on the extent to which they benefit from it. It is known that the poorer a person's social, familial and financial situation is, the less attention he or she pays to health which does not constitute a priority compared with all the person's other problems (apart from in the event of a real emergency). For many citizens, it is not questions of health that are going to excite a wish to participate in the life of the community. Moreover, addressing medical and social questions necessitates a certain mastery of the language and some degree of power with respect to public structures and decision-making bodies. The danger is that the debate will be commandeered by the most outspoken parties, *e.g.* medical experts, trade unions, patient support groups, and other special interest groups which are very active in the field of health.

Placing citizens and health care professionals face to face ignores the fact that the structures that decide on questions of health are dominated by representatives appointed from among the medical community [183]. For most decision-makers and members of the general public, health falls naturally into the field of medicine given that good health is perceived as the absence of disease. This is one of the reasons why the medical approach, a curative attitude to care, has occupied such a dominant position, not only in the field of health care but also in the matter of public health. This has resulted in marginalisation of questions of prevention. It is difficult to initiate any kind of discussion of health which is not in the context of medicine, a problem which enthusiasm about science and medical progress was tending to exacerbate, blunting the critical capacities of the general public and decision-makers alike until fairly recently. Therefore, bringing the private citizen into the decision-making process ultimately boils down to a false dialogue in which one group (the patients and future patients) are asked about their expectations in the matter of health and health care, and the other group (the professionals and experts) find a response to the problem posed; all this under the eye of public decision-makers who decide whether the response is "reasonable" or not, taking into account in their calculations financial considerations and professional interests.

Conditions for meaningful participation

Be it associated with the treatment or the prevention of disease, it has traditionally been seen as normal that specialists be called on to formulate in the most objective, rational way possible decisions which must needs stem from an in-depth understanding of the scientific issues involved. Ideally, their role is to provide an objective viewpoint, free from conflicts of interest and prejudice. However, although decision-making in public health does indeed need to take many technical and scientific parameters into account, the idea that these are the only issues at stake is a false one.

It is vital therefore to establish regulatory mechanisms to control expertise-based processes and guarantee participation on the part of the users, as well as to make sure that all procedures are transparent and ensure that there is genuine discussion of divergent opinions. These points will be dealt with in the following paragraphs.

Citizens ought to be involved in the design of expertise-based processes

Making confrontation possible between the points of view of different experts is necessary if private citizens are to be brought into the process. In many health-related situations, there is disagreement between the experts on what needs to be done and how to do it. Such disagreement is often rooted in differences as to how the scientific data should be interpreted and/or the consequences certain variables may have on health or in society. Thus, instead of trying to arrive at a consensus on the part of the experts, the goal should be to establish a decision-making structure in which arguments are built up in collaboration with private citizens in a co-operative approach to solving public health problems. In introducing the possible alternative technological solutions to a given problem, the expert should emphasise areas of uncertainty, point out any assumptions and approximations, and confess the limitations of his or her knowledge, thereby allowing members into the discussion by giving them a opening to talk about how the various options might affect them personally. This amounts to establishing a real social dialogue about health, exactly what some refer to as "democracy in health". This also amounts to presenting the possible alternatives in order to encourage emergence of disagreement and thereby promote discussion of the central issues.

It is nevertheless important to remember that the various players in the system do not all have the same level of understanding of health information and statistics. Citizens can give a legitimate opinion about the purposes of a public health initiative, about whether the allocated resources are compatible with the objectives, or about the seriousness of possible consequences of proposed solutions. However, they will have more difficulty if the issue in question concerns highly technical questions such as the validity of a theoretical model used to account for scientific data, or the validity of a certain set of results.

The process should be transparent

All participants ought to be aware of any possible conflicts of interest the scientific and medical experts might have in terms of relationships with financial interests and risk managers (*e.g.* the so-called independent expert might have a working or financial relationship with the drug company that produces the drug which he is evaluating [140]). Although such questions are treated with extreme discretion in France, they are treated far more openly in English-speaking countries, especially in the international scientific journals [185].

Total independence is an impossible goal for diverse reasons. Experts tend to approach public health problems from the point of view of a personal representation based on their specialty and their own research. As a result, they make a useful contribution to the decision-making process, as long as their contribution can

A FRAMEWORK TO PROMOTE USER-CITIZEN PARTICIPATION

Work in Quebec in Canada by J.-M. Fourniau [152] has resulted in the "4C" grid which is designed to help in the implementation of measures in the field of public health so that the citizen-user is invited to participate in public action and deliberate on the public health-related decisions, both at the collective and the individual level.

- Communication:
− to allow expression and explanation;
− intended to ensure adherence to choices made;
− may be limited to simple information, or be designed elicit reactions (information/feedback).

- Consultation:
− to allow discussion of proposals;
− intended to provide the necessary information before any choices are made.

- Concertation:
− to allow formulation of a solution in collaboration with the concerned players;
− intended to find common solutions or new knowledge.

- Codecision:
− to allow sharing of the decision between those involved;
− involves negotiation to find common ground.

be seen for what it is and its limitations covered in the discussion, all in the context of a global view of the problem to be resolved [145]. It is important to point out any value systems underlying their methodological approaches, *e.g.* why they preferred a model based on the "price of a human life" or on the "capacity to pay", two very different economic approaches to health problems which imply not only a different attitude to what constitutes a member of society, but also to the weighing of present and future.

Discussion can often obscure the fact that the proposals put forward by experts conceal an interest of which the general public is unaware. Although it is always the preservation of health that is talked about, there are often underlying professional, commercial, social or moral motives which are not necessarily easy to discern in the final decision. Currently, for example, new drugs or new medical systems are regularly launched in the media with the collaboration of important members of the medical community. For certain of these, the goal of the publicity campaign − rather than being to disseminate trustworthy, useful scientific information − is to bring as many people as possible into "medical existence" or, in other words, convince them that they are ill (an approach satirically envisaged by Dr. Knock in Jules Romain's play several decades ago [177]).

Doubt can also be cast on the independence of committees of medical experts appointed directly by the government which hold their meetings on ministerial premises in the presence of an observer from the government. Moreover, the members of such committees are too often nominated by the other members of the committee. The ways in which the decisions of these committees are arrived at do not seem to follow the relevant rules, and the procedures are not always published. All these problems are contributing to the growing mistrust amongst both users and professional health care providers about the way in which the health care system is being managed by the experts. Working methods have to be made transparent which means developing a quality assurance approach to the way in which expert-based regulation of the health care system is functioning; this with a view to improving its performance [168]. Although it is not possible to have 100% confidence in all experts at all times, it should nevertheless be possible to establish a well-controlled "expert-based" regulatory system, the rules and framework of which are clear to all.

Provision should be made for contentious discussion

In public health, most of the scientific information necessary for the decision-making process is generated and provided by public institutions, with few non-governmental sources being capable of competing in this field [187]. In France, the cultural and economic climate is not such that non-governmental groups of experts (be they associated with a commercial organisation or not) are common. Nevertheless, making provision for the possibility of contentious discussion would seem to be an indispensable element if the dialogue is to be genuine.

To encourage critical analysis, organise it at the public level with sustained funding would enhance the general public's understanding of the arguments and promote participation on the part of members of the community. In contentious discussion, divergent opinions are brought out, nothing is left in the dark and everyone learns something. In the same way experts can disagree, there is no reason to suppose that lay people are all going to be of exactly the same opinion on all issues. The confrontation of a variety of different points of view is a precondition for democratic debate: confrontation of different ideas and points of view constitutes the ideal framework for an evaluation and decision-making system in which doubts are given primacy over certainties. If it is to be relevant, such a system must be collective, multidisciplinary and representative of all the various different parts of society.

Role of patient support groups and other associations in discussion forums

In a way, airing doubts about the efficacy of the public decision-making and policy-setting procedures could be seen as paramount to questioning the ability of traditional democratic processes to fulfil the needs of the common citizen. Moreover, the underlying analysis implicitly undermines the "holistic" concept of the public or the people as a single unit composed of individuals, replacing it instead with a very different concept of a whole set of different social groups with highly disparate needs and interests.

From this point of view, it is important to be aware of patient support groups and other associations which claim to be the legitimate representatives of patients and users of the health care system. This type of activity has grown enormously in recent decades and has resulted in wide-scale mobilisation of patients and their friends and families, with a view to either providing a framework for solidarity and mutual support, or to building up political weight in relevant battles, *i.e.* not only so that notice is taken of their constituency but also in order to bring about change in public health practices and policies. This increasingly strong movement perfectly embodies the widely felt desire for democratisation of the health care system. However, such groups are confronted by many difficulties, notably with respect to their selection and legitimisation and in terms of exactly what they are supposed to be doing [144].

The main pitfall to be avoided is to expect such groups to be representative of users, *i.e.* confer democratic legitimacy by their inclusion. What is needed is an alternative viewpoint rather than another power centre which might further spread the distribution of responsibility. An accreditation process is necessary (and accepted in the movement when implemented) if associations are to be granted the right to represent patients and guard their rights, and take a leading part in important discussions. There seems to be broad agreement on two criteria for accreditation:

– justification of effective, public activity in the defence of the rights of the sick, consumers, and users of the health system, since a time to be specified;

– independence from any medical or paramedical commercial organisation, and management structures composed of genuinely independent users.

Citizens and associations ought to be brought into the various stages of the decision-making process to as great an extent as possible, including the earliest stages at which matters for debate and review are selected. In an ideal world, the user would be represented at all stages of this process and, in the absence of specific mechanisms to ensure this, there is a risk that an apparent participation of normal members of the community will be no more than a sham, as has been seen in the "co-management" system for controlling occupational hazards [173]. The need for participation is all the greater by virtue of the novelty and com-

DIFFERENT WAYS OF INVOLVING CITIZENS

The reason for establishing this type of discussion forum is the observation that citizens are demanding more place in the decision-making process. The purpose is to help create a public debate on subjects for which discussion and information are either generally confined to experts or too often dominated by special interest groups. Three forums for such democratic debate are of particular interest:

The citizen jury

The objective is to arrive at an opinion formed by informed citizens (as opposed to experts) on questions of a political or social nature. Twelve to sixteen citizens are recruited randomly to represent their community. The jury meets for four days and works in the following manner:
– experts and interested parties testify to defend their point of view. The members of the jury ask them questions with the help of one or more moderators. Then, the members of the jury deliberate in small groups before a plenary session. In the end, one report is compiled including their conclusions and recommendations, and another with an evaluation of how well the process worked;
– their work is published and broadly diffused via the media.

"Danish-style" consensus conferences

The overall purpose of this method is to allow a panel of citizens to arrive at an opinion or choice on the basis of a maximum amount of common ground.
A consensus conference also has two other objectives:
– to have a group of citizens assess a controversial subject with technological or scientific content;
– to incite discussion throughout society and between all interested parties.
Ten to sixteen citizens are recruited randomly and two weekends are put aside to prepare for the conference. During these, each member presents him or herself and gets to understand the moderator's role. At the same time, the group learns to work together, assimilates the basic knowledge necessary, formulates questions and reviews the type of expert to be called. Two or three weeks later, the panel convenes in a public meeting lasting four days. This is ample time for panel members to put any questions they want to the experts, and discuss the issues with the public. Then, the panel retires for deliberations prior to issuing their results which are published and widely broadcast. A first conference of this type was organised in France by the Parliamentary Office for the Evaluation of Scientific and Technological Choices (OPECST, *Office parlementaire d'évaluation des choix scientifiques et technologiques*) to discuss genetically modified organisms.

Scenario workshops

The purpose of scenario workshops which are common in Nordic countries is to promote the exchange of opinions and knowledge between different players at the local level:
– to identify and discuss points of agreement and disagreement on how to approach the problem and look for an answer;

> – to foster new knowledge, everyone's shared needs and an action plan at the local, regional or national level, and to promote broader local discussion of the resultant recommendations, if such proves necessary.
> The methodology involves bringing together thirty-odd local players from four different backgrounds, namely representatives of citizens and users, technical experts, local decision-makers (politicians and administrators) and business representatives.
> After presentation of the problem, of two or three pertinent questions, and of four scenarios devised by independent experts, workshop sessions in which the players can develop their own perspectives and proposals are alternated with plenary sessions with a view to arriving at a consensus scenario.
>
> *Source: Drees [149].*

plexity of the problems to be tackled, especially the "jump-in-the-dark" aspect of many current questions in public health in which it is necessarily the citizen who is primarily concerned. The presence of citizens at all stages of discussion is all the more vital when it comes to unprecedented questions that are particularly complicated or especially important. Although the "technical" conditions discussed above have been realised, both the place of this dialogue in the formulation of policy and how the work of discussion forums is to be integrated into the public decision-making process remain to be settled. These questions require political consideration which is inextricably linked with the question of how to evaluate public policy in a pluralistic fashion, a topic which is beyond the scope of this working group [163].

Involve users in the running of institutions

We have seen how the question of the place and role of the user in health and health care has changed since the end of the 1980's. It has become clear that members of the community need to be brought into the running and regulation of the system [180] and now, various structures exist in which users are represented, *e.g.* hospital Administrative Councils and the National Agency for Health Accreditation and Evaluation (Anaes, *Agence nationale d'accréditation et d'évaluation en santé*) in which users participate in the groups working on accreditation.

If users are to make a positive contribution, they need to be in possession of a certain amount of reliable, accurate information on how the health care system works. In reality, users are usually poorly informed and, as a result, not really familiar with how the health care system really operates. Such information is necessary to legitimise the user's place in such a structure and help him or her to formulate a valid point of view and thus play a meaningful role alongside the health professionals, administrators and representatives of the authorities. Without this information, the user will not be in a position to formulate any useful judgements or recommendations about how the health care system is working or how it can be evaluated.

In this situation, it seems important to make a distinction between the type of information that the user can expect as a "potential patient" – which centres on the disease and the treatment modalities available (which will be dealt with in the third point) – and that which he or she can expect as a "potential user" of the health care system. It is the latter point that will be developed in the following.

Making sure that the user is adequately informed

For nearly twenty years now in the United States, a whole series of experimental initiatives have been undertaken to provide the general public with comprehensive information on the performance of different health plans and hospitals. Health Maintenance Organizations (providers of "managed care" run by private or public health insurers, offering a full range of services) operate a Report Card system aimed at allowing consumers to compare different insurance plans in terms of the services offered and price so that they can choose the most "efficient" (*i.e.* maximise utility, in the language of economics). In parallel, hospitals participate in a comparative evaluation system heavily focused on the quality of care provision in which details of their performance and outcomes are published. In some States (including Pennsylvania and New York), post-bypass surgery mortality rates are thus published for each hospital and even each surgeon [171].

The benefit hoped for from this large-scale dissemination of information is quite in line with the typical American free market-based way of thinking in which the informed consumer is going to opt for those establishments and doctors with the best performance, so those which perform poorly will inexorably be "squeezed out of the market". Keeping the patient informed is thus a way of improving the quality and efficiency of care provision to the ultimate benefit of the consumer. Of course, such a system does not come free since compiling and broadcasting this information costs.

For this reason, the results of these experiments have been closely assessed [157]. Whatever the specific design of the experiment and whatever the type of evaluation performed, all the results show the same things: firstly, access to this type of infor-

THE CREDOC SURVEY ON THE SOURCES OF HEALTH INFORMATION USED BY FRENCH PEOPLE

The High Committee on Public Health commissioned the Credoc to conduct a survey to determine the sources used by French people to obtain health information, and their opinions of the reliability of the various sources.

For this project, a representative sample of 1,000 people of 18 or over was interviewed in early 2001.

Nearly one-half of all French people had sought information on some specific subject at least once in the previous six months

Of all those interviewed, 44% had sought such information at least once, and 12% had done so frequently.

Two-thirds of these people were looking for information on a specific disease or treatment modality, 21% on preventive behaviour, and 12% on food-related health hazards.

On the other hand, information was only rarely sought on certain other subjects which were specifically mentioned in the questionnaire, including the dangers of smoking and drinking, environmental health risks, and the working of the health care system.

Half of all those who had sought information had experience of the disease in question, and for the other half, the main motivating principle was curiosity – sometimes concerning some specific disease but more commonly a variety of topics, especially those recently mentioned in the media.

The more active the search for information, the more specialised the source used

The people who had sought information in the preceding six months had mainly used relatively targeted sources: half mentioned the media but this tended to be the specialised press (25%) rather than the generalist press (18%) or television (14%).

A health care professional was consulted by 57%, most commonly (40%) the family doctor.

In general, those with experience of the disease consulted their physician whereas those motivated by curiosity sought information in the media.

Other sources of information were not cited by many of the respondents.

Information can also be absorbed passively in the sense that points heard in a variety of contexts can affect behaviour

This type of information is generally relayed by the media, especially in magazine-type programmes on the radio and television. More specialised sources such as programmes about health, specialist magazines and health care professionals were rarely cited.

The French consider themselves relatively well informed on health matters: 17% qualify themselves as well-informed, 62% as fairly well-informed, and only 2% as totally ignorant. However, two-thirds agreed with the statement *"a source of reliable, clear information about health for the general public is lacking"*.

Part four The user, a player in the health care system

> **Professional health care providers appear to be the most credible source**
>
> – Although "passive" information is relayed on the television and in the press, more "active" seeking of information tends to focus on specialist programmes and magazines;
> – Many people who are seeking information about some specific subject consult a professional health care provider;
> – Nearly half of those who had used a variety of different sources judged that professional health care providers are the most reliable source, compared with only one-third who cited any of the various media (the most common of which was some specialist publication).

mation did not significantly change users' behaviour in that they continued to base their choices on information garnered from traditional sources, *i.e.* friends, family and neighbours; secondly, the information had only a marginal effect on the way physicians referred their patients to other services and specialists in the health care system. In fact, the only concrete effect which was definitively identified was a change in the marketing policy of the hospitals considered as the best.

In the name of the pursuit of the benefits of transparency (which is supposed to lead to the shunning of the "worst" establishments by users and their closure in consequence), the magazine *Sciences et avenir* (and many others since) published a ranking of hospitals, clinics and services. Since the initiative was essentially similar to those undertaken in the United States, it is not certain that this publication will have any real impact (other than on magazine sales figures). In France, the question is even more delicate because, although "market values" have certainly gained ground in recent years, in this country there is an idea of public services that does not really exist across the Atlantic, and the health insurance system is based on the principle of collectivism. These ideas continue to weigh heavily on people's behaviour. The key issue which needs to be considered is whether keeping the public informed is to be tackled in a spirit of allowing the market to regulate the health care system, or in order to promote democratic debate to the same end [158]. In other words, information hitherto broadcast with a view to enhancing efficiency by exerting pressure on professional health care providers has not seemed to have much real impact (although this observation continues to escape many decision-makers).

The purposes of information

Extensive research has been conducted (notably by the Drees under the auspices of the Ministry of Employment) into what kind of information about hospitals users expect to be provided with

[138]. In one project designed to ascertain expectations, telephone interviews were used to select a group of fourteen users representing a diversity of experience and knowledge of hospitals. Professional care providers and activists (*e.g.* members of patients support groups) were excluded from the group.

Of course, the discussions of this group were not intended to generate quantitative data and were not even expected to be "representative" of the way users think. Nevertheless, the results of these in-depth discussions deserve examination because they shed significant light on the expectations that users have in the matter of the purposes of information on health-related questions.

- A first purpose is to give users the ability to use the system more rationally and thereby participate more fully in its running and regulation. The group of users brought together by the Drees saw such participation as involving all levels of information – its production, dissemination and control – and this in the general framework of a citizen-based approach.

- A second purpose – one which is very much in vogue in the English-speaking world, as referred to above – is to enable the user to choose the most suitable hospital on the basis of comprehensive information about the quality of services offered at different establishments. Such information constitutes a medium to increase competition between different care providers. For this type of information, it is essential to be able to measure and compare performance levels, and ranking is a primary objective. The users consulted were hesitant about this kind of approach which turns information compiled with a view to evaluating hospital activities for comparative purposes into an instrument for selecting the best accessible department or hospital.

One of the possible reasons for this ambivalence is the problem that lay people have in understanding indicators which do not seem to correspond to their own priorities (and the same goes for many health care professionals). For most people, devising technical indicators is a matter for the experts. Nevertheless, they thought it essential that lay people be given the information necessary to judge and use the indicators, once devised by experts. Another reason can be envisaged, complementary to the first, namely a reticence to believe in the predictive value of quantitative, classified data on relative care quality. Do users really feel in a position to reconsider their choices when confronted by "demonstrated poor outcomes"? Where is the room for manœuvre when it comes to going back on an initial choice? In practice, information about the hospital does not have any direct effect on a user-consumer's attitude to a hospital although it might be taken into account in the making of their decision. This is because, whereas the information expected concerning "global hospital provision" is based on a description of resources and activities, it also depends on knowledge of the links each structure has with people and institutions outside, and relationships it has forged with a whole variety of collaborators which will be of enormous value to the user following discharge.

- This is related to a third purpose of such information, namely that of providing the user-patient with wide-reaching information about the health care system which would make the logic of the treatment and hospital stay easier to understand and therefore make time factors easier to handle. This applies to all aspects of health care, not just hospital treatment.

- The fourth purpose corresponds to information that can be used within the hospital setting, *i.e.* information that would enable the user and/or patient to handle his or her treatment and stay at the establishment.

The wish for greater participation on the part of users during hospital stays has often been related to what can be considered as the fifth purpose of information, namely increasing the user's cognitive resources in order to improve his or her dialogue and relationships with the professionals (doctors, nurses, administrators, etc.) [167]. Such a dialogue is all the more important these days when there is a clear loss of confidence, not only in medical care providers but also, to a certain extent in the administrators and regulators of the health care system. This distrust among users was extensively discussed at the Consultative Assembly on Health and echoed in the Drees working group. However, it also emerged from the discussions at the Consultative Assembly that users are more than willing to make an effort to remedy this situation so that their confidence in professional health care providers is restored. How can better information help this rebuilding of confidence? The information will only be useful if it is presented in a form which the user can exploit. The questions of form and about the contribution that better information about hospitals might be able to make to favour dialogue between patients and care providers are thus put.

Many observers and managers of the health care system attribute to this general feeling of mistrust the desire on the part of users for more information about the safety of treatment modalities. In France as in the United States, when users were asked about this subject, they proved to be more interested in looking for information which might provide evidence that care providers are taking users' questions and points of view into account (which was the yardstick upon which they gauged the establishment) than in information on the safety of treatment. This is because safety seems too technical a field and the users are prepared to place their confidence in the professionals in this respect as long as account is taken of their point of view and some degree of transparency is maintained when it comes to the compilation and dissemination of results.

COMPLAINTS BY THE USERS OF HEALTH CARE TABLISHMENTS

Complaints, notably those expressed by hospital users on the special forms provided, represent a useful source of information about people's expectations, how the relevant laws are being applied, and how health care establishments are working. In this light, particular attention needs to be paid to how complaints are handled because they can be a precious resource in the endeavour to improve the quality of patient care.

Achieving this end is governed by several imperatives:

– *There needs to be a change in how such complaints are perceived* by staff, both administrators and care providers: a complaint should not be seen just as a criticism of how the hospital works, but rather as a means of increasing awareness and understanding, and therefore as an aid to improving how the organisation is functioning.

– *An ideal complaint processing system needs to be defined* to ensure, not only rapid responsiveness but also to include an analysis of the problems which gave rise to the complaint and propose remedial measures.

To this end, complaints have to be classified on the basis of different types. Those which pertain to some general, systematic malfunction of the health care system will have to be dealt with by the Regional Hospital Agency (ARH, *Agence régionale de l'hospitalisation*) or, when there is a major problem in a specific department justifying an administrative enquiry, by the ARH working together with the establishment concerned. However, the establishment alone will be able to deal with the vast majority of complaints, *i.e.* those that concern specific conditions of the patient's hospital stay.

Therefore, a formal complaint processing system needs to be set up in every hospital, with stipulated modalities governing collection, analysis, registration and response. In this respect, the new Bill on modernisation of the health care system replaces the current Conciliation Commission with a commission on relationships with users and the quality of care provision which is designed to be a forum for exchange in which users will be able to "describe their problem to the managers of the establishment, hear the latters' explanations, and be told about the follow-up to their complaint". Moreover, the Commission will be qualified to make recommendations concerning the admission and care policy of the establishment in the light of users' complaints. The Commission will compile an annual report to be discussed by the Administrative Council (or some other qualified body) before being sent to the Regional Hospital Agency and the Regional Health Council.

Therefore, this Commission is to play an essential role in the processing of complaints which is why the Decree of Implementation needs to stipulate its composition and workings to take into account all the implications referred to above. The Decree should also provide for, on the basis of experience with the Conciliation Commissions, flexible, tailored working conditions to make it possible for smaller structures to apply the principles embodied in the Law.

– *Methods – from processing to implementation – will have to be reviewed* in order to ensure better exploitation of the valuable resource constituted by complaints so that concrete measures are implemented to improve the way the hospital functions. To this end, apart from classification of the reasons for complaints (which is

Part four   The user, a player in the health care system

> essentially an evaluation tool), types of organisational breakdown leading to complaints will also have to be classified, which presupposes a review on a complaint-by-complaint basis to deduce the series of events that led to the problem. Common definition of a classification system will contribute to the success of any remedial measures subsequently implemented because it will lead to an overview of the hospital's objectives.
> – *To forestall complaints, measures to be taken further up the line will have to be envisaged*: any measure intended to promote user expression ("users' offices", instruments to promote co-operation between different non-profit-making organisations, etc.) or provide more information (on how hospitals work, departmental organisation structures, the cost of care, etc.) and any organisational measures to, for example, appoint a "resource person" capable of making an immediate response to verbal complaints during a hospital stay. Provision will also have to be made for training staff, and increasing their awareness of the importance of both good relations with patients and the usefulness of the complaint process.
>
> *Directorate for Hospitalisation and Care Logistics (DHOS, Direction de l'hospitalisation et de l'organisation des soins).*

So what are the prerequisites in terms of the information aimed at lay people that will ensure restoration of their confidence about what goes on inside hospitals? Firstly, one can theoretically consider the possibility of "orchestrating" the key elements (essentially qualitative) involved in confidence using a series of appropriate indicators. This corresponds to identifying in the short term concrete elements which can be put into the public arena. Otherwise, it is well recognised that simply producing a piece of information is not enough to bring about any change if the professionals involved in gathering and compiling the information do not actively participate. Improvements in treatment and relationships between patients and care providers depend to a large extent on the professionals, whether they work inside or outside a hospital. Therefore, recognising the usefulness of such an approach to information and involving the health care professionals both constitute key prerequisites if the approach is to be a successful one.

In conclusion, it would seem that, in the light of various studies conducted both in France and abroad, the users of health care systems need concrete information about hospitals, *i.e.* information that will help them imagine the future and organise their lives in a more effective fashion, at the moment when disease is encountered.

Users show themselves to be very attached to the idea of participation to as great an extent as possible in the compilation of various grids so that the indicators reflect their points of view. In order to assimilate the corresponding information, they need it to be disseminated in an interactive fashion, which gives rise to a necessity to invent special systems for relaying such information. Moreover, if it is to be possible to use the information, it will have to be presented in summary form, as is demonstrated by all the research carried out in this field. At the same time, everybody must be able – if he or she so desires – to go back to the source data in order to check how the information was generated.

Therefore, the current priority is to find institutional modalities which will allow users to participate in the generation and control of information disseminated about the working of the system in the context of an initiative jointly developed and managed by lay people, health professionals and the public authorities. These institutions should be so set up that information can be shared, a structure which will enable the system to respond to the population's needs and expectations in any given context. Making it possible for the various players to share information is all the more important now that patient support groups have become such central players in the medical and medico-social fields.

Role of patient support groups

The nature of non-profit-making organisations involved in the field of health has changed over the years with different types dominating at different times, *e.g.* philanthropic, professional-militant, general or disease-specific [161]. Such associations act to defend patients' rights and support their families but they also help design and implement preventive measures and provide funding for research.

The purpose of patient support groups is to provide information to patients and families, catalogue their needs and expectations, defend their interests from a position of solidarity, and collectively seek solutions to encountered problems. The number of associations based on experience of a particular disease or treatment modality (*e.g.* dialysis or ostomies) multiplied in the 1980's. In most cases, the problem or disease is chronic and entails both major upheaval in the organisation of daily life, and sustained contact with medical institutions. One of the association's missions is to lobby society and the public authorities to take more account of patients' interests by implementing tailor-made responses to their health-related questions. Many such associations have been founded based on either a single disease or a single form of disability [141], and some are so heavily contributed to by the general public that the sums that they can disburse endow them with influence in terms of research policy.

Originally, the medical community mastered how to exploit users and citizen-puppets to get them to speak for professional strategies which were not always made clear. Certain patient support groups thus became "Yes-men" for physicians, advocates for the biomedical philosophy of health, or instruments for the collection of research money. However, there has been a major change in this respect and today's movement is characterised by a new climate in which patient support groups are tending to bring physicians and patients together, a context in which an increasing number of doctors are prepared to establish a less technical relationship with their patients and are willing to engage in a collective dialogue.

Moreover, patient support groups are managing to emancipate themselves from their dependence on the medical profession. In recent years, several large associations have appointed a patient or the parent of a patient as president, a post previously always held by a member of the medical profession. Some associations have also begun to pay more attention to the patients' wishes, *e.g.* in terms of the which research programmes to fund, or procedures in clinical trials. A new image of the patient and a new attitude on the part of society at large have been constructed. On behalf of patients, above and beyond the right to be considered, patient support groups are now calling for a right for a part in the decision-making process.

In the area of AIDS, the mobilisation of patients and the early lack of scientific progress both contributed to the accumulation of real power by patients, and to bringing them to the forefront of the debate [178]. Many patients developed and are developing expertise based on their own experience and view of the disease [172]. Although this new type of expert cannot claim to speak on behalf of other victims, they can certainly help bring out the key questions and draw attention to the key problems which concern anyone who is infected with the virus. AIDS activists, for example, have not hesitated to tackle all aspects of medical practice, especially when it comes to the methodologies used in clinical trials.

By virtue of their familiarity with the realities of the situation, their flexibility, their reactivity and their determination, patient support groups have managed to establish themselves as indispensable collaborators in the field of public action, often participating at early stages in the design and implementation of measures intended to address novel or neglected questions. From this perspective, the difficulties encountered by citizen members of hospital Administrative Councils illustrate how important it is that they be afforded the conditions and tools to allow them to make their opinion significant and heard when it comes to how the hospital is being run. Similarly, the time might have come for a review of the place of users in the Anaes, and how they make their contribution to its deliberations, particularly when the new accreditation manual is being compiled.

The moment at which users are being brought into the health care system seems to us a propitious time to examine and redefines roles. *E.g.* that of the director of a health care establishment in

THE COLLECTIVE OF HEALTH-RELATED NON-PROFIT-MAKING ORGANISATIONS

The Collective of Health-Related Non-Profit-Making Organisations (CISS, *Collectif inter-associatif sur la santé*) was created to monitor the 1996 hospital reforms and formulate proposals in the matter of health and social policy. Although the CISS was specifically created in the context of these reforms, its remit is nevertheless seen as covering all aspects of health and the health care system.

One of the novel features of the CISS is that it is composed of a wide variety of different non-profit-making organisations and patient support groups* although all have some kind of interest in the field of health. This pooling of different cultures and experiences affords a far more global approach to health-related problems.
The main objectives are:
- To inform users of the health care system by sharing knowledge about users' needs, regulatory affairs and interesting new developments;
- Training users' representatives on hospital Administrative Councils so that they are no longer marginalised and so that they can make a more valid contribution than simply being a token presence;
- Ongoing monitoring of changes in the health care system, analysis of problem areas, and defining common strategies to improve admission and care in all types of structure;
- Broadcasting CISS findings and claims to the public with a view to establishing it a central spokesman and representative of users of the health care system;

The CISS now includes twenty non-profit-making organisations, from family, consumer and patient support groups to structures representing the disabled and handicapped.

Source: French Review of Social Affairs (Revue française des Affaires sociales) [176].

---

* AFD: Association française des diabétiques (Diabetes); AFH: Association française des hémophiles (Haemophilia); AFLM: Association française de lutte contre la mucoviscidose (Cystic fibrosis); AFM: Association française contre la myopathie (Muscle degeneration); AFP: Association française des polyarthritiques (Arthritis): Aides (Fédération nationale); APF: Association des paralysés de France (Paralysis); CSF: Confédération syndicale des familles (Families); Ffair: Fédération française des associations et amicales d'insuffisants respiratoires (Respiratory failure); Fnamoc: Fédération nationale des associations de malades cardio-vasculaires et opérés du cœur (Heart and cardiovascular disease); Fnap-Psy: Fédération nationale des associations d'ex-patients psy (Mental disease); Fnath: Fédération nationale des accidentés du travail et des handicapés (Disability); Familles rurales (Country families); Le Lien: association de lutte, d'information et d'études des infections nosocomiales (Nosocomial infections); LNCC: Ligue nationale contre le cancer (Cancer); Orgeco: Organisation générale des consommateurs (Consumers); Reshus: Réseau hospitalier des usagers (Hospital users); UFC-Que Choisir?: Union fédérale des consommateurs (Consumers); UFCS: Union féminine civique et sociale (Womens rights); Unaf: Union nationale des associations familiales (Families); Unapej: Union nationale des associations de parents et amis de personnes handicapées mentales (Mental handicap); Unafam: Union nationale des amis et familles de malades mentaux (Mental disease).

the handling of complaints, a role which is quite different from that of monitoring complaints as a means of analysis with a view to improving the quality of the services offered, a role in which the user has a rightful place. Similarly, in medicosocial areas such as institutions set up to care for the severely handicapped, a clear distinction should be made between the role of the families in the associations which manage the establishments, and that of the "spokesman" representing users, which would seem to devolve on them in a natural way.

The democracy in health resulting from the action of patient support groups and other associations active in the field should nevertheless be submitted to the question of the extent and nature of the fields and needs it covers. For various reasons, certain diseases today are associated with dense, powerful networks of associations whereas, in contrast, other diseases are still isolated, because the victims and/or their families and friends are not sufficiently organised. In a real situation of democracy in health, the public authorities are honour bound to support the patient support group movement. To this effect, they should make a point of establishing monitoring and research instruments with a view to setting up procedures and institutions capable of remedying such insufficiencies and eradicating current inequalities.

Therefore, the situation calls for improvement and rationalisation of the instruments designed to enhance user knowledge and participation. This will notably involve seeking to avoid or attenuate possible ruptures and inequalities according to individual capacities to find and understand information. Depending on the efficacy of the support structures and instruments, making sure that the user is adequately informed might become either a new means of arbitration in the arena of dialogue, or a reason for confused confrontation in which user and care provider cannot find any common ground. In the coming years, improving user knowledge – matched to everyone's needs and expectations – will be one of the priority areas for action to promote and reinforce democracy in health: development of the problematic of informing users, notably with respect to their rights, in the context of the initial and ongoing training of health care professionals; contribution of the media to the knowledge of users about health care issues; adaptation of information-related instruments to match the diversity of the general public concerned, and establishment of the necessary support structures; investment on the part of the public authorities in the definition and collection of information intended for the general public.

Ensure balance in the patient/care provider relationship

Conferring on the patient an active role in the health care system is a logical follow-on from reforms begun thirty years ago concerning patients' rights. Legally guaranteed patients rights were superimposed on the system, the regulation of which had hitherto been left up to the self-imposed principles of physicians. Between 1970 and 1999, a whole series of laws pertaining to hospitals embodied the recognition of a variety of rights [147]: the right of a patient to choose his or her physician freely (passed on December 31 1970); a patient's rights as a human being (the Hospitalised Patient's Charter in the Ministerial Communication of May 6 1995); the right to access to medical records (passed on July 31 1991); on the requirement for consent (the so-called Bioethics Laws, passed in July 1994); the right to high-quality care and the establishment of conciliation committees (April 24 1996); on access to health care for the underprivileged (July 29 1998); and on the benefit of palliative treatment and pain relief (June 9 1999).

At the same time as these legislative changes, the prevalence of chronic disease was on the rise (replacing infectious disease in the course of the last half of the 20th Century) leading to a new attitude to the meaning of patient support. In an ideal world, the patient-physician relationship would have smoothly evolved during this period, from one of the doctor taking a person into care in order to "confront" his or her disease, to one more based on a collaborative approach aimed at managing the pathology and providing as much support for the patient as possible. This type of approach is based on treating the individual, a singular and whole person, rather than just the affected organ. Insofar as the care strategy should also maximise the patient's "room for manœuvre", more attention should be paid to patients' expectations, even to the extent of allowing them to make their own independent decisions, if they so wish.

This freedom only makes sense if everyone has equal access to health care resources. The idea of democracy in health is inextricably linked with that of equitable access to the health care system for everyone, wherever they live. But access to health care cannot be reduced to the mere existence of a right to be reimbursed (totally or partially) for a given medical service or procedure. One of the necessary conditions for such access is awareness of the possibilities, which depends on access to comprehensible information about health and the health care system of such a nature as to

Part four The user, a player in the health care system

allow the user to exercise his or her rights of usage more effectively; this is at the heart of the subject of this section.

It is also worth emphasising that providing access to health care necessarily entails creating a propitious climate, *e.g.* by better management of waiting lists so that patients are dealt with more quickly, or making access to specialists more equitable in different parts of France (which remains a serious problem). Finally, for a significant fraction of the sick (either foreigners who do not speak French well or people with impaired hearing), the presence of an interpreter is a prerequisite if any real relationship is to be forged.

The patient-doctor relationship: first and foremost, a meeting

The doctor-patient relationship has to be considered as a meeting between two people involved in an interactive care process based on mutual confidence. The medical approach to disease has become complex because of the extraordinary growth in medical knowledge, therapeutic progress and the huge number of examinations that are possible. The doctor's relationship with his or her patients is still often a paternalistic one with the physician knowing always what is best. The doctor makes decisions in the patient's name without any involvement of the latter, and subjects who seek advice from colleagues or information elsewhere are poorly seen. This type of relationship is at the root of numerous conflicts.

Nevertheless, it is the patient who makes the decision to consult a doctor because something is disturbing the order in his or her life, *e.g.* pain, restricted activity, somebody else noticing some abnormality hitherto seen as minor, etc. The patient expects the doctor to put his or her life back in order. In most cases, patients want to participate in the care process and in any decisions which might affect them. They do not want to be considered as just as a case of some disease but as people.

In the course of the meeting, both the doctor and the patient must participate which means replacing a "medical decision" with an informed interaction, a necessary precondition to negotiated confidence. Joint participation means reflecting on what is important to the person who is expressing a need for treatment and/or understanding of his or her state of health. But the interaction between doctor and patient brings into play rationalities which vary according to the disease and the treatment, and which may be founded on a heterogeneous set of representations, experiences and areas of knowledge.

Looking at a subject, an observer can only see what he is used to seeing. The painter Bonnard described how, when visiting an old, sick friend, he became fascinated by the bluish reflection of a vein in this friend's wasted neck in the oblique light of the setting sun. When confronted with a patient seeking care, each different type of care provider (nurse, doctor, etc.) risks only seeing what is relevant to their own skill, or even worse, worrying about what is beyond their skill. The situation becomes even more complicated if it is known that the person being observed only shows the aspect which is likely to interest the observer. To the doctor, he will talk about disease, to the psychologist about anxiety and phobia, and to the social worker about financial problems. Even if the three are synthesised, it can be difficult to build up a coherent picture.

Once the first contact has been established in a consultation, an attempt must be made to go some way together. At this moment, the meeting starts to make some sense, it starts to become a relationship. This entails discussion, negotiation and accepting compromises without immediately wanting to measure everything using evaluation scales. The doctor does not always know what is going to emerge in the course of a consultation or an evaluation. He can propose stopping, can try to explain, or suggest some kind of help or treatment. But, as therapist and professional, he or she must know how to control the discussion, both in its scope and its length.

Providing the patient with information

Although it may appear useful for the doctor to provide the patient with information, the process raises a number of questions, both practical and theoretical questions. What does the patient expect from such information? What do the doctor and the care provider expect? What type of information is relevant? In what form and how should information be presented? What is the purpose?

Everyone is unanimous: patients want to be kept informed and supported throughout the care process. This presupposes that their opinion was taken into account in the first place. Because any medical action entails possible risks as well as benefits, the patient should be given comprehensive, accurate and suitably presented information about procedures before he is asked to consent to them. This desire for information also applies to the nature, the cause and the severity of the disease, and treatment programmes, the results and effects of diagnostic tests, the progress of the disease, and whether or not it is terminal. These days, the emphasis is on the transmission of medical information from doctor to patient, rather than on a dialogue or an exchange between two different players. Thus, the "aids" produced by learned societies for the purposes of patient information about the dangers associated with certain invasive procedures often seem to be support materials for the physician designed to replace oral communication with the patient. It seems to us that, above and beyond this "objective" information, what patients also want is to be able to position themselves in their care track, *i.e.* find out when, where and why each person involved is going to perform their part of the treatment process with a view to understanding the process as a whole.

Being provided with adequate information is an important part of the confidence a patient has in his or her physician, but it is equally important when it comes to other members of the care providing team; keeping the patient informed is an integral part of the care process.

The obligation to keep the patient informed is by no means new. It follows on from the contractual bond between doctor and patient, as stipulated in a 1936 decision of the Appeals Court which explains that a genuine contract is established between the two parties, and the existence of a contract implies that both parties are consenting. This was affirmed in Article 35 of the Code of Professional Medical Ethics: *"It is the duty of the physician to provide to the person being examined or treated, appropriate, clear and trustworthy information about his or her state of health and any investigations or treatment that is proposed."* Article L. 710-2 of the Public Health Code stipulates that public and private health care establishments are obliged to communicate to those receiving treatment any information contained in their medical records [151]. The 1978 Law on citizens and information created the Commission for Access to Administrative Documents (Cada, *Commission d'accès aux documents administratifs*) and led to the drawing up of the Patient's Charter.

The principles are established but putting them into practice raises many difficulties. Doctors claim to be in a delicate position, notably because of legislative and regulatory changes. They fear increased legal pressure in the context of providing information to patients. A series of Appeals Court rulings in 1997 and 1998 broadened the scope of the will to provide information to patients to encompass the doctor having to furnish proof that such information was communicated. Thus, there exists an obligation to inform patients of serious risks which might result in death or disability, even if such serious consequences are rare. However, in another ruling issued in May 2000, the same Court judged that limitation of the information *"should be founded on a legitimate basis and in the interest of the patient, this interest being assessed in the context of the nature of the disease, its predicted progress, and the patient's personality"* [179].

The issues related to information go well beyond the legal protection of doctors, risking instrumentalisation of the patient and legalism through a reaction on the part of the medical community, a situation which would be to the detriment of care relationships

INFORMING PATIENTS: THE DANGERS ACCORDING TO THE ANAES

Possible pitfalls	Anaes recommendations (quotes)
Taking care of patient information by routinely using written, general texts, especially concerning technical procedures.	*"The discussion incited by information necessitates that it be transmitted verbally. Verbal information is primordial because it can be matched to the individual. It is necessary to devote time to this, and be available..."* Only verbal information gives the patient a chance to ask questions and the physician a chance to reply. *"Verbal information may be complemented by documentation."*
Giving information once and for all.	*"The information pertains to the patient's state of health and treatment, be it a one-off procedure or long-term care. It needs to be updated regularly."*
Concentrating on the possible risks associated with procedures.	Patient information should *"be ranked and based on validated facts"* and should include *"the expected benefits before any disadvantages and risks"*. The information concerns: – the patient's current and foreseeable condition, which means explanations about the disease, and its usual progress with and without treatment; – a description of the nature of and procedures involved in any envisaged examinations, investigations, treatments and interventions, together with information about alternative strategies: – purpose, usefulness, and expected benefits; – consequences and disadvantages, possible complications and risks; – general and particular precautions recommended to patients.
Underplaying rare events or serious risks.	Patient information should *"stipulate the serious risks, including rare events, i.e. those that may be life-threatening or may lead to permanent disability"*.
Providing information using technical terminology and/or in a difficult-to-understand form.	The information given to the patient should be comprehensible. *"The doctor must make sure that the patient has understood the information provided."*
Leaving it up to the patient to choose between multiple alternatives.	The doctor *"points to the solution he/she has in mind, and explains the reasons for the choice"*.

Part four — The user, a player in the health care system

Possible pitfalls	Anaes recommendations (quotes)
Providing information with the primary purpose of obtaining confirmation in writing that information was indeed provided.	*"The only point of the information form is to give the patient information in a written form and this document does not need to be signed by the patient. For this reason, it should not be combined with any form requiring signature."* *"Written documents should state that the patient is invited to ask any questions he/she wants".*

Source: Anaes [137], Prescrire n° 21, 2001, p. 68.

and the confidence required in this relationship [154]. This is why the legal strictures must also take into account characteristics of medical practice in order to allow the medical community to further improve its services to patients. Although these characteristics have sometimes been abused by certain physicians to exonerate themselves from the obligation to provide adequate information, rare instances of aberrant behaviour should not obscure the need to take into account the fact that the act of providing information is associated with a certain number of problems.

Information is a central issue in the patient-doctor relationship. What information should the patient be given? How should it be given? How can it be ascertained that the patient has understood? None of these questions has a simple, obvious answer. At this stage of the discussion of this subject, it seems important to make distinction between the different objectives when providing information. Four such objectives are clear:

- To improve *communication between physician and patient*. It is difficult to imagine in today's world a doctor taking a patient into care without keeping him informed of his diagnostic conclusions, his therapeutic proposals, and even the prognosis, if the doctor thinks that the patient would be better off knowing. For example, the physician might provide the patient with all written documents associated with consultations and hospital stays, as is already the practice in some departments [142]. An advantage of this would be that the physician would be obliged to put his diagnostic hypotheses in writing and consider more carefully the tests that he orders and his proposed therapeutic strategy. But in all cases, it is important to make sure that the patient has understood what is going to be done to him, why, in what order, where and when *(see box)*.

- To improve the *decision-making process when it comes to undertaking complementary examinations or therapeutic procedures*. The purpose of providing the patient with information is to supply enough readily understood details in order to permit the patient to participate in the decision-making process. Information

Ensure balance in the patient/care provider relationship

allows both patient and physician – in a sharing of knowledge – to come to an agreement about the best course of action to follow, taking the patient's desires into account. It may happen that the patient rejects the doctor's proposals once he has appraised the associated risks. This is up to the patient who is making his decision in full knowledge. On the other hand, the patient and the physician cannot share the same values (as has become evident in the discussions about artificial abortion), so the preferences of the patient may lead to a different solution to that arrived at by the doctor on the basis of his personal preferences.

- To improve *compliance*. Providing information is one of the reliable ways of maximising compliance, although in some cases the ultimate effect is counter-productive with the patient choosing to believe the worst.

- To reduce *the patient's anxiety and improve tolerance of invasive procedures and/or treatments*. If the patient knows about possible side effects, it may be possible to deal with them at an earlier stage. However, doctors worry that a greater level of awareness of risks may lay them open to more malpractice suits. The first question concerns the extent of risks which should be revealed to the patient. In two rulings issued in 1998, the Appeals Court stipulated that *"apart from emergency situations, when the patient refuses to be informed, and when it is impossible to give the patient information, the doctor is obliged to provide the patient with clear, trustworthy and appropriate information about any serious risks associated with proposed investigations or treatments, and this obligation is not affected by the eventuality that the adverse consequence concerned occurs only rarely"*. The problem is that the information on risks might obscure the information about possible benefits, *i.e.* "the risk of doing nothing".

From information to consent

Among a doctor's other obligations, that of collecting a patient's informed consent prior to proposed investigations or treatment is crucial. This obligation follows on from "human respect" and consent is therefore an implicit expression of the confidence which must exist between patients and doctors. It is the privileged instrument of expression of a person's independence. Etymologically speaking, consent means reproduce a sense among many, *i.e.* agree on a truth or an interpretation. Requesting consent for treatment and, in the event, accepting the patient's rejection are founded on the principle of respecting the patient's freedom of choice although the latter is sometimes seen as a challenge to the physician's authority.

A certain proportion of physicians consider themselves as their patients' "voice of reason". From their point of view, both the mental capacity and the will of the patient are compromised so that he is not in a position to take an informed, rational decision. Therefore, there is a moral obligation, based on protection of the weak, to take his decisions for him, for his own good, the attitude which underlies medical paternalism [175]. It is essential to recognise that the position of the doctor and that of the patient are completely different. The patient may be in a vulnerable state, and the doctor may be worried about losing a "customer". Recognising the difference makes it possible to reflect about the evolution in the processes governing the patient-doctor relationship. In this perspective, patient information and informed consent are not ends in themselves but rather a way of promoting participation in the decision-making process in which both patient and physician have their own specific roles and responsibilities.

The desire to be informed should not be confused with the desire to take an active part in the making of decisions. In some cases, the patient may wish to unload on the doctor a large part of the psychological stress associated with the uncertainties of treatment. The problem of the inability of certain patients to give informed consent (*e.g.* demented patients) raises the question of delegation of this right. Who should be given the information if the patient is not in a position to understand it? There may, for example, exist conflicts of interest between parents and children. But it has been accepted for a long time (embodied in the code of professional ethics and in jurisprudence) that doctors may act on their own initiative in emergency situations. Is there a need to define what constitutes an emergency or an indispensable medical intervention? The right to leave instructions not to be given any treatment in certain circumstances is recognised in an increasing number of national rights and this might lead doctors to treat the idea of emergency with some caution [143]. The Bill on modernisation of the health care system should review the idea of right of attorney which confers on a third party the right to make decisions when the first party is *"not in a position to express his or her wishes or integrate information to this end"*. This person would be appointed in writing with revocation possible at any moment.

From informed consent to shared decision-making

Providing the patient with information cannot sum up the entire interaction between patient and physician. Why does the information only go from doctor to patient? What place should be made for the patients to talk about their life experience and knowledge, and ask questions? [154] Thus, it is up to patients to ask questions and talk about their emotions, real life and preferences, if they desire to do so. It is up to the doctor to explain his rationale, the risks and benefits associated with such and such a procedure, and alternative medical options. The physician should also be able to distinguish his patient's expectations in the medico-technical register, in the existential register and in the emotional register.

This exchange of information is necessary if the decision-making process is to be shared and lead to acceptance, rejection or adjustment of the strategy to be adopted. It is also necessary to allow the patient to take decisions in the conduct of his existence. Shared decision-making involves several care options and consists of a three-step process: a two-way exchange of information (knowledge/preferences); discussion of the various options (interaction); taking of the decision on how to treat the problem.

Numerous models are proposed in the literature to ascribe a place in the medical decision-making process to the patient:
– the "paternalistic" model in which the doctor makes the decision and the patient consents,
– the "honest broker" model in which the doctor explains his personal preferences to the patient and then makes a decision on his own as the most reliable representative of the patient's best interests,
– the "shared decision-making" model in which information is shared and decisions are taken jointly,
– the "consumer" model in which the role of the physician is limited to providing the necessary information and leaving the patient make the decision on his own.

Each model might have its advantages in different clinical situations and with patients with different expectations, so it is not a question of selecting the single best model. The problem resides in recognising that the patient is always a more or less active player in the field of health and recognising this fact leads to a reshuffling of the relationships between the exercise of medicine and the experience of patients. In other words, the care process appears as a co-construction involving both patient and doctor in different ways [139]. It is nevertheless important to question whether all patients conform to the model of the responsible patient, a player in his disease as represented by patient support groups and the public authorities. Do they all want to participate in the decision-making process? Many patients do not want to feel alone in the face of their disease and their anxiety, and rely on the presence of their physician.

The various responsibilities to be co-ordinated

Most medical decisions – whatever their complexity or import – are taken by physicians in a state of uncertainty which they do not allow the patient to see in any way. The decision is taken on the basis of the doctor's knowledge, beliefs, experience, culture and values. Recognising that everyone has a role in the care process should promote shared responsibility. What does this mean? In an atmosphere of confidence, everyone participates in the decision-making process according to his abilities and knowledge. Thus, the process is founded on a mutual respect of skills, on the knowledge of all concerned, and on a recognition that it is advantageous to pool expertise.

It is important to make a distinction between different types of knowledge and responsibility. The medical decision is ultimately up to one person, he who is legally responsible, *i.e.* the doctor. Although the process can include the sharing of information and negotiation, the burden of liability is the doctor's and can never be shifted onto the patient [154]. But in contrast, the patient is responsible for his own life and that can never be the responsibility of the doctor.

The shared decision-making process should depend on a process of deliberation in which the physician and patient together construct a care space. Many physicians mistrust this type of approach because they are worried about making their patients anxious. They under-estimate their patients, considering that most of them would be unable to integrate and weigh all the diverse elements in the choice to be made. Physicians also point out that the rejection of treatment by an informed patient can be damaging to his health, *e.g.* if a patient with spondylodiscitis refuses a bone biopsy so that an antibiotic must be prescribed on a probabilistic rather than a targeted basis (with a greater risk therefore of therapeutic failure).

In this approach, the doctor's job is to discover the patient's wishes. In order to do this, both knowledge and adequate consultation time are necessary. What information does the patient need? How should the information be presented?

The right of access to medical records has been claimed by patient support groups for many years now, in the name of the responsibility of the patient and also to maintain continuity and efficacy in treatment. Patient support groups persistently claim that the information given to patients is insufficient and incomprehensible: information about state of health and treatment, about devices proposed, about knowledge, about doubts and areas of ignorance, and about risks. However, it seems to us that, above and beyond these "objective" facts, what the patient really needs is to be able to locate himself in the treatment process: know when and why the diverse care providers are going to do what they have to do. In this way the patient would know what is to happen in advance, and would be relieved of certain anxieties associated with the coherence of the actions of the care providing team. In this respect, the patient's medical records (which can also be a medium for procedures aimed at improving the technical quality of care and its organisation: *see box*) have other virtues in that they can provide an indicator for a clear project concerning the patient. This should resolve any "misunderstandings" about access to these records, which are primarily related to an absence of real dialogue. The planned modernisation of the health care system provides for direct access to medical records, with accompaniment if the patient so wishes.

FROM TRADITIONAL MEDICAL RECORDS TO THE UNIQUE COMPUTERISED PATIENT RECORD

For a long term, medical records were not considered as anything more than a tool to help a care provider to follow his/her patient's case, and each practitioner kept – or did not keep – records in the way best suited to his/her own needs.

Since, this idea has evolved and Articles L. 1112-1 and R. 710-2-1 and the following of the Public Health Code stipulate that health care establishments are obliged to maintain medical records, and lay down conditions governing how they are stored and how their contents may be communicated.

Despite such regulations, medical records are far from uniform with respect to format, contents and archiving, and independent practitioners are not even obliged to keep such records, although Article 45 of the Code of Medical Ethics provides for "Personal Observation Sheets" ("fiches d'observation personnelles").

Lack of uniformity entails problems when it comes to using records, whether to record or obtain information. Thus, at a time when medical practice is becoming more technical and more complex, and when patient care necessarily entails a more integrated, global approach, there is a greater need than ever for a formally structured information system with records compiled, handled and shared by all the various players involved in a patient's care.

To this end, more consistency is necessary in both form and content of records within and between different establishments, and it is essential that independent practitioners be included in the system. An ideal system could be based on a "Unique Computerised Patient Record" containing the person's entire medical, psychological and social history which is relevant to care; this would be available to all involved in that patient's treatment.

Experiments carried out in Boston have demonstrated the validity of a "Unique Computerised Patient Record" system with respect to reducing medical mistakes (thanks to software which instantly detects errors and also due to the elimination of errors caused by the misreading of illegible inscriptions) and increased efficiency (no more losing of records, records are immediately and readily available, scheduling is easier, etc.), especially when the electronic record is combined with a computerised prescription system.

However, the fact that this type of system is far from commonplace is not without valid reasons: apart from cultural obstacles (notably a degree of mistrust of such a novel mode of operation on the part of the medical profession), other questions remain to be answered, e.g. financial questions (mainly the cost of computerisation) and legal questions (how is the medical information to be rendered secure, and how is access to the data to be controlled, notably who is to

Part four The user, a player in the health care system

have access and how, is access to be full or partial, and will access be read-only or must the ability to modify the data be an option).

It is worth pointing out that computerising records would solve the problem of archiving insofar as the validity of electronic signatures is already recognised by the Law (Law n° 2000-230 of March 14 2000). However, this too raises questions of security in various areas: in legal terms, *e.g.* how can modification of an electronically signed document be rendered impossible; and with respect to archiving, notably the risk of information being lost in the course of multiple electronic exchanges if hard copies are to be entirely done away with. And finally there is the question of cost, this form of storage being currently two or three times as expensive as conventional paper-based archives.

It is therefore worth considering this opportunity of adopting a unique format for medical records with consistent form and content. Involved in this discussion should be not only hospital-based professionals but also external professionals (independent medical practitioners, nurses and social workers) at a time when integrated hospital-outpatient care is expanding. Moreover, account will have to be taken of the opinions of users' representatives who will soon have a right of direct access to their own records. Currently, a patient only has the right to access his/her own file through the intermediary of a doctor but, in the new law on modernisation of the health care service, provision is made for direct access, in response to a long-standing and growing demand on the part of users and non-profit-making organisations. This provision is included in the name of transparency, patient responsibility, and the continuity and efficacy of care. This new aspect of the Law on its own deserves close inspection for the ethical, legal and practical questions it raises.

It is important that this new initiative does not result in the compilation of records intended as "defensive" instruments by professionals. In contrast, the current change represents a chance to re-think the way information relevant to their own case is provided to patients, and how important information about the patient is communicated to other health care professionals.

Directorate for Hospitalisation and Care Logistics (DHOS, Direction de l'hospitalisation et de l'organisation des soins).

Recommendations

It has long been recognised that users are players in the field of health and especially in the health care system but the preoccupation of public authorities as to how to involve them in the system is new. It is not possible to issue a law that people get more involved. The will stems rather from a number of different questions which have been addressed in this chapter in which distinction was made between various levels of participation: the participation of the citizen in state-sponsored, health-related initiatives; the participation of users in the working of health-related institutions; and the participation of patients in the making of decisions about diagnosis and treatment.

Making the user a player in the health care system – by involving citizens in the choice between possible options at both the collective and the individual level – will depend on certain preconditions:

Establish a policy to bring the user into all structures related to health, with a view to addressing their expectations and taking stock of their suggestions.

In all health-related structures, users and their representatives should be brought in to participate at all levels of the process of deliberation and assessment, notably during the gathering of data, the generation of tools with which to analyse the data, the decision-making process, and the evaluation of results. This does not apply to just those institutions which are part of the health care system but to any structure which makes decisions with a potential impact on health, *e.g.* the Regional Health Councils *(conseils départementaux d'hygiène)* or committees which deal with environmental planning.

Clarify the responsibilities of the various different players in the health care system according to the three different levels of relationship stipulated (populational, institutional and individual).

The responsibilities of each player – the public authorities, the risk managers, the managers of institutions and health care establishments, elected officials, health care professionals, experts and users' groups – need to be clarified if each player is to be empowered to contribute to the dialogue and genuinely participate in the resolution of health-related problems. As with any form of policy, this initiative must include an administrative component with the means of stimulating the dialogue, of converting the conclusions into legislation, and finally of assessing the results of the policy. Consolidating administrative means should be linked to a review process to redefine the place of the administration with respect to the user. Similarly, if users must have their place in the decision-making process, then the elected representatives of the users must preserve their prerogatives when it comes to making health-related choices on behalf of the people.

Encourage initiatives and allow enough time for consolidation of the new relationships between the various players (which were only established for the first time in recent years).

It is important to consolidate existing approaches as well as encouraging new ones, without boxing them in with an over-restrictive legislative framework. This means supporting the players in their initiative to construct a health care system which responds to today's priorities. Methodological support would seem to be important and it might be useful to investigate the opportunity of creating a technical institution with, as objectives, the promotion of innovation in this field, the analysis of associated advantages and difficulties, the synthesis of knowledge and its dissemination to the public, and the production of aids for decision-making and support materials for providing users with information.

To make sure that the novel modes of operation in the health care system tend to diminish rather than exacerbate existing social inequalities in health.

This consideration should be systematically taken into account in any measures aimed at promoting user participation which have to be regularly evaluated. Initiatives favouring those in a psychologically or socially vulnerable position should be encouraged, developed and adapted to this population.

Four directions seem to us to be particularly important to give a new impetus to user participation in the health care system:

- **Guarantee user representation in all structures involved in health and health care.**

This involves supporting users' representatives in these new roles (training, financing, accreditation, etc.).

- **Help health professionals take better stock of the expectations of patients and, in a more general way, of users.**

This might necessitate developing training programmes in relations and communications. Consideration in this context – notably legal and economic reflection – of the doctor-patient relationship is indispensable if user participation is to be stepped up and if the circulation of information between health professionals and users is to be improved.

- **Create new discussion forums to encourage users to express themselves at every level,** *i.e.* local, regional and national.

This will involve the reorganisation of already-existing institutions with a view to democratisation of their ways of working, and the generation of a regulatory system for the decision-making process in the field of health in order to make the process both more effective and more transparent.

- **Provide the health administration with the resources (human, financial and technical) necessary to fulfilling its duties in this field at the national, regional and departmental levels.**

PART FIVE

A critical, prospective analysis of the way the health system is organised

Part five A critical, prospective analysis of the way the health system is organised

Composition of the Working Group

President Bertrand Garros, National Prevention Committee

Members Anne-Carole Bensadon, General Health Directorate,
Ministry of Employment and Solidarity
Jean-Pierre Claveranne, High Committee on Public Health
Anne-Lore Coury, Social Security Directorate,
Ministry of Employment and Solidarity
Jean-François Dodet, High Committee on Public Health
Isabelle Ferrand, High Committee on Public Health
Alain Jourdain, National School of Public Health
Maguy Jean-François, Directorate for Hospitalisation and Care
Logistics, Ministry of Employment and Solidarity
Claudine Parayre, Directorate of Research, Studies, Evaluation
and Statistics, Ministry of Employment and Solidarity
Yvette Ract, National Health Insurance Agency
for Salaried Workers
Myriam Revel, Directorate for Hospitalisation and Care Logistics,
Ministry of Employment and Solidarity
René Roué, High Committee on Public Health
Frédéric Rouillon, Teaching Hospital, Créteil
Bernadette Roussille, French Committee on Health Education
Jean-Claude Sailly, Centre for Economic, Sociological
and Management Research
Roland Sambuc, High Committee on Public Health
Martine Stern, Social Security Directorate,
Ministry of Employment and Solidarity

Co-ordination Marc Duriez, General Secretariat of the High Committee
on Public Health

Acknowledgements Caroline Colmadin, Intern, DESS

Introduction

Undertaking a "critical, prospective analysis" of the way in which the health system is organised necessarily entails putting many different aspects into context. So many that such an exercise, if not unrealistic, is inevitably a complex one which necessitates a great deal of time. From a pragmatic viewpoint, and one quite consistent with HCPH philosophy, the Working Group decided to base its deliberations around a public health approach. Indeed, in its 1994 General Report on "Health in France", the Committee recommended *"focusing first and foremost on public health"*, meaning that *"not only must the funding system be organised on the basis of health targets for entire populations, but also that the organisation of the health care system be subordinate to the idea of public health, i.e. that structural planning, staffing at all levels [...] and in all areas [...], and training orientations should all be conditioned by public health-related considerations"*. Recently the Minister of Health, Bernard Kouchner, lent his unqualified support to this approach. The Working Group has therefore chosen to track the progress made in the logistics of the health care system since these recommendations were issued by trying to answer the following questions:

• Is the way the health care system currently works based on genuine priorities, and does it cater to people's needs?

• Is the health care system organised in a strategic, functional, way?

• Are questions of health dealt with in democratic processes in which the general public can participate?

Part five A critical, prospective analysis of the way the health system is organised

The answers to these three questions have been compiled in such a way as to present first a description of the current situation, and then a critical analysis thereof.

The prospective analysis has been formulated as an answer to a fourth question: **"Is the health care system in a position to respond to future challenges?"** In this answer are contained certain concrete proposals, the number of which has been deliberately kept to a minimum.

Is the way the health care system currently works based on genuine priorities, and does it cater to people's needs?

The current situation: the "public health approach" envisaged in the 1996 Rulings

Prior to the Rulings published in April 1996, various texts were in existence dealing with the need to take people's needs into account when allocating resources. The Law of July 3 1991 pertaining to reform in the hospital sector is an example: this states that the purpose of the health card system and of re-organising health care on a regional basis is *"to meet the demand for health care in as effective a way as possible"* and that the measures are *"based on an assessment of the population's needs"*. Nevertheless, apart from specific provisions introduced over the years, there was no overall, integrated structure to provide a broad vision, as pointed out by the HCPH. Although this objective was not always emphasised, the April 1996 Rulings established a link – for the first time in such a clear, global fashion in France – between funding and health priorities.

At the national level, it is now Parliament which is responsible for setting expenditure targets when it passes the Social Security Funding Laws (Article 1 of the Constitutional Law of February 22 1996). Every year, the Funding Bill submitted to Parliament by the Government must take health policy priorities into account together with any ideas concerning the reimbursement of care costs proposed at the National Health Conference (Article 1 of the April 24 1996 Ruling on Controlling Health Care Expenditure and the Law of July 22 1996). The Funding Bill is submitted to Parliament with two reports, one compiled by the National Health Conference and the other by the High Committee on Public Health.

The targets and management modalities subsequently agreed between the Government and the National Health Insurance Organisations (in accordance with the Funding Laws) must address the long-term direction of the stipulated measures in the field of public health as well as specifying how the measures are to improve the quality of the services provided for users and how the targets relate to general social policy and policy in the matter of prevention (Article 1 of the April 24 1996 Ruling on Organisation of the Social Security system). The way in which these agreements are implemented is subject to regular review by an independent Monitoring Council which reports to Parliament.

Finally, regional hospital expenditure budgets are set on the basis of the population's needs in conjunction with local and national health policy priorities, the over-riding principle being progressive reduction of inequality between different regions (Articles 16 and 21 of the April 24 1996 Ruling on Reform of Public and Private Hospitals).

The health care system reforms contain several provisions aimed at identifying regional health priorities and ensuring that they are effectively addressed.

Firstly, a series of Regional Health Conferences are created with a remit of establishing public health priorities in their own region, and making proposals as to how to improve the population's health status with reference to any measure, be it in the field of health, health care or social policy. The Regional Conference's report is submitted to the National Conference, the Regional Hospital Agency, the Regional Union of Health Insurers, and the Union of Independent Medical Practitioners (Article 1 of the April 24 1996 Ruling on Controlling Health Care Expenditure).

The Regional Hospital Agencies (ARH, *Agence régionale de l'hospitalisation*) draw up long-term contracts specifying objectives and modalities with health care establishments. These contracts cover quality and safety targets, and implement any directions recommended by the Regional Health Conference (Article 8 of the 24 April 1996 Ruling on Reform of Public and Private Hospitals). The Regional Hospital Agency submits an annual report to the Regional Health Conference on measures implemented by health care establishments relevant to the health care priorities identified by the Conference (Article 10 of the 24 April 1996 Ruling on Reform of Public and Private Hospitals).

Regional Unions of the Health Insurance Organisations (Urcam, *Unions régionales des caisses d'assurance maladie*) help oversee the implementation by each of the individual organisations of the measures aimed at prevention and health education entailed by the public health priorities as decreed at the regional level (Article 22 of the 24 April 1996 Ruling on Organisation of the

Social Security system). The Urcams need to co-ordinate in particular with the Regional Unions of Independent Medical Practitioners (URML, *Unions régionales de médecins libéraux*) created in a 1993 Law. The remit of the UMRL is to *"contribute to improving the way the health care system is managed and promote high-quality care"*. These bodies must participate in the following activities:
– analysis and evaluation of the workings of the system in general and independent medical practice in particular as well as conducting epidemiological surveys and assessments of medical needs,
– evaluation of behaviour patterns and professional practices in the perspective of the quality of patient care,
– organisation and regulation of the health care system,
– prevention and general health-related measures,
– co-ordination with other health care professionals,
– educating and informing physicians and users.

Since the July 1998 Law pertaining to social exclusion, a Regional Health Policy Committee (presided over by the Prefect) has been in charge of the overall co-ordination, monitoring and evaluation of measures following on from either the identification of regional health priorities or the implementation of national policies, *e.g.* in the area of cancer screening.

These provisions apply at the national as well as the regional level, to the public as well as the private sector, and to hospitals as well as independent practice. For all sectors, they establish – at least officially – a link between identified health priorities and resource allocation within the health care system.

Critical analysis: health priorities, a successful concept but one which is vague when it comes to action

Publication of the first General Report of the HCPH in 1994, the first Regional Health Conferences, and the 1996 Rulings have all no doubt made major contributions to assimilation of the public health approach and the idea of health priorities. The mode of operation of the Health Conferences – which was inspired by that of consensus conferences, hence the presence of a jury – has been remarkably successful in that it has made it possible for all the regions to follow a more or less consistent approach, and that in a country with no historical experience of the principle of identifying health priorities. However, it is clear that the idea of health priorities remains somewhat vague, both because the concept has never been formally defined and because the methods used to identify and then confirm priorities are still far from robust.

Formulating priorities generally remains a haphazard process, and the relatively non-specific priorities identified tend to reflect no more than a general attitude. As a result, it is often difficult to construct concrete strategy on the basis of the identified priorities. In other words, the way to proceed is only clear if the players concerned are in a position to work out an exact response to the identified problem. The strategic aspect is little mentioned in the Rulings. In the absence of this kind of perspective, there is a risk that any health priority might be perceived as no more than a vain wish, worthy and well-intentioned certainly but quite impossible to do anything about. This situation follows on in part from the vagueness of the ideas involved, which is such that the priorities identified at the national and regional levels cover highly disparate areas. It is also important to emphasise that, while the idea of a population's needs may be easy to grasp at an intuitive level, it is not so useful in concrete, operational terms. Therefore, clarification of these concepts is urgently needed, notably what certain words really mean such as priority, objective, goal, target, level, etc. This is partly to ensure that each means the same thing to everyone. In each region, priorities will have to be reformulated in the light of this review, so that the priorities defined are more precise, more structured, and more operational with respect to devising strategies to be followed in order to attain stated objectives.

The absence of a sufficiently precise, rigorous framework has led many players in the health system to question the validity of a logistical structure based on health priorities. For example, some have imagined that funding is going to be cut off from non-priority areas, significantly if not completely. As a result, the temptation has been to expand the list of priorities to cover as wide a scope as possible – lest anything be left out. Moreover, there has been a serious lack of consistency in the way in which national health priorities are formulated in different contexts, *e.g.* between the High Committee on Public Health, the National Health Conference, the Social Security Laws, and the agreements on targets and management modalities established between the Government and the National Health Insurance Agency for Salaried Workers. Suddenly, where before there were no priorities at all, now we have too many priorities, and everyone knows that too many priorities cannot be priorities at all. This situation has been exacerbated by the parallel existence of processes at both the national and regional level which no one knows how to co-ordinate. Although France is not a federal state, regional players often consider that they are only concerned by regional priorities, and requests from the National Conference to have some common topic discussed at all the Regional Conferences have often been seen as yet another manifestation of Parisian tyranny.

Other questions can be asked about the effective impact of the idea of priorities on resource allocation and investment. According to many analysts, the impact has actually been minimal with the main institutions and players having managed to side-step the essential thrust of the initiative apart from a few token concessions, in the vanguard of which is the establishment of the Regional Health Programmes. There is evidence to support this view. Despite the unacceptable premature mortality rate – many of which deaths could be avoided by measures in areas outside of the care system – and despite the demand of the people having been clearly expressed at the Constitutive Assembly on Health, the amount of resources diverted towards prevention and preventive medicine has been insignificant. In other words, today's Regional Health Programmes are no more than another form of the old Regional Health Promotion Credits *(Crédits régionalisés de promotion de la santé)* and other public health funding sources, the real effect of which has been further marginalisation of the public health approach rather than the generalisation of resource allocation mechanisms. On the other hand, other analysts – without denying the paucity of the resources mobilised in the name of health priorities – point out that the real benefit is to be found in the fact that such high-profile operations can change attitudes. In this perspective, the problem is seen as largely culturally based and, unless perceptions and attitudes evolve, no real change is possible: the rudder is only a small component, but it is enough to change the boat's course and take it into new waters. As is consistently the case, examples from the regions bear witness to the relevance of this voluntarist vision, although the fact that such experiences remain anecdotal tends to point up its limitations. It is therefore important to sustain the commitment of the players by means of attractive incentives, one option being the allocation of significant resources to the regions in the context of the National Health Insurance Expenditure Target (Ondam, *Objectif national des dépenses d'assurance maladie*), as proposed by the HCPH.

Is the health care system organised in a strategic, functional way?

The current situation: the way health determinants are taken into account lacks consistency

In a public approach, assessing the coherence of the health care system means taking stock of two broad aspects: the first is the compatibility of the strategies undertaken with what is known about health determinants; and the second bears on the compatibility of the modus operandi – from both an institutional and financial point of view – with efficient, effective action.

As a result of extensive research, we now have a fairly good idea of what factors are important in determining health status, both at the individual as well as the collective level (although this distinction is rarely absolute). Individual determinants are primarily physiological, largely associated with genetic make-up (which everyone is endowed with at birth and about which nobody can do a great deal, although this picture may change in the future). "Lifestyle" factors represent another set of determinants and these have a major individual component although, in many cases, they are significantly conditioned by collective considerations, *e.g.* dominant values in society. The social environment, the physical environment, living and working conditions, all these are more clearly collective determinants which may promote good health or lead to disease. In the final analysis, it is a combination of individual and collective factors acting synergistically which determine health status and dictate whether disease appears earlier or later, and it is now recognised that the health of a population depends on all these many and various determinants.

Disease cannot always be avoided and, in the event of impaired health, the efficacy of the health care system is an obvious factor involved in determining the patient's ultimate health status after treatment.

In other words, although it is good to have an effective care system when you are sick, even better is to have a system which prevents you becoming sick.

Health policy needs to cover three different levels of strategic intervention:

– at the level of the factors which determine health – above and beyond any considerations to do with care – in order to promote good health and thereby prevent or delay the appearance of health problems;

– once anyone has developed a health problem, to ensure that top quality care is initiated at as early a stage as possible;

– finally, to limit the repercussions of disease on all the various aspects of the patient's life.

These three different levels cannot be considered in isolation but rather as a continuum of "preventive" interventions based on the principle of avoidability. Although this holistic idea is sometimes alluded to in an abstract fashion in France, rarely is anything concrete done about it. Resources and attention are massively concentrated at the second level of intervention, *i.e.* care and treatment. Ever since the end of the Second World War, policy has focused on improving access to health care rather than improving health. Stepping up provision and enhancing accessibility have constituted the dominant strategy in the fight against socially and geographically based inequality in health.

Part five A critical, prospective analysis of the way the health system is organised

Complicated logistics

The logistics of the health care system are characterised by ever-increasing compartmentalisation and overlap between different areas of expertise and activity, and this problem is constantly being compounded. In regulations and procedures pertaining to services, distinction is made between health and the medico-social or social, between the private and public sectors, between profit-making and non-profit-making organisations within the private sector, and between independent or outpatient practice and hospitals. At the national level, the roles of State authorities and health insurers are constantly being re-interpreted and redefined. With respect to care provision, while hospitals are under direct State control, independent practice is under the aegis of the health insurance system (to simplify the situation for reasons of clarity). Otherwise, as a result of fall-out from the HIV-contaminated blood scandal, a multitude of different agencies are now involved in questions that used to be directly handled by the central administration of the Health Ministry.

At the regional, departmental and local levels, decentralisation and devolution together with the 1996 Rulings have resulted in multiplication of structures and institutions acting in the same areas. Devolved State agencies, regional health insurance offices, and local authorities, institutions and players (both administrators and insurers) are all following their own strategies, often in ways which are entirely independent of anyone else. Thus, there exist the State-sponsored Regional Health Programmes (PRS, *Programmes régionaux de santé*), the Regional Health Insurance Programmes (Pram, *Programmes régionaux de l'assurance maladie*), and the plans formulated by departmental councils, among many others. However, in recent years, an effort has been made when defining policy to keep such structures as integrated and multi-disciplinary as possible, especially with respect to the co-ordination of health-related and social services.

The financial logistics of the health care system are entirely based on an annual footing (in order to preserve compatibility with the overall public accounting system). Both the National Health Insurance Expenditure Target (Ondam, *Objectif national des dépenses d'assurance maladie*) and the State budget are thus structured despite the fact that the measures and programmes being financed follow a more long-term rhythm. Some progress has been made in this respect in recent years, at least with respect to the stipulation of long-term objectives, *e.g.* in the context of the National Fund for Prevention, Education and Intervention in Health (FNPEIS, *Fonds national de prévention, d'éducation et d'intervention en santé*). However, the multiplicity of decision-makers is paralleled by a multiplicity of sources of funds, a situation which is compounded by the tendency of individual institutions to have multiple internal sources, each often acting independently without any measure of co-ordination.

Critical analysis: the excess premature death rate is probably due to a deficit in certain types of health strategy

The promulgation of a strategy heavily dependent upon curative medicine and the biomedical approach – in preference to if not at the expense of other strategies to improve health – has resulted in a widely held conviction that good health depends primarily on access to health care, a perspective in which intervention is seen as usually being able to restore the level of health that existed prior to the appearance of the problem being treated. This philosophy stems from situations such as the ability to cure infectious disease with antibiotics, together with the efficacy of some of the new surgical procedures (which are regularly "hyped up" in the media).

This conviction is very widespread, not only among the general public but also among politicians and professional health care providers. Therefore, it is not surprising that increasing care provision, *i.e.* removing obstacles – notably financial – to access to care, should be seen as the most effective way of improving the nation's health. While such a strategy has brought indubitable benefit to sick people, it has not significantly affected the incidence of disease. What is at issue here is not the value of the biomedical strategy but its quasi-exclusive character. In practice, even for health problems which can be completely cured (without any complications) by a given treatment modality, a biomedical strategy is not necessarily the most efficient policy, either in financial terms or, more importantly, in human terms. And the efficacy of treatment is limited in many health problems, *e.g.* diseases associated with smoking and drinking, AIDS, and road accidents, a set of problems which together account for a significant fraction of premature death (*i.e.* death before 65) and which could all be combated by strategies based on prerogatives other than care. Little investment has been made in such strategies, so it is not surprising that the premature death rate in France is one of the highest in the Union Community. In other words, the current predominance of biomedical strategy at the expense of other types of intervention is inconsistent with what is known about what determines health at the population level.

Acting on health determinants involves diverse areas above and beyond that of health itself, including education, farming, the environment, industry and finance, a global dimension which is not always understood. Thus, a crisis like bovine spongiform encephalopathy can place the Minister of Agriculture right at the heart of the health debate! Fragmentation and compartmentalisation in the health care system is incompatible with coherence and consistency. The current administrative structure is built around a whole series of different institutions distinguished according to their:

– function (be it policy making or implementation),
– the level at which they operate (central or local).

Part five A critical, prospective analysis of the way the health system is organised

The 1996 Rulings transferred the power of setting the budget for care provision to Parliament but without stipulating targets or performance objectives. The philosophy behind this type of regulation is first and foremost that of the accountant since it places the emphasis on the financial consequences of any measure rather than its impact on health status. In practice, this type of logic tends to favour those players with more influence at the funding bodies and is prejudicial to any attempt to promote co-ordination.

Numerous provisions in the April 1996 Rulings stipulate that the funding system must take health needs into account but references to "needs" tend to be too abstract, especially when there are insufficient direct links between monitoring and decision-making bodies, and when the information system is inappropriately organised. There are still major areas in which information is lacking (*e.g.* morbidity) or in which the instruments like the PMSI are incapable of assessing the usefulness and efficacy of the care being provided. Moreover, no procedures exist for regular evaluation of how well the strategies are performing with respect to identified health issues and outcomes.

Breaking down the hospital budget on a regional basis has had the effect of making the regulators try to balance the resources allocated to the different regions. But equitable resource allocation is not necessarily compatible with fulfilling specific demands in different regions. This approach is based on the debatable hypothesis that equal resource allocation is equivalent to equal health care "productivity". And anyway, what does equality mean if only hospitals are concerned and similar resources are not attributed to the different regions for independent practice? This paradox is exacerbated by the gap (in some fields) between independent practice and hospital which is at the root of major obstacles both to co-ordination (network creation) and to the generalisation of novel forms of intervention (*e.g.* outpatient surgery). Moreover, it raises problems when it comes to the dynamic process of integrating new technologies into the system.

Annually-based funding is incompatible with the epidemiological picture

It is impossible to address the coherence of the mode of operation of the health care system without emphasising the incompatibility of an annually based funding system with the epidemiological picture in France. Life expectancy is now very high in France and, in general terms, the ageing of the population and reduced mortality have led to a major increase in the incidence of a range of chronic diseases which cannot be cured but which can be controlled for many years. Thus, any measures intended to tackle these problems are necessarily long-term ones, spanning many years, so it is impossible to put all the counters back to zero at the end of every year. Nevertheless, this is how the Ondam works, as if the epidemiological cycle in France was still dominated by infectious diseases rather than by chronic ones. In other words, the books will never be balanced with the current logic of the health care system insofar as the setting of annual expenditure targets bears little relation to the real epidemiological situation. In these circumstances, it is unlikely that the Ondam will ever be met.

Consolidation of regional power through an intricate process

From the point of view of institutions, the recent creation of regional bodies has resulted in a major change in the way health policy is determined and implemented. The region now plays an important role in the initiation and co-ordination of national policy by virtue of its power to determine regional priorities and implement regional measures. In the light of recent experience, it is clear that establishing links between the Regional Hospital Agencies, Urcams and Regional Health Conferences has not really helped break down the resource allocation-based approach which stems from the system of central regulation. Thus, there is still no global sense of health which includes preventive medicine and takes into account all the many and various factors which together determine state of health.

In reality, the multiplication of regional management structures has only increased the complexity of the logistics of the health care system and further reduced its transparency. The process has tended to exacerbate competition and tension at the regional level, not only between different institutions but even within certain institutions, *e.g.* for the State between the Drass and the Regional Hospital Agencies, or for the health insurance system between the Urcams and the Personal Accounts Branches of the National Health Insurance Agency (CPAM).

Nevertheless, the region should constitute an ideal context for co-ordinating priorities, notably in the framework of the Regional Committee for Health Policy. Unfortunately, up until now this body has not really been able to effectively co-ordinate the various players since its authority depends on obtaining a consensus which, as a general rule, corresponds to a very limited area of common ground. In practice, the President of the Committee (the Prefect) has no direct power over the Directors of either the Regional Hospital Agency or the Urcam. As already mentioned, the Urcam compiles a Regional Health Insurance Plan (Pram, *Plan régional de l'assurance maladie*) which includes a hospital-related component (the PRH) in the context of the health insurance system's obligation *"to obtain an overall assessment of the supply of both independent and hospital care and to ensure a unified vision on the part of the health insurers concerning questions about co-ordination between hospitals and independent practice"*. The Regional Hospital Agencies are involved to a greater or lesser extent in the regulation of independent practice in the context of networks which include both hospitals and independent practitioners, or in areas in which there is overlap such as "emergency services". ARH involvement in the independent sector is increased as a result of these agencies being responsible for allocating resources for projects involving independent practitioners under the auspices of bodies such as the Regional Unions of Independent Medical Practitioners (URML, *Unions régionales des médecins libéraux*). The creation of the Fund for the Improvement of the Quality of Independent Care (FAQSV, *Fonds d'amélioration de la qualité des soins de ville*) has somewhat restored the balance by providing the Urcams with specific means of financing their own projects in the independent sector.

Up until now, consolidation of the role of the region in the organisation and management of the health system has occurred in the context of a process of devolution rather than one of decentralisation. In reality, this process has been exclusively focused on health care. In contrast, policies pertaining to health determinants (living conditions, environmental factors, education, social measures, transportation, etc.) come under the auspices of decentralisation and the transfer of power. The implementation of global health programmes – integrating care with prevention and action at the level of determinants – will necessitate co-ordinating highly disparate institutions with diverse areas of expertise.

Finally, although despite all this, efforts to broaden the approach in the field of policy-making are bearing fruit, it should be pointed out that, when it comes to implementation the system is as compartmentalised as ever (with a very small number of exceptions). This is a genuine contradiction which leads to inefficient functioning and under-exploitation of the various available resources, be they human, financial or material.

The difficulty of co-ordinating between the national, regional and local levels

Moreover, co-ordination between the various geographical levels – national, regional, departmental and sub-departmental – is often very inefficient, if there is any at all. As a result of French cultural and legal traditions, we are used to the principle of non-hierarchical functioning at different levels of the administration, with power being distributed down through the various levels. Thus, no hierarchy exists between local institutions, rather each has its own specific powers. The Director of a Regional Health and Social Affairs office is not the "boss" of all the Departmental Directors in the region, just as the heads of Personal Accounts Branches do not answer to the Director of a Regional Health Insurance office. Each level of power tends therefore to develop its own policy in "its" territory without having to worry too much about its neighbours' policies. This is particularly true in social and medico-social policy where no regionally-based process is currently in place to even discuss co-ordination (let alone co-ordinate) between different departments in a region. In the context of hospitals, the creation of the Regional Hospital Agencies was an attempt to address this problem.

Co-ordinating between the regional and national levels is no more simple. One of the main effects of implementing the 1996 Rulings has been to establish processes to identify regional health priorities in the framework of the Regional Health Conferences, an initiative undertaken to bring local players into the process. In parallel, the National Health Conference proposes its own priorities, as do both the Ministry of Health and the different National Health Insurance Agencies. At this time, national priorities are not really compiled in the context of an ascendant process which would make integration with regional priorities possible. There are no processes in existence whereby national policies can be adapted to suit regional particularities other than routine administrative procedures whose future is not certain. As a result, regional players tend to consider only those priorities identified locally as worthy of their interest.

Are questions of health dealt with in democratic processes in which the general public can participate?

The current situation: the possibility of involving on-formalised regional structures

The term "democracy in health" usually refers to the involvement of people or users in the formulation of health policy. But the first issue when considering the democratic and participatory nature of decision-making processes in the field of public health concerns how democratically elected political bodies – Parliament, and the Regional, Departmental and Municipal Councils – deal with health-related problems.

At the national level, the April 1996 Rulings made Parliament responsible for dictating the macro-economic balance of the health care system and, when setting the Ondam, Parliament has been directed to take health priorities into account. The transfer of this responsibility to Parliament required a change in the Constitution, which is in itself a demonstration of the force of political will behind the initiative. Once a year, the Parliamentary debate on the Social Security Funding Bill provides a chance to tackle health-related questions in a global fashion, with reference to the conclusions of both the National Health Conference and the High Committee on Public Health.

Since decentralisation, Regional Councils have been endowed with a general power to promote improved health at the regional level although they have not been specifically commissioned to act in any particular areas. Nor are they absolutely required to come to any decisions in the matter of health – the Law only stipulates that they be consulted about regional organisation of the system, if only for an opinion.

Departmental Councils have been entrusted with more power in the areas of social and medico-social services, especially with respect to certain populations, namely those living in precariousness, young people in difficulty, disabled adults and the elderly. The Departmental Council also has power in the field of preventive medicine, especially with respect to the health and protection of mothers and children, sexually transmitted disease, and tuberculosis. Curiously, by putting the region in charge of the funding of consultations at Cancer Centres, the Government has also theoretically transferred the responsibility for cancer prevention to the Departmental Councils. Every year during the budget debate (or at longer intervals if other planning schedules are adopted), the various Departmental Assemblies are convened to vote on the policies adopted by the standing majority in all these fields.

The commune is deeply involved in various environmental questions (*e.g.* water and air quality, noise pollution, etc.) as well as in many socially based health determinants. Within the framework of the World Health Organisation's "Town-Health" initiative, some communes have developed their own full-blown public health policy, voted in by the municipal council after consultation with the electors. These new directions are in response to urgent and insistent demands from inhabitants, and are evidence of an increased general consciousness of public health as an issue as well as of the need for close co-operation to find solutions tailored to local needs. These directions also show the value of placing any initiative in the context of a global approach to health in general, instead of confining the consideration to the care system. This represents an emerging public consciousness of the need to both address the factors which determine a population's health status, and oblige elected representatives to take the necessary steps.

New processes to involve the general public

In a democratic country like France, any elected official – members of Parliament and of Regional, Departmental and Municipal Councils – has an indubitable claim to represent the people and their interests at whatever is the relevant administrative level. Nevertheless, other forms of representation and expression exist. These may be based on socio-occupational structures such as the national and regional economic and social councils, or in the co-management framework of the Administrative Councils of National Health Insurance Organisations, *e.g.* in the French *Mutualité sociale agricole* as in the mutual societies providing complementary insurance, delegates and administrators are elected, and the Annual General Assembly is often an opportunity for in-depth discussion of topics of interest).

The 1996 Rulings expanded this framework by setting up the National and Regional Health Conferences in order to create new forums for discussion between the various players in the health care system, including users. This initiative was in response to an emerging demand from citizens after profound changes which began in the mid-1980's. The spread of AIDS followed by that of Hepatitis C, the recrudescence of diseases believed to have been more or less conquered, and the emergence of new diseases, all revived the spectre of massive epidemics such as had not been seen in France for many decades. These phenomena sounded the death knell for a health system based exclusively on care and dependent on biomedical invincibility and relentless technological progress.

People came to appreciate that such a system may be fallible and began to ask whether those in charge were in a position to respond to the new problems. This consciousness was spurred by a series of scandals such as those associated with the contamination of both transfused blood and therapeutically administered Human Growth Hormone. What emerged from this movement was the need to implement preventive strategies, to find ways of helping patients, and to develop a complaint system within the non-profit-making organisation framework. Patients are now tending to assume the responsibility for management of their disease, while claiming help from the authorities to do so, a tendency which started with AIDS groups.

In 1998-1999, the authorities launched the Constitutive Assembly on Health, the most significant advance in direct public consultation and in ascertaining the man in the street's expectations. The Constitutive Assembly has provided a forum for direct contact between health professionals and users at the regional level, the purpose being to bring all parties together into the discussion of how well the health care system is working, and to encourage the emergence of real democracy in the matter of health. The primary aim was to identify people's expectations in order to define directions for health policy. Discussions took place at "citizens' forums" (based on Scandinavian and Rhine models) in the regions. For the first time in France, true democracy in health was being practised, an entirely novel experience in a system quite unaccustomed to such a process. It should be emphasised that this type of process is widespread in Scandinavia (and in the Rhineland in Germany) where it has become routine. Experts and citizens discuss together some complex topic in which both socio-political issues and societal values are at stake; the role of the citizen is to contribute a "lay but informed" opinion to the debate.

Health thus becomes a truly public concern insofar as everyone in society – citizens as well as politicians, administrators, professional health care providers and experts – feels involved. Raised awareness among members of the general public generates a new dynamic which has resulted in significant changes over the last fifteen years. This new dynamic has not only resulted in stimulating politicians to action, but has also affected public opinion on major health problems, has accelerated the decision-making process, and has resulted in more attention being paid to crucial social aspects of disease.

Critical analysis: the public health approach poses problems for elected bodies

It might be thought that conferring on Parliament a central role in regulation of the health care system would have brought citizens into the decision-making process but this is going to remain far from the reality as long as the parliamentary debates are unapproachably abstract and seem to be accessible to only a select few. Do delegates still need a clear explanation of what the issues are? Between having to find their way around a new field of legislation and the complexity of health-related questions, the delegates have no doubt not been given enough time to prepare for and fulfil their role properly. It is not sure that the preliminary work of the National Health Conference and the High Committee is sufficient to inform their debate, and it will probably be necessary to improve co-ordination between structures responsible for the evaluation and analysis of needs, and structures responsible for making decisions and setting strategies. This is because the delegates are experiencing difficulty in making the link between their decisions and the data provided by the experts.

In addition, *"a real contradiction exists when it comes to discussing questions of public health in the context of a law pertaining to funding, the primary objective of which is not to define health policy but rather to fix an expenditure target,* i.e. *a predominantly financial undertaking"*[1]. Moreover, the per annum basis of expen-

---

1. Cour des comptes. La sécurité sociale, september 2000, 633 p.

diture targets makes for an accountant's approach to problems which, by their nature, warrant policies and resource allocation mechanisms based on a longer time frame.

At the regional level, the real paradox is that the choices made are never validated by any democratically elected body. Despite all the effort made to bring users or people together with the politicians, the decision-making process is still dominated by a technocratic approach. This is particularly flagrant in hospital policy, in which area, in the absence of any formalised role for users, any claims or complaints – and they are frequent – have to come from "the street". Even though such demonstrations obviously correspond to "community participation", they nevertheless bear witness to the complete absence of democratically elected structures in the decision-making process in this area.

However, as is clear at the level of the department and the commune, the handling of health-related issues at smaller democratic scales is not always simple. The fragmentation of authority and the predominance of financial questions often make it difficult to arrive at holistic, integrated conclusions. The field of health is often perceived in a simplistic fashion. The specific health consequences of measures implemented in a wide variety of different areas are rarely included in the local decision-making process and in fact, more consideration is usually given to a measure's environmental impact than to its impact on health.

Meetings are too irregular to ensure genuine public participation

The Regional Health Conferences have a number of defects – only teething problems, one hopes – which heavily compromise their ability to encourage structured discussion at the regional level and thereby bring the citizen into the decision-making process. The Regional Conferences do not usually convene for more than one day a year, and the amount of preliminary, preparatory work varies enormously from region to region. It is obviously true that one day is not enough to understand and assimilate all the dense, complex information necessary and then draw valid conclusions. In other words, the only people who are in a position to make a valid contribution are those who are already in possession of the relevant materials, *i.e.* those who are already participants in the process (as members of Commissions, committees, etc.); this basically corresponds to experts, health administrators and professional care providers. Broadly speaking, despite a demonstrated will to avoid excluding private citizens from the health policy-making process, in the current situation, experts still play the dominant role. Moreover, there has been criticism of the fact that proceedings of the evaluation agencies (on which the debates of the National and Regional Health Conferences are based) are held in camera. Therefore, in France, public opinion still remains a marginal influence on health policy.

Convocation of the Constitutive Assembly represented a response to this situation. However, it is now necessary to await the next assembly at which a long-term view might be possible with an evaluation of the extent to which the conclusions of these bodies are taken on board by politicians and decision-makers. The irregular nature of the meetings of the Constitutive Assembly makes it difficult to evaluate the impact of the Assembly's conclusions on the way in which public health priorities are defined in the context of a more inclusive approach. Moreover, questions can be asked about the mutual roles of the Constitutive Assembly and that of the Regional Health Conferences.

Consolidating democracy in health, a key component in building a democracy of proximity

This new expression on the part of citizens calls for institutionalisation of democracy in health. This necessitates emergence of the idea of the responsible citizen, an idea which implies promoting transparency in both activities and decisions, the right to the truth, and the right to hear and be heard, all of which are necessary before genuine participation can be possible.

Democracy in health should lead to the establishment of a series of close relationships between various groups of participants. Apart from the citizen, there is the State (as the overall structure responsible for all decisions), experts and professionals (as those "in the know"). The idea should lead to a re-balancing of the roles of these various players in the decision-making process.

Citizen participation can be envisaged in a number of different ways. Up until recently, this idea did not correspond to anything more than patient support groups which came into action whenever there was disagreement on a particular issue. The modernisation of the health care system bill mentions users' groups but the new public health vision is tending to broaden the idea to include individuals and elevate participation to the level of a broadly inclusive public debate.

Any coming together will have to be co-ordinated around health system institutions as a forum for public discussion, the conclusions of which process can then be relayed to decision-makers. Recent directions in health system regulation have elevated the role of the region in the monitoring and analysis of health determinants, and in the management of health-related structures. Nevertheless, questions remain as to the democratic legitimacy of the region.

But democracy in health must not and cannot be seen in a fragmented manner. Today, new channels are opening in the context of the growing movement towards a democracy of proximity. The emergence of the County Development Councils and Neighbourhood Councils in the bigger towns should encourage expression on the part of citizens and genuine co-ordination with the deliberative assemblies. In the same way, restricting the accumulation of mandates and improving the conditions in which local mandates are exercised should increase the possibilities of politicians so that they can better perform their ever-increasingly complex jobs from a more informed position.

Is the health care system organised in such a way as to enable it to respond to future challenges?

Clarification of the challenges from a public health perspective

From reports published and analyses carried out over the last ten years, the fundamental challenges confronting the health system are emerging in an increasingly clear fashion. They are not many in number and they need not be difficult to grasp. Broadly speaking, there are five major challenges.

The ageing of the population and increased longevity

In a number of French departments, the number of people of 60 years of age and over now exceeds for the first time in history the number of people of under 20. Although this is not yet true for France as a whole, this should come to pass in about 2025, according to the Insee. Even though healthy life expectancy is rising, the simple increase in the numbers of the elderly and very old is going to mean a higher absolute number of people living with chronic disease (although these will not all necessarily be dependent). New therapeutic possibilities – of varying cost and inconvenience – already mean that many lives are already being preserved in sufficiently positive conditions, *e.g.* many patients suffering from heart failure are today living independent lives whereas just ten or twenty years ago, they would either have been dead or in a far more debilitated condition. The number of dependent people will therefore not rise in proportion to the increase in the total number of old people, although the corollary of this is that there will be an increased demand for treatment.

However, in many cases, treatment cannot entirely prevent the loss of independence. This means that managing the consequences of disease is becoming an across-the-board priority in health policy, at least as important as the actual treatment of disease. In order to cope with an ageing population and increased longevity, risk management is going to be a key component, on the one hand to prevent or delay the onset of chronic disease, and on the other hand to ensure the early, holistic and effective treatment of such disease in order to preclude as many of its adverse consequences as possible.

Reducing premature death and inequality in health

The premature death rate is high in France, compared with that in other developed countries, notably those of the European Union. At the same time, inequality in health – both socially and geographically-based inequality – is more pronounced. If the factors underlying this picture are examined, it is always the same ones which emerge, and they are factors which can be more effectively addressed by strategies and measures which are not directly related to the care system. Indeed, steady expansion in recent years of both care provision and the accessibility of treatment have not made any great inroads into either premature mortality or inequality.

The available data amply demonstrate that there exists clear inequality at the level of health determinants. In other words, the chance of falling ill is more subject to social and geographical variables than is the chance of obtaining effective treatment once ill.

The falling number of professional health care providers

In coming years, the overall number of doctors is going to drop; when the decline will begin and the ultimate magnitude of the decrease depend on discipline and geographical area. For logistical reasons, the effects will be different in different sectors, be it public or private medicine, hospital or independent practice. The trend has been exacerbated by both implementation of the thirty-five hour week and new norms on staff numbers established to enhance safety. This situation applies to all professional care providers, not just doctors. Although the numbers of certain qualified personnel are dictated by special circumstances such as the number of students admitted for training, it is important not to forget that the changes being predicted are also part of a general demographic pattern of the number of those in work reaching retirement age exceeding the number coming onto the job market.

The question is not so much whether there is going to be insufficient professional health care providers in France to meet the population's needs, but rather whether the health care system will be able to continue to operate in the same way with fewer staff without major changes being made to the way it is organised. This question is a particularly acute one in the hospital sector where infrastructural considerations pre-suppose a certain minimum number of staff for acceptable performance. And already today, the situation in this respect is not perfect, even before the real drops in numbers of care providers have begun. Therefore, the challenge is to achieve reform of the health system in such a way as to care with the new demographics. Fierce competition between the various sectors which employ professional health care providers? Or controlled re-organisation of the entire system?

Territorial dynamics

The discussion of health in recent years has centred on the role of the Regions. As has already been mentioned, it is around the regional level that it was chosen to re-organise the health care system in the framework of the devolution of State services. In contrast, the Region has been virtually ignored in the process of decentralisation but significant power had been transferred to smaller-scale administrative entities in numerous fields related to health determinants and prevention. Because of the absence of a global public health vision, this counter-productive dissociation has passed almost unnoticed. The current debate on regionalisation of the health system fails to address this aspect of the problem, and has not recognised the need for consistent decision-making and implementation instruments to overcome this artificial compartmentalisation.

The new-found importance of the Region should not obscure the current emergence of new entities in the form of the "communities of communes" and urban communities. This reformulation of the basic "administrative" instrument is going ahead extremely rapidly and the power of these bodies is bound to increase if, as many demand, the delegates to these new institutions are directly elected by universal suffrage. Policies will be increasingly based on such territorial entities in a global, integrated framework. As has already been seen with the first territorial diagnoses, it is clear that health will be included in this movement.

Cultural assimilation and democracy

It is a commonplace to point out that doctors are given insufficient training in the field of public health. However, the reality is that there is a generalised lack of a public health culture which is not just confined to the medical profession. It cannot be otherwise as long as the topic is ignored in school and very little information about it is directed at the general public. It is true that AIDS drew attention to a number of important issues, notably concerning preventive strategy, but there is still a major inadequacy with respect to provision of the information necessary for a more comprehensive understanding of current health-related issues and challenges.

As long as access to care is seen as the over-riding component in the health equation, it will be difficult to implement the kind of deep-seated re-organisation which our health care system requires – and which will in the end be inevitable anyway. A series of politicians of all colours have experienced how difficult it is to get their message over, be it to health professionals or the general public. This is partly because, in the absence of adequate knowledge or understanding, the discussion tends to get bogged down in emotional arguments. Notwithstanding, the recent experience of the Constitutive Assembly on Health showed that knowledge and information can be assimilated by all as long as the specialists and experts make an effort to be comprehensible.

Thus, in a first phase (constructed in an appropriate framework), a consensus can be arrived at as to which are the key social values and the priority problems. In a second phase, the agreement of the various groups of the population concerned will be sought on concrete policy, how to implement it and then how it can be adequately regulated. Each stage of this "collective learning process" will have to be conducted in the spirit of consensus.

In other words, devising equitable policy means basing it on reasoned principles which are agreed on or at least approved by all the various players concerned. These principles need to be pragmatic, measurable and solid enough to induce significant change even in the face of the opposition which will inevitably be encountered when they are applied.

The current irregular convocation of the Constitutive Assembly on Health, and the inadequacy of the one-day Regional Health Conferences do not make for a genuinely constructive and self-propagating process to encourage structured public discussion involving citizens and users, professional health care providers, decision-makers, politicians and administrators. However, the generalisation of such discussions – be it at the local, regional or national level – constitutes one of the essential conditions for genuine democracy in health.

Inevitable changes

The above-mentioned issues obviously represent formidable challenges and it is vital that the difficulties to be encountered are not under-estimated. It is exactly for this reason that the way that the health care system is organised should not compound the difficulties or lead to problems which could otherwise be avoided.

Broaden the scope of the strategies implemented

Before any of these challenges – the ageing of the population, premature death or inequality in health – can be confronted, questions have to be asked about current health strategy in France. It is clear that strategy must include a biomedical component but that this is not of itself sufficient. For each of the challenges, action needs to be taken before care becomes an issue, *i.e.* to prevent or delay the development of health problems.

In the case of ageing and, in a broader sense, disability in general, the consequences of the problem also need to be taken into account. However, as has been regularly pointed out by the HCPH, it is exactly strategy in these areas – management prior to and following care – which is most lacking in France. As a result, the French health system is inappropriately organised for coping with today's challenges.

Act at the cultural level

Changing this situation is going to mean modifying culturally based perceptions. In practice, the inadequacy of the strategies being implemented to deal with the problems encountered largely stems from an under-estimate of the importance of health determinants. Unfortunately, practically whenever this question is raised, it is taken by health professionals as a denigration of their place and utility, thus inciting radically defensive positions which fail to advance matters in any direction. Pointing out the importance of determinants unrelated to the care system does not in any way undermine the relevance of that system. There will always be patients who will need high-quality care, and that distributed in as equitable a way as possible in both geographical and social terms.

To convey the importance of other types of health determinant, it might be useful to require a preliminary evaluation of the impact on health of any proposed public decision, analogous to the present system vis-à-vis the environment. This approach would encompass all State legislation and policies, as well as any regulatory measures being proposed by local authorities.

Change the perspective to one based on a continuum of prevention, treatment, rehabilitation, and return to normal life

Devising strategies intended to prevent or delay the development of health problems constitutes an obligation, both on ethical grounds and in the name of efficiency. In this light, it is vital that the division between preventive and curative medicine be broken down, a form of compartmentalisation which is at the root of counter-productive discontinuity and artificial dispersion. In reality, the situation is a continuum, throughout which various types of health professional can intervene. Preventing the avoidable is the key concept when it comes to the measures to be implemented in the framework of this continuum: act on health determinants to prevent disease, avoid failure to treat or delays in commencing treatment, prevent exacerbation or complications, avoid the repercussions of disease on patients' normal lives. Such an approach is entirely compatible with a quality-based vision encompassing every field of action which can affect health instead of one which exclusively focuses on care provision.

Unfortunately, the way today's health system works is not organised on the basis of the logic and consistency of such a continuum which makes it very difficult to devise strategies designed to cope with the challenges to come. A new, compatible set of strategies

Part five   A critical, prospective analysis of the way the health system is organised

can only be conceived in the context of longer-term funding mechanisms associated with the ideas of investment and return on investment.

Simplify logistics and enhance co-ordination

As has already been discussed, the organisation of our health care system is characterised by a multiplicity of different levels and structures which massively complicates operations and the implementation of measures. This situation probably results in over-investment on human and financial resources. This would go some way to accounting for why our expenditure is so high and why we need more professional care providers and medical equipment than many other countries of a similar degree of economic development, countries in which health status is comparable. At least this equivalence shows that France remains a rich country which is able to make up for any defects in the organisation of its care system by paying out.

It is clear that this situation is unsustainable, even if health expenditure does not have to be cut in the future. The number of professional health care providers – especially doctors and nurses – is going to decrease: coping with this predicted, more or less inevitable decline is going to mean having to reorganise to make better use of the available human resources. To this end, rather than increasing the number of administrations as is currently the routine solution to problems, we need to establish regionally based structures with shared logistical means to regulate a variety of different institutions responsible for implementing health policy. The objectives are simplicity and efficiency, especially with respect to co-ordinating networks operating together in a genuinely synergistic fashion. This, rather than trying to patch up a fragmented, compartmentalised system governed by institutional rather than functional imperatives. Such simplification could be carried out in the context of the new territorial entities which are now emerging. However, unless co-ordination between all these new geographical entities is formalised in new, clarified procedures, any gain in efficacy could be entirely nullified, with the end result of disruption of the resource distribution system exacerbating existing problems rather than solving them.

Finally, not only must there be a discussion process preliminary to any decision being taken, but the debate should be open and involve as broad a spectrum of interested parties as possible. This means that the conditions in which decisions are arrived at and responsibilities for implementing those decisions need to be defined more clearly, more precisely and more restrictively.

Acknowledgements

- Association for Socioeconomic Questions and Health (Argses)
- European Regional Office of the World Health Organisation (WHO)
- National Health Insurance Agency for Salaried Workers (Cnamts)
- Centre for Research into Medicine, Disease and Social Science (Cermes)
- Centre for Research and Documentation on the Economics of Health (Credes)
- Centre for Research into Living Conditions (Credoc)
- Centre for Economic, Sociological and Management Research (Cresge)
- French Committee on Health Education (CFES)
- National Prevention Committee (CNP)
- National Council of the Order of Physicians
- General Health Directorate (DGS)
- Social Action Directorate (DGAS)
- Directorate for Hospitalisation and Care Logistics (DHOS)
- Directorate of Research, Studies, Evaluation and Statistics (Drees)
- Social Security Directorate (DSS)
- National School of Public Health (ENSP)
- National Federation of French Mutual Societies (FNMF)
- National Federation of Regional Health Surveillance Centres (Fnors)
- Humanitarian Institute
- National Institute for Health and Medical Research (Inserm)
- National Institute for Economic Studies and Statistics (Insee)
- Institute for Public Health Surveillance (InVS)
- Space, Health and Territory Laboratory, Université Paris X
- Pays-de-la-Loire Regional Health Surveillance Centre
- IMS-Health Company

References

Part one
Data about health status

1. Arènes J., Baudier F., Janvrin M.-P. *Baromètre santé Jeunes 97/98*. Vanves: CFES, 1998.
2. Bajos N. *et al. Les échecs de contraception en France*. Paris: Inserm, juin 2001.
3. Blondel B., Bréart G. "Le système d'information en périnatalité en France: situation au niveau national". *J Gynecol Obst Biol Reprod*, 1998, 27: 573-76.
4. Bolignini M., Plancherel B., Nunez R., Bettschart W. (dir.). *Préadolescence, théorie, recherche et clinique*. Paris: ESF, 1994.
5. Calvez M. *La sélection culturelle des risques du sida*. Rennes: IRTS de Bretagne, 1992.
6. Cohen S. Y. *et al.* "Le vieillissement de l'œil et de ses annexes. Rapport annuel des Sociétés d'ophtalmologie de France". *Bull Soc Ophtamol Fr*, 1999; XCIX: 1-324.
7. Comité national d'experts sur la mortalité maternelle. *Rapport 1995-2001*. Paris: Ministère délégué à la Santé, mai 2001.
8. Dartigues J.-F., Gagnon M., Michel P., Letenneur L., Commenges D., Barberger-Gateau P., Auriacombe S., Rigal B., Bedry R., Alpérovitch A., Orgogozo J.-M., Henry P., Loiseau P., Salamon R. "Le programme de recherche Paquid sur l'épidémiologie de la démence. Méthodes et résultats initiaux". *Rev Neurol*, 1991, 147: 225-230.
9. Dressen C. et Navarro F. (dir.), Godeau E. *Les années collège: Enquête HBSC 1998 auprès des 11-15 ans en France*. Vanves: CFES, 2000.
10. Fagnagni F., Everhard F., Buteau L., Detournay B., Sourgen C., Dartigues J.-F. "Coût et retentissement de la maladie d'Alzheimer en France: une extrapolation des données de l'étude Paquid". *Rev Gériatr*, 1999, 24: 1-7.
11. Forette F., Seux M.-L., Staessen J.-A., Thijs L., Birkenhager W. H., Babarskiene M. R., *et al.* "Prevention of dementia in randomised double-blind placebo-controlled systolic hypertension in Europe (Syst-Eur) trial". *Lancet*, 1998, 352 (9137): 1347-1351.
12. Fratiglioni L., Launer L.-J., Andersen K., Breteler M. M. B., Copeland J. R. M., Dartigues J.-F., Lobo A., Martinez-Lage J., Soininen H., Hofman A. "Incidence of dementia and major subtypes in Europe: a collaborative study of population-based cohorts". *Neurology*, 2000, 54 (Suppl 5): S10-S15.

13. Hassoun D. *Rapport sur la pratique de l'IVG en France*. Paris: Ined, 1993.
14. HCPH. *La souffrance psychique des adolescents et des jeunes adultes*. Rennes: ENSP, 2000, 116 p.
15. Inserm. *Santé et conditions de travail, une recherche à développer*. Paris: La Documentation française, coll. Analyses et prospective, 1985.
16. Jodelet D. *Folie et représentations sociales*. Paris: PUF, 1989.
17. Klaver C. W., Wolfs R. C. W., Vingerging JR, *et al.* "Age-specific prevalence and causes of blindness and visual impairment in an older population". *The Rotterdam Study Arch. Ophthalmol.*, 1998; 116: 653-658.
18. Kogevinas M., Pearce N., Susser M., Boffetta P. *(eds)*. *Social inequalities and cancer*. Lyon: IARC, coll. IARC Scientific Publication, n° 138, 1997.
19. Lagrange H., Lhomond B. *et al. L'entrée dans la sexualité*. Paris: La Découverte, 1997.
20. Laumon B., Martin J.-L., Collet P. *et al. A French Road Accident Trauma Registry: First Results. 41st annual proceedings*. Orlando, Floride: Association for the advancement of automotive medicine, 10 et 11 novembre 1997.
21. Le Van C. *Les grossesses à l'adolescence. Normes sociales et réalités vécues*. Paris: L'Harmattan, 1998.
22. Lévy-Rosenwald M. *Rapport de la Commission instituée par l'article D 176-1 du Code de la sécurité sociale*. septembre 1999.
23. Lobo A., Launer L. J., Fratiglioni L., Andersen K., Di Carlo A., Breteler M. M. B., Copeland J. R. M., Dartigues J.-F., Jagger C., Martinez-Lage J., Soininen H., Hofman A. "Prevalence of dementia and major subtypes in Europe: a collaborative study of population-based cohorts". *Neurology*, 2000, 54 (Suppl 5): S4-S9.
24. Marmot M. G., Theorell T. "Social class and cardiovascular diseases: the contribution of work". *Int J Health Serv* 1988; 18: 659-674.
25. Marot J.-P. *La cécité et la malvoyance en France. Rassemblement et critical analysisdes données épidémiologiques. Étude préalable à des actions de prévention. DEA Sciences et techniques appliquées au handicap et à la réadaptation*. Paris: Inserm, 1989.
26. Michel E., Jougla E. "Mortalité liée à l'imprégnation alcoolique en France et étude comparative France/Angleterre". In: *Alcool, effets sur la santé*. Paris: Inserm, coll. Expertises collectives, 2001.
27. Michel J.-P., Gold G., Brennenstuhl P. *et al.* "L'impact du déficit visuel dans la vie du sujet âgé". In: *Le handicap visuel. Déficits ignorés et troubles associés*. Safran A. B. et Assimacopoulos A. Paris: Masson, 1997; 118-125.

References

28. Ministère de l'Emploi et de la Solidarité, General Health Directorate. *Rapport sur la démographie médicale*, Juin 2001.
29. Moreau C., Bajos N., Bouyer J. *Les conditions d'accès à l'IVG en France*. Rapport Inserm-Cnamts, septembre 2001.
30. Nisand I. *L'IVG en France. Propositions pour diminuer les difficultés que rencontrent les femmes*. Rapport à la ministre des Affaires sociales, février 1999.
31. Observatoire national interministériel de sécurité routière. *Bilan annuel. Statistiques et commentaires. Année 2000*. Paris: La Documentation française, juin 2001.
32. Observatoire régional de la santé Franche-Comté. *Le devenir des 15-24 ans accidentés de la route en Franche-Comté*. Besançon: Observatoire régional de sécurité routière de Franche-Comté, 1998.
33. Oddoux K. (coord.). *La communication sur la santé auprès des jeunes*. Vanves: CFES, coll. Dossiers techniques, 2000.
34. OMS. *Health Behavior School-Aged Children (HBSC)*. Copenhague: Ed. OMS, Bureau régional de l'Europe, 2001, 50 p.
35. *Organisation mondiale de la santé. Rapport sur la santé dans le monde 2001. La santé mentale: nouvelle conception, nouveaux espoirs*. Genève: OMS, 2001.
36. Parquet P.-J. (coord.). *Itinéraires de déprimés: réflexion sur leurs trajectoires en France*. Rapport d'un groupe d'experts, 2001.
37. Piel E., Roelandt J.-L. *De la psychiatrie vers la santé mentale.* Rapport de mission, ministère de l'Emploi et de la Solidarité. ministère délégué à la Santé, juillet 2001.
38. Rossignol M., Stock S., Patry L., Amstrong B. "Carpal tunnel syndrome: what is attribuable to work?" *The Montreal study. Occup Env Med*, 1997; 54: 519-523.
39. Rumeau-Rouquette C., Du Mazaubrun C., Verrier A., Mlika A. *Prévalence des handicaps. Évolution dans trois générations d'enfants 1972, 1976, 1981*. Paris: Doin-Inserm, 1994, 178 p.
40. Salive M. E. "Functional blindness and visual impairment in older adults from three communities". *Ophthalmology*, 1992; 99: 1840-1847.
41. Schulz R., Beach S. R. "Caregiving as a risk factor for mortality. The caregiver health effects study". *JAMA*, 1999, 282: 2215-2219.
42. Tursz A., Gerbouin-Rérolle P. *Les accidents de l'enfant en France*. Paris: Inserm, 2001.
43. Unafam et associations partenaires. *Le livre blanc des partenaires de santé mentale France*. Paris: juin 2001.

Part two
Health inequalities and disparities in France

44. Aiach P. "De la mesure des inégalités: enjeux sociopolitiques et théoriques". In: Leclerc A., Fassin D., Grandjean H., Kaminski M., Lang T. (eds). *Les inégalités sociales de santé*. Paris: Inserm-La Découverte, 2000, 83-92.
45. Appay B. "Précarité, précarisation: réflexions épistémologiques?". In: Joubert M., Chauvin P., Facy F., Ringa V. (eds). *Précarisation, risque et santé*. Paris: Inserm, 2001, 15-27.
46. Appay B., Thebaud-Mony A. (eds). *Précarisation sociale, travail et santé*. Paris: Iresco/CNRS, 1997.
47. Atkinson T., Glaude M., Olier L., Piketty T. *Inégalités économiques*. Paris: La Documentation Française, 2001.
48. Bazely P., Catteau C. *État de santé, offre de soins dans les départements d'Outre-Mer (Guadeloupe, Guyane, Martinique, Réunion)*. Paris: Drees, coll. Série études, Document de travail, 14, juin 2001.
49. Benamouzig D. "Des mots pour le dire: exclusion et précarité, catégories d'action publique". In: Lebas J, Chauvin P (eds), *Précarité et santé*. Paris: Flammarion, coll. Médecine Sciences, 1998, 23-32.
50. Berkman L. F., Glass T. "Social integration, social networks, social support, and health". In: Berkman L. F., Kawachi I. (eds). *Social epidemiology*. New York: Oxford University Press, 2000, 137-173.
51. Berthod-Wurmser M. "Postface: quelles orientations pour la recherche?". In: Joubert M., Chauvin P., Facy F., Ringa V. (eds). *Précarisation, risque et santé*. Paris: Inserm, 2001, 467-472.
52. Bouhnik P., Touze S. "Précarisation et consommation de drogues illicites: amplification des prises de risque à l'ère de la substitution". In: Joubert M., Chauvin P., Facy F., Ringa V. (eds). *Précarisation, risque et santé*. Paris: Inserm, 2001, 395-414.
53. Bourgeois D., Berger P., Hescot P., Leclercq M.-H., Doury J. "Oral health status in 65-74 years old adults in France, 1995". *Revue d'épidémiologie et de santé publique*, 1999, 47: 55-59.
54. Brunner E., Marmot M. "Social organization, stress and health". In: Marmot M., Wilkinson R. (eds). *Social determinants of health*. Oxford: 2000, Oxford University Press, 17-44.
55. Caisse nationale d'assurance maladie des travailleurs salariés. *Statistiques financières et technologiques des accidents du travail. Années 1996-1997-1998*. Paris: Cnamts, 2000.
56. Calot G., Febvay M. "La mortalité différentielle selon le milieu social". *Études et conjoncture*, 1965, 11: 75-159.
57. Calvez M. "Le sida". In: Leclerc A., Fassin D., Grandjean H., Kaminski M., Lang T. (eds). *Les inégalités sociales de santé*. Paris: Inserm-La Découverte, 2000, 283-294.

References

58. Castel R. "Les marginaux dans l'histoire". In: Paugam S. (ed). *L'exclusion, l'état des savoirs*. Paris: La Découverte, 1996, 32-41.
59. Castel R. *Les métamorphoses de la question sociale, une chronique du salariat*. Paris: Fayard, 1995.
60. Cavelaars A. E., Kunst A. E., Geurts J. J. et al. "Morbidity differences by occupational class among men in seven European countries: an application of the Erikson-Goldthorpe social class scheme". *International Journal of Epidemiology*, 1998, 27: 222-230.
61. Chauvin P. "État de santé, recours aux soins et modes de fréquentation des personnes en situation précaire consultant des centres de soins gratuits: le projet Précar". In: Joubert M., Chauvin P., Facy F., Ringa V. (eds), *Précarisation, risque et santé*. Paris: Inserm, 2001, 99-117.
62. Chauvin P. "Précarisation sociale et état de santé: le renouvellement d'un paradigme épidémiologique". In: Lebas J., Chauvin P. (eds). *Précarité et santé*. Paris: Flammarion, coll. Médecine Sciences, 1998, 59-74.
63. Chauvin P. "Santé et inégalités sociales: de nouvelles approches épidémiologiques". In: Parizot I., Chauvin P., Lebas J. (eds). *Actes de la Conférence Hexapolis Unesco, novembre 2000*. Paris: Flammarion, coll. Médecine-Sciences, sous presse.
64. Collectif. *Santé, soins et protection sociale en 1998*. Paris: Credes, 1998, n° 1282.
65. Dargent-Paré C., Bourgeois D. "La santé bucco-dentaire". In: Leclerc A., Fassin D., Grandjean H., Kaminski M., Lang T. (eds). *Les inégalités sociales de santé*. Paris: Inserm-La Découverte, 2000, 267-282.
66. Davey Smith G., Hart C., Watt G., Hole D., Hawthorne V. "Individual social class, area-based deprivation, cardiovascular disease risk factors and mortality: the Renfrew and Paisley study". *J Epidemiol Community Health*, 1998, 52: 399-405.
67. Desplanques G. "L'inégalité sociale devant la mort". *Économie et Statistiques*, 1984, 162: 29-50.
68. Desplanques G., Mizrahi A., Mizrahi A. "Mortalité et morbidité par catégorie sociale". *Solidarité Santé*, 1996, 4: 75-85.
69. Diez-Roux A. "On genes, individuals, society, and epidemiology". *Am J Epidemiol*, 1998, 148, 1027-1032.
70. Diez-Roux A. V., Nieto F. J., Muntaner C. et al. "Neighbourhood environments and coronary heart disease: a multilevel analysis". *Am J Epidemiol*, 1997, 146, 48-63.
71. Ducan C., Jones K., Moon G. "Do places matter: a multilevel analysis of regional variations in health-related behaviour in Britain". *Soc Sci Med*, 1993, 37, 725-733.
72. Dumesnil S., Grandfils N., Le Fur P. *Méthode et déroule-*

ment de l'enquête sur la santé et la protection sociale. Paris: Credes, 1998, 1234.

73. Dumesnil S., Grandfils N., Le Fur P., Mizrahi A., Mizrahi A. *Santé, soins et protection sociale en 1996*. Paris: Credes, 1997, n° 1204.

74. Duncan O. D. "A socio-economic index for all occupations". In: Reiss AG (ed). *Occupation and social status*. New York: Free Press, 1961, 109-138.

75. *Effets sur la santé des principaux types d'exposition à l'amiante*. Paris: Inserm, coll. Expertises collectives, 1997.

76. Evans R. G., Stoddart G. L. "Produire de la santé, consommer des soins". In: Evans R. G., Barer M. L., Marmor T. R. (éds.). *Être ou ne pas être en bonne santé, biologie et déterminants sociaux de la maladie*. Montréal (Québec), Paris: Presses de l'Université de Montréal et John Libbey Eurotext, 1996.

77. Fassin D. "La santé des immigrés et des étrangers: méconnaissance de l'objet de reconnaissance". In: M. Joubert, Chauvin P., Facy F., Ringa V. (eds). *Précarisation, risque et santé*. Paris: Inserm, 2001.

78. Firdion J.-M., Marpsat M., Lecomte T., Mizrahi A., Mizrahi A. "Vie et santé des personnes sans domicile à Paris". In: Joubert M., Chauvin P., Facy F., Ringa V. (eds). *Précarisation, risque et santé*. Paris: Inserm, 2001, 167-186.

79. Girard F., Cohidon C., Briançon S. Les indicateurs globaux de santé. In: Leclerc A., Fassin D., Grandjean H., Kaminski M., Lang T. (eds). *Les inégalités sociales de santé*. Paris: Inserm-La Découverte, 2000, 163-172.

80. Gochman D. S. (ed). *Handbook of health behavior research, Vol I: personal and social determinants*. New York: Plenum Press, 1987.

81. Goldberg M., Goldberg S., Luce D. "Disparités régionales de la reconnaissance du mésothéliome de la plèvre comme maladie professionnelle en France (1986-1993)". *Rev Epidemiol Santé Publ*, 1999, 47: 421-431.

82. Haan M., Kaplan G. A., Camacho T. "Poverty and health: prospective evidence from the Alameda County Study". *Am J Epidemiol*, 1997, 125: 898.

83. Herbert C., Launoy G. "Les cancers". In: Leclerc A Fassin D Grandjean H., Kaminski M., Lang T. (eds). *Les inégalités sociales de santé*. Paris: Inserm-La Découverte, 2000, 239-250.

84. Hescot P., Bourgeois D., Doury J. "Oral health in 35-44 years old adults in France". *International Dental Journal*, 1997, 47: 94-99.

85. Hescot P., Roland E. *La santé dentaire en France, 1993. Le CAO des enfants de 6, 9 et 12 ans*. Paris: Union française pour la santé bucco-dentaire, 1994, 128 p.

References

86. Hescot P., Roland E. *La santé dentaire en France*. Paris: Union française pour la santé bucco-dentaire, 1998.
87. Jamouille P. "Limitation des dommages liés aux drogues et accès aux dispositifs socio-sanitaires. Perceptions et représentations de personnes qui sont ou ont été toxicomanes". In: Joubert M., Chauvin P., Facy F., Ringa V. (eds). *Précarisation, risque et santé*. Paris: Inserm, 2001, 415-436.
88. Joubert M. "Précarisation et santé mentale, déterminants sociaux de la fatigue et des troubles dépressifs ordinaires". In: Joubert M., Chauvin P., Facy F., Ringa V. (eds). *Précarisation, risque et santé*. Paris: Inserm, 2001, 69-95.
89. Jougla E. "La mortalité". In: Leclerc A., Fassin D., Grandjean H., Kaminski M., Lang T. (eds). *Les inégalités sociales de santé*. Paris: Inserm-La Découverte, 2000.
90. Jougla E. "Relation entre le niveau de l'état de santé et le niveau des densités médicales", *Revue du praticien*, 1990, 86: 71-80.
91. Jougla E., Rican S., Le Toullec A. "Disparités sociales de mortalité en France". In: Leclerc A., Fassin D., Grandjean H., Kaminski M., Lang T. (eds). *Les inégalités sociales de santé*. Paris: Inserm-La Découverte, 2000, 147-162.
92. Kaminski M., Blondel B., Saurel-Cubizolles M.-J. "La santé périnatale". In: Leclerc A., Fassin D., Grandjean H., Kaminski M., Lang T. (eds). *Les inégalités sociales de santé*. Paris: Inserm-La Découverte, 2000, 173-192.
93. Kaplan G.-A., Lynch J.-W. "Whither studies on the socioeconomic foundations of population health? (editorial)". *Am J Public Health*, 1997, 87, p. 1409-1411.
94. Karasek R. A., Baker D., Marxer F., Ahlbom A., Theorell T. "Job decision latitude, job demands, and cardiovascular disease: a prospective study of Swedish men". *Am J Public Health*, 1981, 71, 694-705.
95. Kogevinas M., Pearce N., Susser M., Boffetta P. (eds). *Social inequalities and cancer*. Lyon: IARC, 1997, IARC Scientific Publication n° 138.
96. Kovess V., Gysens S., Chanoit P.-F. "Une enquête de santé mentale: l'enquête des Franciliens". *Annales médico-psychologiques*, 1993, 151, 624-633.
97. Krieger N. "Discrimination and health". In: Berkman L.-F., Kawachi I. (eds), *Social epidemiology*. New York: Oxford University Press, 2000, 36-75.
98. Krieger N. "Society, biology and the logic of social epidemiology", *Int J Epidemiol*, 2001, 30, 44-46.
99. Kunst A. E., Groenhof F., Mackenbach J. P. "Inégalités sociales de mortalité prématurée: la France comparée aux autres pays européens". In: Leclerc A., Fassin D., Grandjean H., Kaminski M., Lang T. (eds), *Les inégalités sociales de santé*, Paris: Inserm-La Découverte, 2000, 53-68.

100. Kunst A. E., Groenhof F., Mackenbach J. P. "Occupational Class and Mortality among Men 30 to 64 years in eleven European Countries". *Social Science medecine*, 1998, 1459-1474.
101. Lang T., Ribet C. "Les maladies cardio-vasculaires". In: Leclerc A., Fassin D., Grandjean H., Kaminski M., Lang T. (eds), *Les inégalités sociales de santé*, Paris: Inserm-La Découverte, 2000, 223-238.
102. Leclerc A., Fassin D., Grandjean H., Kaminski M., Lang T. *Les inégalités sociales de santé*. Paris: Inserm-La Découverte, 2000.
103. Legrand-Cattan K., Chouaïd C., Monnet I., et coll. "Évaluation des expositions professionnelles et cancer bronchopulmonaire". *Rev Mal Respir* (sous presse).
104. Lovell A. "Les troubles mentaux". In: Leclerc A., Fassin D., Grandjean H., Kaminski M., Lang T. (eds). *Les inégalités sociales de santé*. Paris: Inserm-La Découverte, 2000, 223-238.
105. Lynch J., Kaplan G. "Socioeconomic position". In: Berkman LF, Kawachi I (eds). *Social epidemiology*. New York: Oxford University Press, 2000, 13-35.
106. Macintyre S., Ellaway A. "Ecological approaches: rediscovering the role of the physical and social environment". In: Marmot M., Wilkinson R. G. (eds). *Social determinants of health.* Oxford: Oxford University Press, 2000, 211-239.
107. Mackenbach J. P. *et al.* "Socioeconomic inequalities in morbidity and mortality in western Europe". *Lancet*, 1996, 349: 1655-1659.
108. Maisondieu J. "Psychiatrie et exclusion". In: Lebas J., Chauvin P. (eds). *Précarité et santé*. Paris: Flammarion, coll. Médecine Sciences, 1998, 23-32.
109. Maisondieu J. *L'idole et l'abject*. Paris: Bayard, 1995.
110. Marmot M. "Improvement of social environment to improve health". *Lancet*, 1998, 351, 57-60.
111. Math A. "Protection sociale et inégalités: les débats européens". In: Daniel C., Le Clainche C. (eds). *Réduire les inégalités, quel rôle pour la protection sociale?* Paris: Mission Recherche Drees, ministère de l'Emploi et de la Solidarité, 2001, 59-70.
112. Menahem G. *Problèmes de l'enfance, statut social et santé des adultes*. Paris: Credes, 1994, n° 2010, 221 p.
113. Mesrine A. "Les différences de mortalité par milieu social restent fortes". In: *Données sociales. La société française*. Paris: Insee, 1999, 228-235.
114. Mormiche P. "Inégalités de santé et inéquité du système de soins". In: Jacobzone S. (ed). *Économie de santé, trajectoires du futur*. Paris: Insee Méthodes, 1997, n° 64-65, 84-94.

References

115. Mormiche P. *et al. Inégalités et handicaps*. Colloque Montpellier 30 novembre-1er décembre 2000.
116. Mormiche P., Ravaud J.-F. "Premiers résultats de l'enquête HID", *Insee première*, 2001, 742.
117. Najman J. M. "Class inequalities in health and lifestyle". In: Waddell C., Petersen A. R. (eds). *Just health: inequalities in illness, care and prevention*. Melbourne: Churchill Livingston, 1994, 27-46.
118. Nam C. B., Terrie E. W. *Comparing the 1980 Nam-Powers and Duncan SEI occupational scores*. Tallahassee, Florida: Sate University, Center for the Study of Population, 1986.
119. Navarro V. "The new conventional wisdom: an evaluation of the WHO report Health systems: improving performance", *Int J Health Services*, 2001, 31, 23-33.
120. Niedhammer I., Goldberg M., Leclerc A., Bugel I., David S. "Psychosocial factors at work and subsequent depressive symptoms in the GAZEL cohort". *Scand J Work Environmental Health*, 1998, 24: 1-9.
121. OMS. *Rapport sur la santé dans le monde 2000: pour un système de santé plus performant*. Genève: OMS, 2001.
122. Paugam S. *La disqualification sociale, essai sur la nouvelle pauvreté* (édition revue et augmentée). Paris: Presses Universitaires de France, 1994.
123. *Programme national de surveillance du mésothéliome*. Rapport au comité scientifique, année 1999. Saint-Maurice: Institut de veille sanitaire, 1999.
124. Ravaud J.-F., Mormiche P. "Handicaps et incapacités". In: Leclerc A., Fassin D., Grandjean H., Kaminski M., Lang T. (eds). *Les inégalités sociales de santé*. Paris: Inserm-La Découverte, 2000, 147-162.
125. Reijneveld S., Schene A. "Higher prevalence of mental disorder in socio-economically deprived urban areas in the Netherlands: community or personal disadvantage?" *J Epidemiol Community Health*, 1998, 52: 2-7.
126. Salem G., Rican S., Jougla E. *Atlas de la santé en France, volume I: les causes de décès*. Montrouge: John Libbey-Eurotext, 2000, 189 p.
127. Shaw M., Dorling D., Davey Smith G. "Poverty, social exclusion, and minorities". In: Berkman LF, Kawachi I (eds). *Social epidemiology*. New York: Oxford University Press, 2001, 13-35.
128. Siegrist J., Peter J., Junge A., Cremer A., Seidel D. "Low status control, high effort at work and ischemic heart disease: prospective evidence from blue-collar men", *Soc Sc Med*, 1990, 31: 1127-1134
129. Sureau P. *L'inégalité devant la mort*. Paris: Economica, 1979.
130. Townsend P., Phillimore P., Beattie A. *Health and deprivation, inequality in the North*. London: Croom Helm, 1988.

131. Tronchet C. *Synthèse des programmes régionaux d'accès à la prévention et aux soins élaborés en application de l'article 71 de la loi du 29 juillet 1998 d'orientation relative à la lutte contre les exclusions.* Paris: General Health Directorate, 2001, 113 p.
132. Turk D. C., Kerns R. D. (eds). *Health, illness, and families: a life-span perspective.* New York: Wiley, 1985.
133. Tursz A. et Gerbouin-Rérolle P. *Les accidents de l'enfant en France.* Paris: Inserm, 2001.
134. Vogt T. M., Mullooly J. P., Ernst D., Pope C. R., Hollis J. F. "Social networks as predictors of ischemic heart disease, cancer, stroke and hypertension: incidence, survival and mortality". *J Clin Epidemiol*, 1992, 45: 659-66.
135. Von Korff M., Koepsell T., Curry S., Diehr P. "Multilevel analysis in epidemiologic research on health behaviours and outcomes". *Am J Epidemiol*, 1992, 135: 1077-1082.
136. Weigers M. E., Drilea S. K. *Health status and limitations: a comparison of Hispanics, blacks and whites.* Rockville: Agency for Health Care Policy and Research, 1999.

Part four
The user, a player in the health care system

137. Agence nationale d'accréditation et d'évaluation en santé. *Information des patients. Recommandations et références destinées aux médecins.* Paris: Anaes, Service des recommandations et références professionnelles, mars 2000, 64 p.
138. Amar L., Bachimont J, Bremond M *et al.* "Une approche expérimentale de consultation des usagers sur les informations relatives à l'hospitalisation". *Solidarité Santé*, Études et résultats, n° 115, mai 2001.
139. Amar L., Minvielle E. "L'action publique en faveur de l'usager: de la dynamique institutionnelle aux pratiques quotidiennes de travail". In: *Vous avez dit "public"?* Lévy E. (dir.). Paris: L'Harmattan, 2001, 91-127.
140. AMM. "L'expertise de l'Agence du médicament: santé publique ou santé des entreprises?" In: Cassou B., Schiff M., *Qui décide de notre santé? Le citoyen face aux experts.* Paris: Syros, 1998, 64-76.
141. B. Tricot Consultant. *Annuaire des associations de santé: patients-famille/information, éducation, soutien.* Gignac: 2000, 505 p.
142. Boutron I., Dougados M. "L'information du patient". *Synoviale*, 2001, numéro spécial arthrose.
143. Byk C. "Le consentement à l'acte médical dans la relation médecin-patient en Europe". In: Lemaire F *et al. Consentement aux soins: vers une réglementation.* Paris: Flammarion, coll. Médecine-Sciences, 1995, 30-42.
144. Caniard E. *La place des usagers dans le système de santé.*

References

Rapport et propositions du groupe de travail auprès du secrétariat d'État à la Santé et à l'Action sociale. Rapport ronéoté, 2000.
145. Cassou B., Schiff M. *Qui décide de notre santé? Le citoyen face aux experts*. Paris: Syros, 1998.
146. Chandernagor P., Dumond J.-P. "L'hôpital des années quatre-vingt-dix et ses médecins". In: Contandriopoulos A. P., Souteyrand Y. (dir.). *L'hôpital stratège: dynamiques locales et offre de soins*. Paris: John Libbey Eurotext, 1996, 203-214.
147. Clément J.-M. *1900-2000: la mutation de l'hôpital*. Bordeaux: Les études hospitalières, 2001.
148. Comité national d'orientation des Constitutive Assembly on Health 1998-1999. *Les citoyens ont la parole*. Document ronéoté.
149. *Études et résultats*. Drees: 2001, n° 115, p. 2.
150. Evans R. *Être ou ne pas être en bonne santé: biologie et déterminants de la santé*. Paris: John Libbey Eurotext, 1996.
151. Folscheid B. "Le consentement éclairé en France". In: Durand-Zaleski I. (dir.). *L'information du patient: du consentement éclairé à la décision partagée*. Paris: Flammarion, coll. Médecine-Sciences, 1999, 3-6.
152. Fourniau J.-M. "Projet d'infrastructure et débat public: Transparence des décisions et participation des citoyens". In: *Technique, territoires et sociétés*. Paris: Ministère de l'Aménagement du territoire, de l'Équipement et des Transports, Drast, mai 1996, 9-47.
153. Fourniau J.-M. "Transparence des crises et participation des citoyens". In: *Projet d'infrastructure et débat public, collection techniques, territoires et santé*. Paris: Éditeur Meltt, 1996, 31: 9-47.
154. Frattini M.-O. *Place du patient et du médecin dans le processus décisionnel en médecine: pour une amélioration des interactions entre deux personnes, patient et médecin*. Paris: Fondation de l'avenir, rapport ronéoté, 2000.
155. Gaille M. *Le citoyen*. Paris: Flammarion, 1998.
156. Ghadi V., Naiditch M. "Le patient et le système de soins". *Actualité et dossier en santé publique*, 2000, 33: 33-36.
157. Ghadi V., Naiditch M. *L'information de l'usager-consommateur sur la performance du système de soins*. Document de travail, n° 13, mai 2001, Drees, série Études.
158. Ghadi V., Polton D. "Le marché ou le débat comme instrument de la démocratie". *Revue française des affaires sociales*, 2000; 54: 15-32.
159. Gucher C. "Citoyenneté et insertion sociale". In: *Retraite et citoyenneté: actualité d'une question paradoxale*. Grenoble: Presses universitaires de Grenoble, 2001, 7-18.

160. Jarno P. "Critical analysisde la détermination des priorités de santé en France". *Santé publique*, 2000, 15: 529-544.
161. Jobert B. *Les usagers comme acteurs dans la gestion des services collectifs: analyse des processus dans le secteur sanitaire*. Rapport au Commissariat général du plan. Grenoble: Cerat, Institut d'études politiques, Université des sciences sociales de Grenoble, 1990, document ronéoté.
162. Joly P.-B. "Quand les 'candides' évaluent les OGM: la conférence de citoyens, nouveau modèle de démocratie technique ou manipulation médiatique". In: *L'opinion publique face aux plantes transgéniques, Colloque de la Villette, Paris: 24 novembre 1998*. Paris: Albin Michel, 1999.
163. Kessler M. L. *et al*. *Évaluation des politiques publiques*. Paris: L'Harmattan, 1998.
164. Koubi G. "Droits de l'Homme et droits de la Personne: réflexions sur l'imprudence d'une indistinction". *Revue internationale de psychosociologie*, 2000, 6, 35-43.
165. Lahoute C. "Droits des usagers du système de santé: de la réglementation à la pratique". In: Cresson G., Schweyer F.-X. *Les usagers du système de soins*. Rennes: ENSP, 2000, 17-24.
166. Lascoumes P. *L'information, arcane politique paradoxale*. Actes du séminaire sur les risques collectifs et situations de crise de l'École nationale supérieure des Mines de Paris. Paris: École nationale supérieure des Mines de Paris, 1998, 15-34.
167. Letourmy A., Naiditch M. "L'information des usagers sur le système de soins: rhétorique et enjeux". *Revue française des affaires sociales*, 2000; 54: 45-60.
168. Martin A. *et al*. "L'expertise est-elle codifiable?". *La Recherche*, février 2001, 339, 46-50.
169. Moatti J.-P. "Éthique médicale, économie de la santé: les choix implicites". *Annales des Mines*, 1991, juillet-août, 74-80.
170. Morelle A. *La défaite de la santé publique*. Paris: Flammarion, 1996.
171. Naiditch M. "Partage de l'information médicale: l'exemple de la chirurgie cardiaque dans l'État de New York". *La Recherche*, octobre 1999.
172. Paterson F., Barral C. "L'association française contre les myopathies: trajectoire d'une association d'usagers et construction associative d'une maladie". *Sciences sociales et santé*, 1994, 12.
173. Pezerat H. "Un lieu d'expertise paralysé: l'Institut national de recherche et de sécurité (INRS)". In: Cassou B., Schiff M. *Qui décide de notre santé? Le citoyen face aux experts*. Paris: Syros, 1998, 50-63.
174. Polton D. *Quel système de santé à l'horizon 2020*. Rapport

References

préparatoire au schéma des services collectifs sanitaires. Paris: La Documentation Française, 2000, 99-105.
175. Rameix S. "Du paternalisme à l'autonomie des patients: l'exemple du consentement aux soins en réanimation". In: Lemaire F. et al., *Consentement aux soins: vers une réglementation*. Paris: Flammarion, coll. Médecine-Sciences, 1995.
176. *Revue française des Affaires sociales*, 2000, n° 2, juin, 101-102.
177. Romain J. *Le triomphe de la médecine*. Paris: Gallimard, coll. Folio, 1972.
178. Rosman S. "Entre engagement militant et efficacité professionnelle: naissance et développement d'une association d'aide aux malades du sida". *Sciences sociales et santé*, 1994, 12.
179. Sargos P. "L'actualité du droit de la responsabilité médicale dans la jurisprudence de la Cour de cassation". *Droit et patrimoine*, 2001, 92, 18-27.
180. Schweyer F. X. "Genèse et dimensions des usagers de l'hôpital public". In: Cresson G., Schweyer F. X. *Les usagers du système de soins*. Rennes: ENSP, 2000, 37-54.
181. Setbon M. "Le consentement éclairé en France: le point de vue du sociologue". In: Durand-Zaleski I. (dir.). *L'information du patient: du consentement éclairé à la décision partagée*. Paris: Flammarion, coll. Médecine-Sciences, 1999, 11-14.
182. Setbon M. *Pouvoir contre sida*. Paris: Le Seuil, 1993.
183. Steffen M. "La santé: les bénéficiaires en dehors des réformes". In: Warrin P. *Quelle modernisation des services publics? Les usagers au cœur des réformes*. Paris: La Découverte, 1997.
184. Supiot A. "La fonction anthropologique du droit". *Esprit*, février 2001, 151-173.
185. The McCormick Tribune Foundation. "Intérêts financiers et publication d'informations médicales". *Prescrire*, 2000, 20, 705-706.
186. Vedelago F. "L'usager comme atout stratégique du changement dans le système de santé". In: Cresson G., Schweyer F. X. *Les usagers du système de soins*. Rennes: ENSP, 2000, 55-73.
187. Zerbib J.-C. "Santé: les citoyens face aux experts". In: Cassou B., Schiff M. *Qui décide de notre santé? Le citoyen face aux experts*. Paris: Syros, 1998, 224-233.

Abbreviations

afssa	French Agency for Safe Food *(Agence française de sécurité sanitaire des aliments)*
anaes	National Agency for Health Acreditation and Evaluation *(Agence nationale d'accréditation et d'évaluation en santé)*
ARH	Regional Hospital Agency *(Agence Regionale de l'hospitalisation)*
AYLL	Attributable years of life lost
BMI	Body mass index
cada	Commission for Access to Administrative Documents *(Commission d'accès aux documents administratifs)*
canam	National Health Insurance Agency for the Self-Employed *(Caisse nationale d'assurance maladie des professions indépendantes)*
CCAA	Outpatient Alcohol Severance Centre *(Centre de cure ambulatoire en alcoologie)*
CCAM	Common Classification of Medical Procedures *(Classification commune des actes médicaux)*
cermes	Centre for Research into Medicine, Disease and Social Science *(Centre d'études et de recherches sur la médecine, les maladies et les sciences sociales)*
cetima	Mediterranean and International Study Centre *(Centre d'études méditerranéennes et internationales)*
CFES	French Committee on Health Education *(Comité français d'éducation pour la santé)*
CHAA	Safe Food and Alcohol Centre *(Centre d'hygiène alimentaire et d'alcoologie)*
CISS	Collective of Health-Related Non-Profit-Making Organisations *(Collectif inter-associatif sur la santé)*
CLCC	Committee for the Fight against Cancer *(Comité de lutte contre le cancer)*
CLIC	Local Geriatric Care Information and Co-ordination Centre *(Centre local d'information et de coordination gérontologique)*
CLIN	Committee for the Fight against Nosocomial Infection *(Comité de lutte contre les infections nosocomiales)*
CMU	Universal Health Insurance Coverage *(Couverture maladie universelle)*
cnamts	National Health Insurance Agency for Salaried Workers *(Caisse Nationale de l'assurance maladie des travailleurs salariés)*

Abbreviations

CNS	National Health Conference *(Conférence nationale de santé)*
CPAM	Personal Accounts Branch of the National Health Insurance Agency *(Caisse primaire de l'assurance maladie)*
Credes	Centre for Research and Documentation on the Economics of Health *(Centre de recherche, d'étude et documentation en économie de la santé)*
Credoc	Centre for Research into Living Conditions *(Centre de recherche pour l'étude et l'observation des conditions de vie)*
CRS	Regional Health Conference *(Conférence régionale de santé)*
CSG	Generalised Social Contribution *(Contribution sociale généralisée)*
Ddass	Departmental Directorate of Health and Social Affairs *(Direction départementale des affaires sanitaires et sociales)*
DGAS	Social Action Directorate *(Direction générale de l'action sociale)*
DGS	General Health Directorate *(Direction générale de la santé)*
DHOS	Directorate for Hospitalisation and Care Logistics *(Direction de l'hospitalisation et de l'organisation de soins)*
Drass	Regional Directorate of Health and Social Affairs *(Direction régionale des affaires sanitaires et sociales)*
Drees	Directorate of Research, Studies, Evaluation and Statistics *(Direction de la recherche, des études, de l'évaluation et des statistiques)*
DSS	Social Security Directorate *(Direction de la sécurité sociale)*
EGS	Constitutive Assembly on Health *(États généraux de la santé)*
ENSP	National School of Public Health *(École nationale de la santé publique)*
EPPM	Permanent Medical Prescription Survey *(Enquête permanente sur la prescription médicale)*
ESPS	Health and Social Coverage Survey *(Enquête santé protection sociale)*
FAQSV	Fund for the Improvement of the Quality of Independent Care *(Fonds d'amélioration de la qualité des soins de ville)*
FMC	Ongoing medical training *(Formation médicale continue)*
Fnors	National Federation of Regional Health Surveillance Centres *(Fédération nationale des observatoires régionaux de la santé)*
FNPEIS	National Fund for Prevention, Education and Intervention in Health *(Fonds national de prévention, d'éducation et d'intervention en santé)*

Francim	French Network of Cancer Registries *(Réseau français des registres des cancers)*
GMO	Genetically modified organism
GNP	Gross national product
HBSC	Health Behavior in School-Aged Children
HID	Handicap, Disability and Dependency *(Handicaps, incapacités, dépendances)*
ICD	International Classification of Diseases
IFRH	Federative Institute on Disability Research *(Institut fédératif de recherche sur le handicap)*
Igas	Health and Social Affairs Inspection Bureau *(Inspection générale des affaires sociales)*
Inrets	National Institute for Research on Transport and Safety *(Institut national de recherche sur les transports et leur sécurité)*
Insee	National Institute for Econmic Studies and Statistics *(Institut national de la statistique et des études économiques)*
Inserm	National Institute for Health and Medical Research *(Institut national de la santé et de la recherche médicale)*
InVS	Institute for Public Health Surveillance *(Institut de veille sanitaire)*
LFSS	Social Security Funding Law *(Loi de financement de la sécurité sociale)*
LTC	Long-term condition
MA	Marketing Authorisation
Mildt	Interdepartmental Mission for the Fight against Drugs and Drugs Addiction *(Mission interministérielle de lutte contre la drogue et la toxicomanie)*
Mire	Research Experiment Mission *(Mission recherche expérimentation)*
MSA	Agricultural Employees Health Insurance Agency *(Mutualité sociale agricole)*
OECD	Organisation for Economic Co-operation and Development
Ondam	National Health Insurance Expenditure Target *(Objectif national des dépenses d'assurance maladie)*
ONISR	Ministerial Road Safety Surveillance Centre *(Observatoire national interministériel de sécurité routière)*
OPECST	Parliamentary Office for the Evaluation of Scientific and Technological Choices *(Office parlementaire d'évaluation des choix scientifiques et technologiques)*

Abbreviations

OQN	Quantified National Target *(Objectif quantifié national)*
ORS	Regional Health Surveillance Centre *(Observatoire régional de la santé)*
Pass	Health Care Access Office *(Permanence d'accès aux soins de santé)*
PHRC	Hospital Clinical Research Programme *(Programme hospitalier de recherche clinique)*
PMI	Mother and Child Protection Service *(Protection maternelle et infantile)*
PMSI	Hospital Medical Information Systems Programme *(Programme de médicalisation des systèmes d'information)*
Pram	Regional Health Insurance Plan *(Plan régional d'assurance maladie)*
Praps	Regional Programme for Access to Prevention and Care *(Programme régional d'accès à la prévention et aux soins)*
PRS	Regional Health Insurance Programme *(Programme régional de santé)*
RMI	Minimum Reintegration Income *(Revenu minimum d'insertion)*
Satu	Emergency Reception and Treatment Service *(Service d'accueil et de traitement des urgences)*
SOC	Socio-occupational class
Sros	Regional Health Organisation Scheme *(Schéma régional d'organisation sanitaire)*
STD	Sexually transmitted disease
Unafam	National Union of the Friends and Families of Mental Patients *(Union nationale des amis et familles de malades mentaux)*
Upatu	Neighbourhood Emergency Reception and Treatment Unit *(Unité de proximité d'accueil et de traitement des urgences)*
Urcam	Regional Unions of the Health Insurance Organisations *(Union régionale des caisses d'assurance maladie)*
URML	Regional Union of Independent Medical Practitioners *(Union régionale de médecins libéraux)*
WHO	World Health Organisation

List of tables

Part one **Data about** **health status**	1 Number of deaths on the roads in 2000	100
	2 Accidents broken down according to level of urbanisation and day of the week	101
	3 Main causes of death for men and women	142
	4 Life expectancy at birth and at 60 years of age for men and women	142
Part two **Health** **inequalities** **and disparities** **in France**	1 Life expectancy and death probability by socio-occupational class in France (Insee cohort 1982-1996)	149
	2 Changes in mortality in men of different socio-occupational classes between 1975 and 1995	150
	3 Relative mortality rates in manual and non-manual workers of between 45 and 59 in different European countries	152
	4 Life-threatening risk factors and disability in different socio-occupational classes in France (after normalisation for age and sex). 1996	153
	5 Differential between workers and the population as a whole in different European countries with respect to the question "Do you consider your state of health as less than good?"	153
	6 Premature birth and low weight broken down according to the parents' social status in France. 1995	156
	7 Percentage of 12-year-old children without any caries at 12 years, by the parents' socio-occupational class	157
	8 Mean number of adults with teeth with carries or fillings and missing teeth, according to socio-occupational class: subjects of 35-44 years of age (1993) and 65-74 years of age (1995) living in the Rhône-Alpes region	157
	9 Seriousness of injuries to the driver in road accidents according to socio-occupational class. 1997	158
	10 Body weight profiles among conscripts presenting between 1987 and 1996	174
	11 Prevalence of excess body weight (BMI $\geqslant$ 25) in conscripts presenting between 1987 and 1996, according to the size of their commune of origin	175
	12 Life expectancy in mainland France and its overseas departments. 1990 and 1997	209
	13 Premature birth and low birth weight in mainland France and its overseas departments (1998 National Perinatal Survey)	210
	14 Possible years of life lost (PYLL) (1993-1997)	211
	15 Rates broken down between men and women and causes of death (1993-1997)	212

List of tables

Part three
Resource allocation in the health system

1	Changes in the density of different professional health care providers	228
2	Some figures on hospital equipment and activity	232
3	Pieces of equipment which have to be approved prior to installation	234
4	The Ondam and health insurance expenditure (1997-2001)	238
5	Projected number of physicians in 2004 according to 2000 age brackets	253

List of figures

Part one
Data about health status

1	Main declared conditions among boys and girls of under 15 years of age. 1998	64
2	Main reasons for consultation with an independent practitioner among boys and girls of under 15 years of age. 1992. 1998	65
3	Main diseases of boys and girls of under 15 years of age treated in short-stay hospital departments. 1998	66
4	Main long-term conditions in boys and girls of under 15 years of age covered by the health insurance system. 1998	68
5	Main causes of death in boys and girls of between 1 and 15 years of age. 1997	69
6	Main declared conditions among men and women of between 15 and 44 years of age. 1998	84
7	Main reasons for consultation with an independent practitioner among men and women of between 15 and 44 years of age. 1992. 1998	85
8	Main diseases of men and women of between 15 and 44 years of age treated in short-stay hospital departments. 1998	87
9	Main long-term conditions in men and women of between 15 and 44 years of age covered by the health insurance system. 1998	89
10	Main causes of death among men and women of between 15 and 44 years of age. 1997	90
11	Main declared conditions among men and women of between 45 and 74 years of age. 1998	104
12	Main reasons for consultation with an independent practitioner among men and women of between 45 and 74 years of age. 1992. 1998	106
13	Main diseases of men and women of between 45 and 74 years of age treated in short-stay hospital departments. 1998	107
14	Main long-term conditions in men and women of between 45 and 74 years of age covered by the health insurance system. 1998	109
15	Main causes of death among men and women of between 45 and 74 years of age. 1997	110
16	Main declared conditions among men and women of 75 and over. 1998	126
17	Main reasons for consultation with an independent practioner among men and women of 75 and over. 1992. 1998	128
18	Main diseases of men and women of 75 years and over treated in short-stay hospital departments. 1998	129

List of figures

19 Main long-term conditions in men and women of over 75 covered by the health insurance system. 1998 — 131
20 Main causes of death among men and women of 75 and over. 1997 — 133

Part two
Health inequalities and disparities in France

1 Proportion of individuals in different social classes declaring deficiency (matched for age and sex) — 154
2 Life expectancy at birth for both sexes during the periods 1973-1977 and 1988-1992 in France (scale: employment zone) — 161
3 Life expectancy at 65 years of age for both sexes during the period 1988-1992 in France (scales: employment zone and towns with more than 20,000 inhabitants) — 163
4 Standardised mortality ratios for the period 1988-1992 (scale: canton; integrated figures) — 164
5 Employment zone profiles based on mortality rates during the period 1988-1992 (by five-year age brackets from 15 to 59 years of age) — 166
6 Town profiles based on mortality rates during the period 1988-1992 (by five-year age brackets from 15 to 59 years of age) — 169
7 Employment zone profiles based on comparative mortality rates and cause of death for both sexes (1988-1992) — 171
8 Prevalence of obesity (BMI $\geqslant$ 25) in men of between 17 and 25 years of age in 1987 and 1996 (scales: region and towns of over 20,000 inhabitants) — 176
9 Comparative mortality rates among people of between 25 and 54 years of age between 1987 and 1993 (all causes of death); broken down according to social class at the regional level — 179
10 Ratios between comparative mortality rates for the "worker/employee" class and the "executive/professional" class — 179
11 Standardised mortality rates per 100,000 inhabitants in England and Wales for the richest percentile of the population and the poorest percentile between 1921 and 1983 — 182
12 Declaration of poor state of health: odds ratio estimated by multivariate analysis — 185
13 Theoritical outline of health-related social and psychosocial factors — 186
14 From a simple model based on feedback between state of health and the health care system, to models which incorporate social determinants of health — 192
15 Infant mortality in mainland France and its overseas departments — 209
16 Perinatal mortality in mainland France and its overseas departments — 210

Part three
Resource allocation in the health system

1 Expenditure on medical materials and services (1970-2000)   227
2 Density of physicians and specialists in 1999   229
3 Density of short-stay beds in 1998   233
4 Per capita expenditure on health (1998) ($)   250

List of inserts

Part one **Data about** **health status**	Rationalising perinatal care: an epidemiologist's point of view	71
	Paediatric allergy	75
	The young and health: images, fears and expectations	80
	Drinking in the young	81
	Contraception, abortion and public health	95
	Roads accidents	100
	Premature death which can be avoided in France	112
	Occupational hazards: factors which remain significantly under-estimated	115
	Cardiovascular mortality in France	118
	Mental health: realities and issues	120
	Alzheimer's disease	135
	Vision and the elderly	139
Part two **Health** **inequalities** **and disparities** **in France**	An instance of geographically-based inequality in morbidity: obesity in the young	174
	An instance of socio-geographical inequality: occupational hazards and cancer	180
	Mental health, social inequality and living conditions	196
	Health and inequality/health and poverty: the need for a unified approach	199
	The relationship between poverty, health and health care	201
	Health in French overseas departments	209
Part three **Resource** **allocation in the** **health system**	Ondam case on 2001	238
Part four **The user, a player** **in the health** **care system**	Some semantics	266
	Some legislative and regulatory landmarks	271
	The Bill on modernisation of the health care system	275
	The democraty in Health Office of the General Health Directorate-Employment Ministry	280
	A framework to promote user-citizen participation	283
	Different ways of involving citizens	286
	The Credoc Survey on the sources of health information used by French people	289
	Complaints by the users of health care establishments	293
	The Collective of Health-Related Non-Profit-Making Organisations	297
	Informing patients: the dangers according to the Anaes	303
	From traditional medical records to the Unique Computerised Patient Record	309

List of contents

Preface	5
Foreword	11

Recommended strategic directions

The French paradox

Overall positive results make certain situations all the more difficult to accept	18
• Good overall health indicators	18
• Positive trends	19
• A significant fraction of the Gross National Product is invested in health	19
• Paradoxical situations	20
• Outmoded strategies and logistics	21
Health care issues to be addressed in the medium-term	22
• Dealing with increased life expectancy and an ageing population	22
• Cut down premature death and promote equitable health	24
• Prepare for reduced numbers of health professionals	25
• Take local dynamics into account	26
• Improve performance in the health care system	27
• Promote community involvement and democracy	29
Health policy issues: short-term objectives	30
• 1. Provide information about the situation and explain the issues	31
. Organise national and regional debates	31
. Include systematic evaluation of the impact on health in the public decision-making process	31
• 2. More recognition to restore confidence	31
. Improve mutual understanding of how the institutions and health care professionals operate	32
. Develop new avenues of individual communication between different professionals	32
. Help players make the most of their skills and their institutional affiliations	33
• 3. Simplify the instruments and clarify responsibilities	33
. Cut down the redundancy of procedures	33
. Encourage the centralisation of services	33
. Exploit existing administrative means to enhance budgetary flexibility	34
. Create institutional mediators to implement health-related programmes and actions	34
. Increase the transparency of the procedures which regulate the relationship between the State and the health insurance system	34
• 4. Develop logistics and introduce more flexibility into resource management	35

List of contents

. Develop and harmonise information and assessment systems	35
. Promote the design and running of projects by establishing regional logistical support units	36
. Establish common structures in the form of flexible, innovative legal instruments	37
. To allow genuine mobility between the public and private sectors or between different levels of the administrative structure	37
• 5. Anticipate	38
. Extend vigilance procedures and structures by exploiting the knowledge of the players on the ground	38
. Develop prospective reflection and multidisciplinary approach	39

Part one
Data about health status

Composition of the Working Group	41
Introduction	43
Summary and issues	46
• Improving the working of the health information system	47
• Providing the general public and decision-makers with a more accurate picture of key public health issues	51
• Capitalising on and consolidating the considerable progress made in the matter of health, and making every effort to ensure that this progress is equitably accessible to all	52
• Escalating the fight against avoidable causes of premature death, both within and outside the remit of the health care system	53
• Promoting the development of tertiary prevention modalities, notably for the elderly	54
Methodology	55
• Interpreting health indicators	55
• The data sources used	59
. The Credes Health and Social Coverage Survey (ESPS, *Enquête Santé protection sociale*)	59
. IMS-Health Permanent Survey of Medical Prescription (EPPM, *L'Enquête permanente sur la prescription médicale*)	59
. Hospital Medical Information Systems Programme (PMSI, *Programme de médicalisation des systèmes d'information*)	
– Short-term MSO care	60
. Recognised long-term conditions	61
. Medical cause of death	61
Young people of under 15 years of age	63
• Declared morbidity	63
• Reasons for consulting an independent physician	64
• Reasons for admission into hospital-based medicine, surgery and obstetrics services	67
• Long-term conditions	68
• Medical causes of death	69

• Main health-related issues in children of under 15 years of age	70
People of between 15 and 44 years of age	83
• Declared morbidity	83
• Reasons for consulting an independent physician	85
• Reasons for admission into hospital-based medicine, surgery and obstetrics services	86
• Long-term conditions	88
• Medical causes of death	89
• Main health-related issues in people of between 15 and 44 years of age	91
People of between 45 and 74 years of age	103
• Declared morbidity	103
• Reasons for consulting an independent physician	105
• Reasons for admission into hospital-based medicine, surgery and obstetrics services	106
• Long-term conditions	108
• Medical causes of death	110
• Main health-related issues in people of between 45 and 74 years of age	113
Those of 75 and over	124
• Declared morbidity	125
• Reasons for consulting an independent physician	127
• Reasons for admission into hospital-based medicine and surgery services	128
• Long-term conditions	130
• Medical causes of death	131
• Main health-related issues in people of 75 years of age and over	133
Annexe	142

Part two
Health inequalities and disparities in France

Composition of the Working Group	144
Introduction	145
Socially-based inequality in health	147
• Mortality between 25 and 65 years of age	148
. An executive can expect to live more than six years longer than a worker	148
. Less inequality amongst women?	149
. Are socially-based mortality differentials increasing?	149
. Social differences and medical causes of death	151
. France and other European countries	151
• Social inequality and morbidity	152
. Life-threatening risk factors, handicaps, disability, deficiencies	152
. Inequality begins at birth	155
. Taking dental health as an example	155
. An unknown relationship: social differences and accidents	158
Geographical inequalities in health	160

List of contents

- Differential life expectancy: growing disparities — 160
. Life expectancy at birth — 160
. A similar pattern of disparity for life expectancy at 65 years of age — 162
. Disparities between town and country (and the relevance of the parent region) — 162
- Differences in the age at which people die — 165
. Disparities between different regions and within regions — 166
. Disparities between large and small towns — 168
- Differences in terms of cause of death — 168
. Seven different mortality profiles which follow a clear geographical pattern — 169
. Female mortality gives a far less clear-cut geographical pattern — 172
. Region is a major factor — 172
Socio-geographical inequality in health — 178
Understanding and correcting socially-based inequality in health — 181
- Review the social classes used and identify other determinants — 182
. The classes usually used — 182
. Fragmentary appreciation of the situation — 183
. The limitations of these approaches — 184
. The need to take other determinants into account — 185
. An unknown factor in France: the health status of immigrants — 187
- Consider health determinants at the level of both the individual and the community — 188
. Multi-level analysis... — 188
. ... for comparing different countries or different regions — 189
- Integrate inequality in health into the analysis of precariousness and exclusion — 189
. Exclusion, precariousness and inequality — 189
. An integrated approach based on "social determinants of health status" in the broadest sense — 190
- Broaden the theoretical model of health and its determinants — 191
. Beyond seeking medical advice and treatment — 191
. The role of psychosocial and behavioural characteristics — 191
. The value of the longitudinal approach — 193
- Understanding and prevention — 193
. The "grey area" of personal inequality in health — 193
. Scientific... and political challenges — 194
- Take-home lessons now — 195
Public policy to mitigate inequality in health — 203
. Creation of the *Revenu Minimum d'Insertion* — 204
. The Law against exclusion (July 29 1998) — 204
. Universal Health Insurance Coverage (the Law of July 27 1999) — 207

	. More attention to health in municipal policy	207
	. Support groups	208
	Summary and recommendations	215
	• Recognition of the problem	216
	• Monitoring	216
	• Understanding	216
	• Implementation	217
	• Providing sustained support	217
Part three	Composition of the Working Group	220
Resource	Introduction	221
allocation	Health system resources: the current situation	223
in the health	• General remarks	223
system	• Health accounts: an instrument of macroeconomic analysis	224
	• Production factors	228
	. Physicians	229
	. Other professional health care providers	230
	. Hospitals	231
	. Equipment	233
	. Pharmaceuticals	234
	How resources are estimated and allocated	234
	• What should the level of health insurance funding be? The Ondam	236
	. Setting the Ondam	237
	• Components of the overall Ondam	238
	• Hospital sector resources	239
	. Public hospital sector (included affiliated private establishments)	239
	. Private hospital sector (non-affiliated establishments)	240
	• Independent practice	241
	• Drugs	242
	• Funding of general and specific measures	242
	• Human resources	242
	. Physician numbers	242
	. Other professional health care providers	244
	. Numbers compatible with provision	244
	• The hospital sector	246
	• The pharmaceutical sector	247
	• Clinical research	247
	• The role of crises in implicit and explicit decisions pertaining to resource allocation	248
	• The new role of patients in resource allocation in the health care system: from informed consent to shared decision-making	249
	Discussion	249
	• Health expenditure	249
	• Hospitals	252
	• Care providers	253

List of contents

	• Would other professionals be able to compensate for a shortfall in physicians?	255
	Recommendations	255
	• Resource levels	255
	. Short-term	255
	• Demographics of care providers	256
	• Medium-term	257
	. Short-term measures for long-term effects	257
	• Resource allocation	258
	. Short-term	258
	. Short-term measures for medium-term effects	259
	. Short-term measures for long-term effects	259
	• Monitoring the use of resources	260
	. Short-term	260
	. Medium-term	261
	. Long-term	262
Part four **The user, a player in the health care system**	Composition of the Working Group	264
	Introduction	265
	• Citizenship and democracy in health	267
	• A changing health care system	268
	• The user, a player in the health care system	270
	• Keeping users informed: a vital public health issue	273
	Participation in the formulation of public health policy	276
	• Discussion forums: under construction	277
	• The place of the citizen in discussion forums	279
	• Conditions for meaningful participation	281
	. Citizens ought to be involved in the design of expertise-based processes	282
	. The process should be transparent	282
	. Provision should be made for contentious discussion	284
	• Role of patient support groups and other associations in discussion forums	285
	Involve users in the running of institutions	287
	• Making sure that the user is adequately informed	288
	• The purposes of information	290
	• Role of patient support groups	295
	Ensure balance in the patient/care provider relationship	299
	• The patient-doctor relationship: first and foremost, a meeting	300
	• Providing the patient with information	301
	• From information to consent	305
	• From informed consent to shared decision-making	306
	• The various responsibilities to be co-ordinated	307
	Recommendations	310

Part five
A critical, prospective analysis of the way the health system is organised

Composition of the Working Group	314
Introduction	315
Is the way the health care system currently works based on genuine priorities, and does it cater to people's needs?	316
• The current situation: the "public health approach" envisaged in the 1996 Rulings	316
• Critical analysis: health priorities, a successful concept but one which is vague when it comes to action	318
Is the health care system organised in a strategic, functional way?	320
• The current situation: the way health determinants are taken into account lacks consistency	320
• Complicated logistics	322
• Critical analysis: the excess premature death rate is probably due to a deficit in certain types of health strategy	323
• Annually-based funding is incompatible with the epidemiological picture	324
• Consolidation of regional power through an intricate process	325
• The difficulty of co-ordinating between the national, regional and local levels	326
Are questions of health dealt with in democratic processes in which the general public can participate?	327
• The current situation: the possibility of involving non-formalised regional structures	327
• New processes to involve the general public	329
• Critical analysis: the public health approach poses problems for elected bodies	330
• Meetings are too irregular to ensure genuine public participation	331
• Consolidating democracy in health, a key component in building a democracy of proximity	332
Is the health care system organised in such a way as to enable it to respond to future challenges?	333
• Clarification of the challenges from a public health perspective	333
. The ageing of the population and increased longevity	333
. Reducing premature death and inequality in health	334
. The falling number of professional health care providers	334
. Territorial dynamics	335
. Cultural assimilation and democracy	335
• Inevitable changes	336
. Broaden the scope of the strategies implemented	336
. Act at the cultural level	336
. Change the perspective to one based on a continuum of prevention, treatment, rehabilitation, and return to normal life	337
. Simplify logistics and enhance co-ordination	338

List of contents

Acknowledgements	339
References	340
Abbreviations	353
List of tables	357
List of figures	359
List of inserts	362
Table of contents	363

Achevé d'imprimer par Corlet, Imprimeur, S.A.
14110 Condé-sur-Noireau
N° d'Imprimeur : 70134 - Dépôt légal : octobre 2003
Imprimé en France